Complications of Cardiac Catheterization and Angiography:

Prevention and Management

Complications of Cardiac Catheterization and Angiography:

Prevention and Management

Edited by

Jack Kron, M.D.
Assistant Professor of Medicine
Division of Cardiology
Oregon Health Sciences University

and

Mark J. Morton, M.D.
Associate Professor of Medicine
Division of Cardiology
Oregon Health Sciences University

Futura Publishing Company
Mount Kisco, New York
1989

i

Library of Congress Cataloging-in-Publication Data

Complications of cardiac catheterization and angiography.

   Includes index.
   1. Cardiac catheterization—Complications and
sequelae. 2. Angiography—Complications and sequelae.
I. Kron, Jack. II. Morton, Mark J. [DNLM:
1. Angiocardiography—adverse effects. 2. Heart
Catheterization—adverse effects. WG 141.5.C2 C737]
RC683.5.C25C635   1989   616.1'07572   88-31043
ISBN 0-87993-338-0

Published by
Futura Publishing Company, Inc.
P.O. Box 330,
Mount Kisco, New York 10549

L.C. No.: 88-31043
ISBN No.: 0-87993-338-0

Printed in the United States of America

To my parents, Bella and David Kron, whose devoted support and sacrifice made my medical education possible.

Contributors

J. David Bristow, M.D.   Professor of Medicine, Division of Cardiology, Oregon Health Sciences University, Portland, Oregon

Henry DeMots, M.D.   Professor of Medicine, Head, Division of Cardiology, Oregon Health Sciences University, Portland, Oregon

Lawrence Elzinga, M.D.   Instructor of Medicine, Division of Cardiology, Oregon Health Sciences University, Portland, Oregon

Thomas A. Golper, M.D.   Associate Professor of Medicine, Division of Nephrology, Oregon Health Sciences University, Portland, Oregon

Jeffrey D. Hosenpud, M.D.   Associate Professor of Medicine, Division of Cardiology, Oregon Health Sciences University, Portland, Oregon

Fred S. Keller, M.D.   Professor of Radiology, Chief of Angiography and Interventional Radiology, University of Alabama Medical School at Birmingham, Birmingham, Alabama

Blaine E. Kozak, M.D.   Assistant Professor of Diagnostic Radiology, Division of Radiology, Oregon Health Sciences University, Portland, Oregon

Irving L. Kron, M.D.   Professor of Surgery, Department of Surgery, University of Virginia Medical Center, Charlottesville, Virginia

Jack Kron, M.D.   Assistant Professor of Medicine, Division of Cardiology, Oregon Health Sciences University, Portland, Oregon

Peter J. Kudenchuk, M.D.   Assistant Professor of Medicine, Division of Cardiology, University of Washington School of Medicine, Seattle, Washington

Greg C. Larsen, M.D.   Fellow in Cardiology, Division of Cardiology, Oregon Health Sciences University, Portland, Oregon

Stephen A. Malone, M.D.   Fellow in Cardiology; Division of Cardiology, Oregon Health Sciences University, Portland, Oregon

James L. McCullough, Jr., M.D.   Resident in Cardiothoracic Surgery, University of Virginia Medical Center, Charlottesville, Virginia

Mark J. Morton, M.D.   Associate Professor of Medicine Division of Cardiology, Oregon Health Sciences University, Portland, Oregon

Edward Murphy, M.D.   Associate Professor of Medicine, Division of Cardiology, Oregon Health Sciences University, Portland, Oregon

Robert Palac, M.D.   Assistant Professor of Medicine, Division of Cardiology, Oregon Health Sciences University, Portland, Oregon

Josef Rosch, M.D.   Professor of Diagnostic Radiology, Division of Radiology, Oregon Health Sciences University, Portland, Oregon

Michael J. Silka, M.D.   Assistant Professor of Pediatrics, Oregon Health Sciences University, Portland, Oregon

Richard A. Wilson, M.D.   Associate Professor of Medicine, Division of Cardiology, Oregon Health Sciences University, Portland, Oregon

Acknowledgment: We would like to thank Kimberly D. Pence and Kelli L. Conachan Brock for their secretarial support in the preparation of this manuscript.

Contents

Chapter 1

Introduction

J. David Bristow

Recently, there has been an amazing expansion in the use of vascular catheterization. Patients now come to the cardiac laboratory for management of problems felt in the past to be contraindications to catheterization, such as unstable rhythm, myocardial infarction or shock. As these new therapeutic and diagnostic procedures are applied, and as the indications for established ones expand, it is inevitable that complications of several types will be encountered.

There have been recommendations about standards of performance and acceptable complication rates in catheterization laboratories previously,[1,2] but we have lacked a comprehensive treatise on complications and their management in this new era. This book outlines, in detail, these problems for a wide-ranging group of procedures and, of great importance, tells us how to avoid them and how to manage them.

As new developments are being assessed and integrated into practice, established procedures continue to be performed in ever increasing numbers. For example, the number of coronary angiograms is increasing each year, as is the use of bedside hemodynamic monitoring, which long ago became routine for many clinical problems. Despite extensive national experience with these techniques, complications still occur, a problem that must be addressed. There may remain, in some centers, the "occasional" cardiac catheterizer, analogous to early experience with heart surgery.[3] In fact, there is recent evidence of a proliferation of centers with a low volume of

From *Complications of Cardiac Catheterization and Angiography: Prevention and Management* edited by Jack Kron, M.D. and Mark J. Morton, M.D. © 1989, Futura Publishing Inc., Mount Kisco, NY.

procedures, as competition has increased.[4] This seems undesirable, as it is generally believed that the frequency of complications for procedures is inversely related to experience. For example, in 1968 a difference in complication rates for coronary angiography of 6.7% versus 0.9% was observed in groups with less versus much experience.[5] In a survey in 1973, the mortality risk of coronary angiography was eightfold larger in hospitals with fewer than 200 cases per year.[6] The continuing problem of complications resulting from established, routine procedures has not gone unnoticed.[7] Thus, the appropriate development and utilization of laboratories is a factor in complication rates, and deserves our attention.

An entirely new set of catheterization procedures has been developed in the past few years, each with its own set of potential problems. Included are intracoronary administration of thrombolytic agents such as streptokinase and tissue plasminogen activator. These agents, by their very therapeutic actions, can set the stage for catastrophic hemorrhage, if errors in technique or unnecessary vascular invasion have occurred. Percutaneous transluminal coronary angioplasty has also been explosive in numbers, including its use in some patients with acute myocardial infarction. We now see manipulation of catheters and guidewires in proximal and distal coronary vessels which, at times, will produce significant vascular injury. Such damage may assert itself as acute thrombosis or, conceivably, as an acceleration of the sclerotic process.[8]

The new phenomenon of cardiac transplantation has brought with it the need for repeated entry into the vascular system for right ventricular myocardial biopsies to evaluate the immune rejection process. The patient's life depends on the safe performance of repeated venous access and biopsy.

An obvious feature of the newer uses of intravascular catheterization is that many of the problems so treated reflect severe, often capricious, life-threatening illness. For example, unstable angina is a relatively common indication for coronary angiography, with some patients arriving in the catheterization laboratory while receiving intravenous nitroglycerin, or occasionally, with an intra-aortic balloon pump operating. The acute myocardial infarction population is seen in the laboratory with increasing frequency for angioplasty, lytic therapy, or evaluation for coronary bypass surgery. Some of these patients are hemodynamically unstable to the extreme. Meticulous attention to technique and hemodynamic management are essential in these people, as any complication could be lethal.

New approaches to the management of valvular heart disease have become reality. Balloon inflation can be used to dilate the mitral, aortic, or pulmonic valves or coarctation of the aorta. The patients are likely to be those too fragile to be subjected to a cardiac operation, and are also at substantial risk for the complications of catheterization. Large catheters, sometimes multiple, are required. The pediatric cardiologic community, always faced with very ill infants with heart disease, has also added valvuloplasty to its repertoire of therapeutic procedures performed by catheterization, which already includes atrial septostomy.

As a more assertive approach has been taken to the large population of people at known risk for sudden cardiac death, electrophysiologic testing and arrhythmia induction with catheters have become relatively commonplace in many hospitals.[9] These evaluations may span many days and require repeated insertion of catheters or indwelling catheters for protracted periods. The use of several energy modalities to treat arrhythmias (electricity, laser) also brings the possibility of unwanted cardiac injury.

As a result of therapeutic advances, there are also new populations of people who must be evaluated by intravascular catheterization. The need to study prosthetic valve function in some patients requires a transseptal catheterization, a technique that clearly demands skill and attention to detail. Transthoracic left ventricular puncture is needed in others. The cardiac transplantation population was mentioned previously.

As complications have arisen with the broadened use of catheterization, new methods have been devised for managing and preventing the problems. Ingenious techniques for removal of broken catheters, surgery for vascular complications, and new radiographic contrast agents provide more options for the operator facing complex problems.

The foregoing points exemplify the expanding role of vascular catheterization and remind us that growing numbers of patients with severe disease will have procedures of considerable complexity. Some of these will be lengthy and may require large catheters and manipulation of truly vital structures. The patients may be very ill, and sometimes the procedure must be repeated. The potential for complications, therefore, is great and exceedingly important to assess as well as prevent by practiced techniques.

Given the inherent risks and some unknown factors about new or evolving techniques, it is timely that the problems and complications of vascular catheterization and their prevention be discussed comprehensively. This volume addresses these difficulties directly and offers guidance that should improve the safety of cardiovascular catheterization during changing, challenging times.

References

1. Judkins MP, Gander MP: Prevention of complications of coronary arteriography. Circulation 44:599, 1974.
2. Judkins MP, Abrams HL, Bristow JD, et al: Report of the Intersociety Commission for Heart Disease Resources. Optimal resources for examination of the chest and cardiovascular system. Circulation 53:A1, 1976.
3. Hotchkiss WS: Patent ductus arteriosus and the occasional cardiac surgeon. J Am Med Assoc 173:244, 1960.
4. Robinson JC, Garnick DW, McPhee SJ: Market and regulatory influences on the availability of coronary angioplasty and bypass surgery in US hospitals. New Engl J Med 317:85, 1987.
5. Ross RS, Gorlin R: Coronary arteriography. In Baunwald E, Swan HJC (eds): Cooperative Study on Cardiac Catheterization. American Heart Assoc Monograph 20, 1968, pp III 67-III 73.
6. Adams DF, Fraser DB, Abrams HL: The complications of coronary arteriography. Circulation 48:609, 1973.
7. Schroeder SA: The complications of coronary arteriography: A problem that won't go away. Am Heart J 99:139, 1980.
8. Waller BF, Pinkerton CA, Foster LN: Morphologic evidence of accelerated left main coronary artery stenosis: A Late complication of percutaneous transluminal balloon anigoplasty of the proximal left anterior descending artery. J Am Coll Cardiol 9:1019, 1987.
9. Horowitz LN, Kay HR, Kutalek SP, et al: Risks and complications of clinical electrophysiologic studies. A prospective analysis of 1,000 consecutive patients. J Am Coll Cardiol 9:1261, 1987.

Chapter 2

Complications of Central Venous and Right Heart Catheterization

Jack Kron

Historical Aspects

The first successful right heart catheterization was performed by Werner Forssman, a German medical student, on himself in 1929.[1] Since that time, a vast experience has accumulated, which has contributed extensively to the understanding of cardiovascular physiology.[2] The central venous circulation can be catheterized antegrade from a peripheral vein or directly by proximal venous puncture. Peripheral veins can be entered percutaneously or by direct surgical exposure (cutdown). Generally, central venous access is attained by direct percutaneous puncture of a large central vein (e.g., subclavian, femoral, internal jugular) or a peripheral vein.

The percutaneous approach to the subclavian vein was introduced in the 1950s[3,4] and has since become a frequently used access to the central circulation.[5] The percutaneous internal jugular approach was introduced in the late 1960s and early 1970s,[6,7] partly because of concerns raised by increasingly frequent complications of subclavian venipuncture.[8] Two other significant developments were (1) the introduction of the transvenous approach to temporary and permanent pacemaking in the late 1950s,[9] and (2) the use of balloon flow-directed pulmonary artery catheters in the early 1970s.[10] The latter two developments revolutionized the care of crit-

From *Complications of Cardiac Catheterization and Angiography: Prevention and Management* edited by Jack Kron, M.D. and Mark J. Morton, M.D. © 1989, Futura Publishing Inc., Mount Kisco, NY.

ically ill patients and are now used routinely at most medical centers. There are numerous case reports and review articles documenting the various complications associated with routine balloon pulmonary artery catheters.[6,11-31] This discussion reviews the complications of central venous and right heart catheterization and provides guidelines to maximize the safety of the various procedures.

Indications for Central Venous and Right Heart Catheterization (Table 1)

Central venous catheterization with pressure measurement allows the physician to quickly assess a critically ill patient's filling pressures and facilitates the administration of large volumes of fluid in trauma or fluid loss of any etiology. Central catheters also have

---

Table 1
Indications for Central Venous and Right Heart Catheterization

1. Rapid administration of fluids to hypovolemic patients
2. Chronic administration of sclerotic medications (e.g., antibiotics or chemotherapy)
3. Hyperalimentation
4. Hemodialysis or continuous hemofiltration
5. Plasmapheresis
6. Insertion of temporary or permanent pacemakers
7. Monitoring of central venous pressure
8. Pulmonary artery catheter placement
   a. Management of complicated myocardial infarction
   b. Diagnosis of cardiac tamponade
   c. Detection of left to right shunt
   d. Differentiate between respiratory distress due to pulmonary versus cardiac disease
   e. Management of ventilator patients receiving positive end expiratory pressure
   f. Differential diagnosis and management of shock
9. Access for endomyocardial biopsy, right ventricular or pulmonary angiography, transseptal catheterization, and electrophysiologic studies

---

greatly expedited the administration of medications to chronically ill patients who would otherwise require multiple venipunctures during hospitalization. Any health care provider who has managed burn victims, patients receiving chemotherapy, or patients with chronic infections knows that loss of vascular access and patient discomfort from multiple punctures quickly become major problems. For these reasons, a chronic indwelling silicone catheter, the Hickman catheter, with good tissue compatibility and ease of access was developed. This catheter is placed via the percutaneous puncture of the subclavian vein, tunneled subcutaneously, and brought out through a skin incision on the chest wall. The use of Hickman catheters, although causing some risk, has become widespread in the 1980s.

Perhaps the most common indication for central venous acess is hemodynamic monitoring. First introduced by Swan et al. in 1970,[10] pulmonary artery catheters play an integral role in the management of patients with complicated myocardial infarctions, cardiac patients undergoing noncardiac or cardiac surgery and patients with combined respiratory and cardiac disease. Other situations in which pulmonary artery catheters are helpful include the differential diagnosis and management of shock of any etiology, the detection of left to right shunts (e.g., ventricular septal defect after myocardial infarction), and the diagnosis of cardiac tamponade.

Temporary pacemakers are indicated for patients presenting with symptomatic bradyarrhythmias as well as those at risk for severe bradyarrhythmias (e.g., acute myocardial infarction with high-grade atrioventricular block or new bundle branch block). Occasionally, temporary pacemaking is also useful for the management of difficult supraventricular or ventricular tachyarrhythmias. Percutaneous venous access has been the standard approach to temporary placement. Complications of temporary pacing are discussed in detail in Chapter 5. Although developed and applied 35 years ago, temporary external noninvasive cardiac pacing has been recently reintroduced as a clinically feasible method of temporary pacemaking.[32] The widespread availability of this technique will help to minimize the frequency of emergency pacemaker placement in acutely ill patients, in whom venous access and sterile technique may be difficult. The urgent care of such patients (i.e., cardiopulmonary resuscitation) may preclude the use of fluoroscopy for proper pacemaker lead placement. External noninvasive pacemaking may alleviate many of these difficulties.

Central venous catheterization frequently is used for patients who require acute hemodialysis or hemofiltration for acute renal failure, volume overload, or drug toxicity. Similarly, plasmapheresis has become a valuable form of therapy for a variety of disease states, including myasthenia gravis, Guillain-Barré syndrome, hyperviscosity states, idiopathic thrombocytopenia purpura, Goodpasture's syndrome, and other autoimmune diseases. These procedures all require large, centrally placed intravenous catheters to maintain adequate flow volumes for maximum exchange.

Right heart catheterization, in the cardiac catheterization laboratory, plays an integral role in the complete hemodynamic evaluation of patients with complex congenital or acquired heart disease. It is employed for shunt determination, measurement of cardiac output, determination of vascular resistance, access for electrophysiologic studies, and right ventricular and pulmonary angiography. More recently, endomyocardial biopsy has become an important diagnostic modality after cardiac transplantation and for patients with heart failure of unknown etiology. This subject is discussed more fully in Chapter 6.

Choice of Access Sites

The site selected for catheter insertion depends on multiple factors, including the operator's experience, the anticipated duration of catheterization, the specific anatomy of the patient (e.g., obesity or prior head and neck, groin, or cardiac surgery), and the availability of fluoroscopy (Table 2). For example, patients who require several days of temporary pacemaking or pulmonary artery catheterization are best served by the subclavian approach (Fig. 1). Sterility is easier to maintain at this site as opposed to the groin, where urinary or fecal incontinence may contaminate the catheter. Furthermore, the subclavian site facilitates patient comfort, as movement of the arm or neck in patients with antecubital or internal jugular catheters may be painful. This has to be balanced against the higher incidence of pneumothorax or hemothorax from this approach because of the proximity of the pleura to the subclavian vein. In situations where fluoroscopy is not readily available,

Table 2
Advantages and Disadvantages of Sites for Central Venous and
Right Heart Catheterization

	Advantages	*Disadvantages*
Antecubital vein	1. Ease of access	1. Tortuous route to right heart (especially if lateral vein)
	2. Minimal risk of hemorrhage (site of choice in patient with coagulopathy)	2. High risk of spasm
	3. Avoids risk of pneumothorax	3. Phlebitis and patient discomfort if left in place for > few hours
	4. Patient does not have to lie flat	4. Higher risk of catheter movement or cardiac perforation with arm motion
External jugular vein	1. Ease of access	1. Tortuous anatomy
	2. Low risk of pneumothorax or inadvertent carotid puncture	2. Discomfort in patients with respiratory distress or CHF
Subclavian vein	1. Best site for catheter stability	1. Highest risk of pneumothorax especially in COPD
	2. Easy site to maintain sterility	2. Difficult to control bleeding (e.g., coagulopathy; streptokinase
	3. Avoids carotid artery	3. Avoid in agitated patient or if unable to lie supine
		4. Risk of air embolus
Internal jugular vein	1. "Straight shot" to right heart; best site if fluoroscopy not available	1. Avoid in patients with carotid hypersensitivity or cerebrovascular disease
	2. Lower risk of pneumothorax than subclavian	2. Vein prone to "collapse"

Table 2—(Cont'd)

	Advantages	Disadvantages
	3. Site of choice for endomyocardial biopsy	3. Avoid with coagulopathy or streptokinase
		4. Avoid if patient unable to lie flat (e.g., CHF)
		5. Avoid in obesity or poor landmarks
		6. Higher risk of cardiac perforation because of proximity to the heart
		7. Patient discomfort
		8. Air embolus
Femoral vein	1. Good choice for patients with coagulopathy or streptokinase (ability to apply direct pressure)	1. Branching anatomy (fluoroscopy essential)
	2. Landmarks reliable in most patients	2. Difficult to maintain sterility
		3. Avoid with venous disease or history of deep venous thrombosis
		4. Vein may be difficult to localize with prior vascular surgery
		5. Avoid in extreme obesity
		6. Risk of retroperitoneal hemorrhage

the internal jugular vein (Fig. 2) provides the most reliable access to the right heart as opposed to the antecubital (Fig. 3) or femoral vein route (Fig. 4), where multiple side branches, which the catheter may enter, may be a major problem. The subclavian vein, although superior to the latter routes, does not always result in easy "blind" access to the right heart. When observed under fluoroscopy, it is not unusual to visualize the guidewire going up the ipsilateral internal jugular vein, or out the contralateral subclavian vein. The availability of high quality pressure monitoring may, in some cases, obviate the need for fluoroscopy. Unfortunately, however, misin-

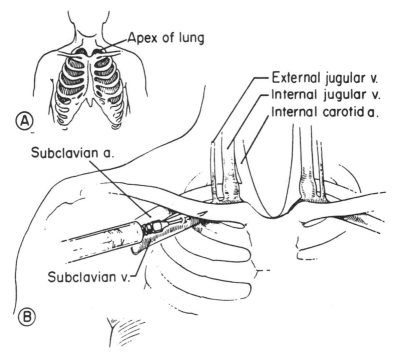

Figure 1. *Upper thoracic and cervical anatomy with structures as labeled. The subclavian vein enters the thorax anterior and slightly caudad to the subclavian artery, between the first rib and clavicle. The external jugular vein passes superficial to the sternocleidomastoid muscle (not depicted) before entering the subclavian vein. The internal jugular vein is superficial and lateral to the internal carotid artery, joining the subclavian vein to form the right brachiocephalic (innominate) vein. Note the proximity of the apex of the lung (A) to the vascular structures and first rib. B. The subclavian vein is entered, with continuous aspiration, at the junction of the proximal and middle third of the clavicle with the axis of the needle directed parallel to the vein. The guidewire should only be advanced if free-flowing non-pulsatile blood is readily withdrawn.*

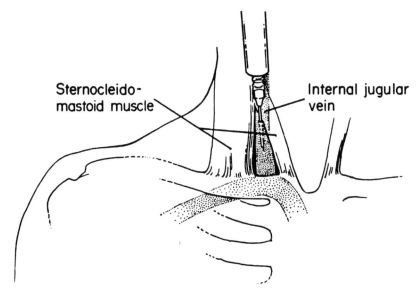

Sternocleido-
mastoid muscle

Internal jugular
vein

Figure 2. *Entry of needle into internal jugular vein. The internal jugular vein is entered just below the junction of the sternal and clavicular heads of the sternocleidomastoid muscle, with the needle directed superficial and lateral to the internal carotid artery.*

terpretation of pressure data may lead to inappropriate catheter placement. A damped pressure waveform, caused by an air bubble in the line, a thrombus at the catheter tip, or inappropriate wedging in the right ventricular outflow tract can be confused with a pulmonary artery wedge tracing. A potential pitfall of the left subclavian or internal jugular approach is a persistent left superior vena cava, a congenital abnormality that occurs in 0.3% of the general population[33] (Fig. 5). In most cases, the left superior vena cava empties into the coronary sinus; however, its presence will confuse the most experienced operator, if fluoroscopy is not used.

The presence of a bleeding disorder (e.g., coagulopathy related to the patient's underlying disease, warfarin therapy, or after streptokinase therapy) is a reason to avoid the subclavian or internal jugular approach. Direct pressure can only rarely be successfully applied to these sites. If the subclavian vein is lacerated or the subclavian artery is entered inadvertently, the patient with coag-

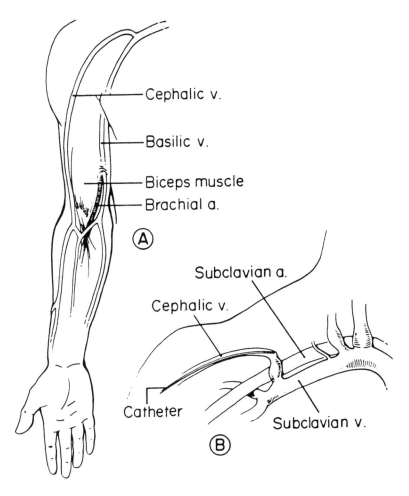

Figure 3. *A. Anatomy of the vascular structures of the arm with structures as labeled. The basilic system runs superficial and medial to the brachial artery and is the preferred approach for central venous catheterization from the arm. The cephalic system drains the lateral structures of the arm. B. The cephalic vein enters the subclavian vein at an acute angle, often resulting in difficult and painful catheterization from this site.*

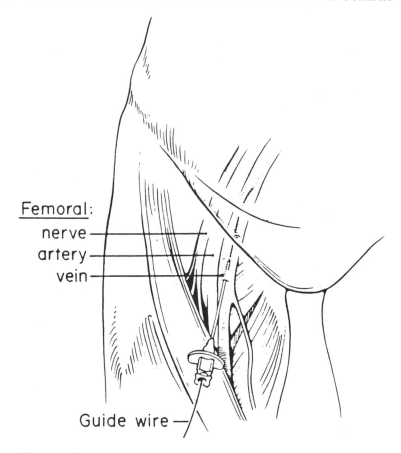

Figure 4. *Anatomy of femoral triangle with structures as labeled. The femoral vein lies medial to the nerve and artery. It is entered with continuous aspiration approximately 2 cm below the inguinal ligament (not labeled). The guidewire should be advanced under fluoroscopic guidance only if free-flowing nonpulsatile blood is withdrawn.*

ulopathy may exsanguinate or develop a severe hemothorax. During internal jugular puncture, inadvertent entry of the carotid artery in patients with coagulopathy, produces severe hemorrhage which may result in tracheal compression or cause neurologic damage (Horner's syndrome). Therefore, sites that can be compressed locally, such as the antecubital, external jugular, or femoral veins

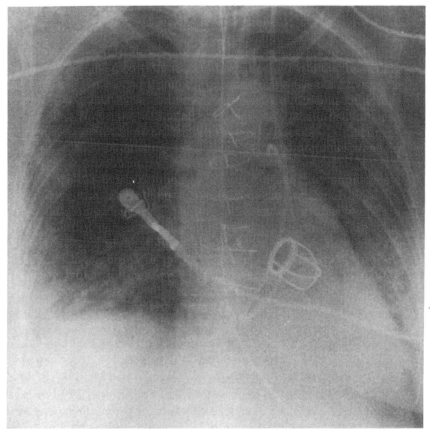

Figure 5. *Pulmonary artery catheter placed via a persistent left superior vena cava from the left internal jugular approach.*

become the access of choice in the presence of a severe bleeding disorder.

Finally, the subclavian access should be avoided in patients receiving assisted ventilation (especially positive end-expiratory pressure). In these patients, even a small air leak will result in a large pneumothorax for which a chest tube must be inserted. Although cases of pneumothorax have been reported with the internal jugular approach, the risk is lower than that with the subclavian, especially if a "high" approach is used. When landmarks for internal jugular cannulation are poor (e.g., obesity, or prior head and neck surgery), another site, such as the femoral or antecubital vein, should be used.

The external jugular vein, if clearly visualized, is a reliable site of entry for central venous cannulation with a reported success rate of 90%.[34] Complications from this site are rare, and this approach is probably underutilized. Catheterization of the right heart, however, may be difficult from this route due to tortuosity and side branches. The use of fluoroscopy with dilute contrast test injection to visualize the anatomy may enhance the success rate of this route in some patients. In addition, the patient must be able to lie flat with his or her head tipped back to extend the external jugular vein if this approach is to be successful.

The percutaneous antecubital approach to central venous catheterization has the advantage of easy access, minimal patient discomfort with insertion, and no risk of pneumothorax. Control of hemorrhage is rarely an issue and in cases of severe coagulopathy, this risk can be further minimized by a cutdown. The anatomy of the venous drainage of the arm is characterized by multiple branches and varies between patients (Fig. 3), however, entry to the central circulation can be greatly facilitated by using a median basilic vein and by direct visualization with contrast injections under fluoroscopy. Lateral veins drain via the cephalic system, which makes a rather acute bend before entering the axillary vein. Although one can often be successful using this approach, its success rate is much lower than that of the medial approach and it often results in considerable patient discomfort from venospasm and traction on the vein. The left antecubital vein is the entry site of choice for placement of catheters into the coronary sinus during electrophysiologic studies. This is because the os of the coronary sinus is best entered by reflecting the catheter with a gentle arc off the opposite wall of the right atrium.

There are caveats to the antecubital approach. The large superficial veins are prone to spasm, which can be extremely difficult to overcome. Injections of intraluminal lidocaine, cold saline, and nitroglycerin occasionally may be useful in overcoming venospasm. Inadvertent entry of the brachial artery, especially in patients in shock with low-volume pulses and desaturated arterial blood, may occur and result in dissection or occlusion of the brachial artery.

The antecubital site may be extremely uncomfortable, if a catheter is left in place for more than a few hours. Furthermore, arm movement can cause the catheter tip to migrate, which could result in myocardial perforation. The subsequent infusion of fluid or bleeding into the pericardium has been reported to cause death in rare cases.[35] Therefore, when using the antecubital approach, the position of the catheter must be documented carefully by chest x-ray and checked daily for tip migration. Because of the concern about tip migration causing perforation, central venous catheters should be left high in the superior vena cava. If a temporary pacemaker is required for several days, then another entry site (i.e., subclavian or internal jugular vein) should be considered to avoid the risks of perforation, chemical phlebitis, or infection, which may be more common from the antecubital route.

The femoral vein (Fig. 4) is an excellent route in patients with coagulopathy or recent thrombolytic therapy, assisted ventilation, distorted chest anatomy, and in patients unable to lie supine. Reasons to avoid the femoral approach include a history of deep venous thrombosis, prior vascular or pelvic surgery which may distort venous anatomy, and morbid obesity which renders this approach more difficult. Furthermore, there are multiple venous branches between the femoral vein and right atrium, which the catheter may enter. This problem will be overcome by fluoroscopy in most cases. The femoral triangle is a difficult site to keep sterile, particularly in obese or incontinent patients. Therefore, if prolonged catheterization is contemplated, another entry site should be used. The proximity of the femoral vein to the femoral artery is another potential hazard that will result in hematoma formation, if the artery is inadvertently punctured. If the femoral vein (or artery) is entered above the inguinal ligament, especially in patients with bleeding disorders, retroperitoneal hemorrhage may occur and should be considered in the diagnosis of unexplained blood loss or abdominal pain following femoral vein catheterization.

Another complication reported during femoral vein catheterization is arteriovenous fistula.[36] Although more common in patients undergoing simultaneous ipsilateral arterial and venous catheterization, it may also occur in patients undergoing femoral venipuncture alone, because of unrecognized arterial puncture. Chronic anticoagulation therapy may be a predisposing factor for this complication.

Complications of Right Heart Catheterization

The multitude of complications[8,31] that can occur during right heart catheterization brings further credence to Murphy's Law, which states: "Anything which can go wrong will go wrong.[37]" Certainly operator experience is a major factor in minimizing the incidence of complications.[38] However, in a recent prospective study of pulmonary artery catheterization, [17] the overall incidence of complications was 24%, with serious complications in 4.4% of the patients. The risk of death directly attributable to the procedure remains quite low, however, with reported mortality in the 1 to 2 in 10,000 range.[25] In critically ill patients, mortality has been reported to be as high as 4%.[39] This section of the discussion focuses on the specific complications of right heart catheterization. Guide-

---

Table 3
Complications of Central Venous and Right Heart Catheterization Related to Access Site

---

Internal Jugular or Subclavian
> Pneumothorax
> Hemothorax / hydrothorax
> Horner's syndrome (more common from internal jugular)
> Air embolus
> Inadvertent carotid or subclavian artery cannulation
> Puncture of aorta (internal jugular approach)
> Hydromediastinum
> Thoracic duct laceration (left internal jugular)
> Cerebrovascular accident (internal jugular)
> Damage to cranial, phrenic, or brachial nerves
> Superior vena cava syndrome
> A-V fistula
> Clavicular osteomyelitis (subclavian)
> Cardiac tamponade secondary to perforation of RA, RV, or SVC
> Cardiac arrhythmias
>   sinus bradycardia (from inadvertent carotid sinus massage or vasovagal reaction)
> PVCs; ventricular tachycardia or fibrillation

Table—(Cont'd)

Internal Jugular or Subclavian—(Cont'd)
  Complete heart block
  Bilateral vocal cord paralysis (internal jugular)
Femoral Vein
  Infection
  Thrombophlebitis
  Retroperitoneal hemorrhage
  Inadvertent puncture of bladder
  Vasovagal reaction
  A-V fistula
  Femoral artery thrombosis or embolus
Antecubital Vein
  Phlebitis
  Brachial artery dissection or thrombosis
  Cardiac perforation
  Inability to advance catheter
  Spasm of antecubital vein
Common to all Access Sites
  Infection or sepsis
  Cardiac perforation
  A-V fistula
  Thrombophlebitis
  Hematoma
  Arrhythmias
  Death

Complications Related to Pulmonary Artery Catheterization

Endocardial damage (RA, RV, tricuspid, and pulmonic valves)
Pulmonary infiltrates
Pulmonary artery rupture or dissection
Hypotension secondary to increased RV afterload with balloon
  inflation in patients with single lung
Catheter looping and knotting
Pulmonary emboli or infarction
Catheter related sepsis
Arrhythmias: PVCs, ventricular tachycardia and fibrillation, complete
  heart block, new bundle branch block, supraventricular
  tachycardia
Death
Erroneous data

lines that will faciliate the safe performance of right heart catheterization in most patients are given.

Pneumothorax

The most frequent serious complication of subclavian venous puncture for right heart catheterization is pneumothorax, the incidence of which ranges from 0% to 6%.[8] The proximity of the subclavian vein to the lungs and pleura is responsible for this complication (Fig. 1), which may also occur during internal jugular vein puncture, especially if a "low" approach is taken. The use of a higher approach (e.g., at the apex of the triangle formed by the two heads of the sternocleidomastoid muscle) at least 2 inches above the clavicle,[40] with the needle aimed at a 30° angle towards the junction of the middle and medial thirds of the clavicle will minimize the risk of pneumothorax from this approach.

Similarly, the risk of pneumothorax from the subclavian route can be minimized, if the operator has a thorough understanding of the anatomy of the subclavian vein (Fig. 1).[41] The subclavian vein crosses under the clavicle approximately one third the length of the clavicle lateral to the sternoclavicular joint. Placing a rolled-up towel under the cervicothoracic vertebrae, with the patient in the Trendelenburg position, drops the shoulder to open access to the subclavian vein between the clavicle and first rib. The needle should be aspirated continuously as it is advanced, and never redirected during insertion. Lateral movement of the needle in the region of the subclavian vein may lacerate the vein, artery, or pleura. Following catheter placement, x-ray visualization is essential to confirm its position and to rule out pneumothorax which is rarely fatal if it is recognized promptly or, if it is small, it generally can be managed conservatively with serial physical examinations and chest x-rays. A pneumothorax greater than 30%, or one that is increasing in size, or even a small pneumothorax in a patient receiving assisted ventilation, requires a chest tube be placed.

In addition to air, blood or other fluids may enter the pleural space or mediastinum. Such complications include hemothorax, usually from laceration of the subclavian vein or artery, and hydrothorax or hydromediastinum (from infusion of fluid into the pleural space and mediastinum, respectively). The latter complication can be avoided by ensuring the catheter is in the intravascular space. Aspiration of free-flowing blood from the catheter at the time it is placed and carefully scrutinizing its position by chest x-ray study help to confirm its intravascular location.

Air Embolus

Although fatal air embolus is a rare complication of right heart catheterization, it should never occur if a few simple precautions are taken. Air may enter the central venous circulation at the time of the initial procedure or if tubing connections inadvertently become disconnected some time after catheterization. Routinely placing patients in the Trendelenburg position, especially those with a low central venous pressure and end-expiratory apnea during guidewire exchanges will minimize the risk of this complication. Needle hubs should not be exposed to air once the intravascular space has been entered (i.e., occluded with the thumb before the guidewire is inserted). If symptomatic air embolus is suspected, the patient should be quickly turned onto his/her left side and the air aspirated.

Cardiac Tamponade

This complication of right heart catheterization is still highly lethal;[35,42-44] mortality ranges from 65% to 95%. The frequent inadvertent insertion of 30-cm polyurethane triple lumen catheters into the beating right atrium or ventricle for concurrent central venous pressure monitoring and fluid infusions may actually be increasing the incidence of this complication. If the patient does not develop tamponade from bleeding into the pericardium at the time of perforation, direct infusion of fluid into the pericardial space will quickly result in tamponade physiology. A case seen recently at our institution illustrates the typical clinical setting.

A 43-year-old male with a recent history of anorexia, nausea, emesis, and progressive abdominal pain was admitted; acute pancreatitis was diagnosed. Two weeks later, a 7 French triple-lumen catheter was placed percutaneously, via the right subclavian vein. Blood was easily aspirated from the catheter and initial chest x-ray studies showed the catheter tip lay in the right atrium. One day later, the patient developed tachycardia and was diaphoretic. His systolic blood pressure was 70 mmHg. A pulmonary artery catheter was placed, and showed intracardiac diastolic pressures equalized in the range of 18– 20 mm. A two-dimensional echocardiogram demonstrated a large pericardial effusion. The patient underwent emergency pericardiocentesis at which time approximately 250 mL of clear fluid was withdrawn from the pericardial space; right heart and systemic pressures promptly returned to normal. The patient subsequently had an uneventful hospital course.

Cardiac perforation can occur from any access route and with any catheter material. In collected series,[42] 53% of perforations occurred in the right atrium, 33% in the right ventricle, and 7% each in the subclavian vein and vena cava. The antecubital approach may be a problem because of catheter-tip migration of up to 7 cm with changing arm position,[44] which may result in myocardial perforation. Tamponade may occur in minutes to days following catheter placement. The diagnosis should be suspected in any patient with a central venous catheter, who develops hypotension and rising central venous pressure. Clinical clues include increasing cardiac size on chest x-ray films; pulsus paradoxus, tachycardia, tachypnea, and low voltage on electrocardiogram. Elevation and equalization of diastolic pressures on pulmonary artery catheterization is confirmatory. Echocardiography demonstrates a large pericardial effusion and diastolic collapse of the right atrium and ventricle. Initial treatment measures include intravenous fluid and inotropic support, followed by emergency pericardiocentesis. Once hemodynamic stability is achieved, the catheter should be withdrawn. A pericardial catheter may be required for several days to monitor for continued hemorrhage and to prevent additional fluid accumulation. Occasionally, a patient will require surgery to close the defect.

Cardiac tamponade can be minimized by fluoroscopy or chest x-ray to confirm the position of the catheter after it has been placed. At the time it is inserted, easy withdrawal of blood is mandatory. Catheters not used for pacemaking or for measuring pulmonary artery pressures should be maintained above the pericardial reflection (i.e., high in the superior vena cava or innominate vein). The antecubital site should be avoided if the catheter is expected to be in place for several days. Whenever possible, soft, nontapered catheters should be used.

Thromboembolic Complications

The occurence of thromboembolic events complicating right heart catheterization is related to the intrinsic thrombogenicity of the foreign body in the vascular space, vessel perforation, duration of catheter placement, and mechnical factors such as distal placement of pulmonary artery catheters with vessel occlusion. The incidence of clinically significant thromboembolic events in the pulmonary vascular bed has been reported to be as high as 7%,[11] however, the incidence has been lower in other series.[17,25] If looked for carefully, the incidence of subclinical catheter-related thrombosis is very high, ranging from 66% to 100%.[45,46] Furthermore, mural thrombi are present in approximately 30% of patients with pulmonary artery catheters examined at autopsy.[27] Thrombosis does not appear to be decreased by low-dose heparin therapy, however, the use of heparin-bonded catheters significantly decreases the incidence of catheter-related thrombosis.[47] In addition to clinically significant thromboembolic events, the accumulation of thrombus at the catheter tip leads to erroneous data, and the inability to infuse fluid or to inject solutions for thermodilution cardiac output. This can be minimized by frequently flushing the catheter and by the continuous infusion of fluids at very slow rates.

Access vein thrombosis is a rare complication, more common in certain patient subgroups, i.e., chronic venous disease, polycythemia, patients undergoing multiple catheterizations, and pediatric patients where it may occur in as many as 2.1% of children undergoing serial catheterization.[48] Although rarely a cause of pulmonary embolus, prompt recognition and management is mandatory. These patients generally present with a swollen, painful extremity, which may not be apparent for several days to weeks after catheterization. Infection must be excluded as an exacerbating factor and if present, may require local venous excision. Thrombosis of the upper extremity generally can be managed with a relatively short course of anticoagulation. Involvement of the femoral or iliac veins generally requires long-term anticoagulation with warfarin.

Superior Vena Cava Syndrome

This syndrome[29] occurs when the vena cava is blocked. It is characterized by swelling of the upper extremity and face, distension of the neck veins, cyanosis, cough, dyspnea, and dysphagia. It is associated with malignancy in 80% of cases.[49] However, the presence of a catheter in the superior vena cava should be implicated immediately as a possible etiologic factor in any patient who develops this syndrome immediately after catheterization. The incidence of pulmonary emboli complicating this syndrome is very high,[50] and once suspected, the catheter should be removed immediately. Treatment consists of heparinization, followed by anticoagulation with warfarin for 3 to 6 months. Intravenous streptokinase may be useful in some cases.[51]

Horner's Syndrome

A rare complication of right heart catheterization,[24] Horner's syndrome is characterized by ipsilateral ptosis, miosis, and anhidrosis. It is more common after internal jugular puncture, but can be seen after subclavian puncture as well. The syndrome probably results from direct damage to the second order (preganglionic) sympathetic neurons which exit the spinal cord through the ventral roots to the paravertebral sympathetic chain. The fibers terminate in the superior cervical ganglion outside the carotid sheath and medial to the carotid artery at the level of the angle of the jaw. There is no specific treatment for this syndrome. Some cases resolve with time, whereas other patients are left with permanent neurologic damage.

Pulmonary Artery Rupture and Pulmonary Infarctions

With an overall incidence of 0.1% to 0.2%, rupture of the pulmonary artery with hemorrhage[14,17,19,25] is probably the most common cause of death in patients undergoing pulmonary artery catheterization. Peripheral pulmonary artery catheter placement into a small vessel and subsequent balloon inflation probably accounts for most of the cases. The outcome is fatal in approximately 50% of patients. Patients with known pulmonary hypertension or those receiving chronic anticoagulation or glucocorticoid therapy may be at greatest risk. The complication may be more frequent during cardiac surgery,[19] secondary to catheter-tip migration in the decompressed heart. Pulmonary infarction due to pulmonary artery thrombosis caused by arterial trauma or persistent obstruction by the catheter, can be seen in as many as 7% of patients. The appearance of a new infiltrate on chest x-ray films or unexplained, worsening hypoxemia should lead one to entertain the diagnosis. The incidence of pulmonary artery rupture or dissection can be minimized by placing balloon catheters in more central rather than peripheral pulmonary artery segments, avoiding balloon overinflation, and by daily monitoring the patient with chest x-ray studies. When possible, pulmonary artery catheters should be avoided in patients with known pulmonary hypertension. In these patients, catheter placement should be guided by fluoroscopy. Since the heart tends to shrink while patients are undergoing cardiopulmonary bypass, the catheter tip migrates further into the pulmonary vasculature, suggesting that catheters be retracted into sterile protective sleeves during the bypass and then readvanced when normal circulation is restored.[52]

Infectious Complications

Catheter-related infections run the gamut from inflamed insertion sites treated simply by catheter removal to sepsis requiring intravenous antibiotics. The latter complication may occur in as many as 2% of patients undergoing central monitoring.[53] When cultures are made routinely from the catheter tip, the incidence of positive cultures is approximately 6%; most are related to primary foci of infection at sites remote from and unrelated to the catheter. Nevertheless, the incidence of unsuspected endocarditis, as a consequence of prolonged pulmonary artery catheterization may be as high as 2% of patients autopsied.[24] The increasing use of Hickman catheters in patients receiving chronic chemotherapy for malignancy[54] has resulted in an increased incidence of catheter-related sepsis, which can be minimized if proper catheter care (i.e., sterile technique when infusing medication and avoiding catheter-related trauma) is exercised.

In most cases, the risk of catheter-related infection can be minimized by not leaving the catheter in place for more than 72 hours.[55] The site should be cleaned meticulously and inspected daily. Catheters should be manipulated under sterile conditions, although protective sleeves may decrease the overall incidence of infection. Once withdrawn a catheter that has been in place for several hours should not be readvanced. Unexpected fever in a patient with a central venous or right heart catheter should immediately heighten the physician's index of suspicion for catheter-related sepsis. Catheter removal must seriously be considered in patients with unexplained fever or positive blood cultures, who have no other apparent source of infection. Catheters should not be left in place for more than several hours in patients with prosthetic heart valves unless absolutely necessary. It has been our practice to administer prophylactic antibiotics in such cases. Mortality from prosthetic valve endocarditis ranges from 50% to 70%. Although there is no clear evidence that prophylactic antibiotics in this setting prevent prosthetic valve endocarditis, the consequences of infection are so great we err on the side of treatment in these high-risk patients.

Arrhythmias and Conduction Disturbances

Atrial and ventricular arrhythmias may occur as a consequence of mechanical irritation of the atrium or ventricle during right heart catheterization or if the guidewire is advanced too far at the time of central venous catheterization. These arrhythmias are usually transient in nature and best treated by withdrawing or repositioning the catheter. The incidence of "advanced" ventricular arrhythmias complicating pulmonary artery catheterization ranges from 12.5% to 30%,[18,31] with up to 3% of patients having sustained ventricular tachycardia or fibrillation. Although it has been reported that lidocaine prophylaxis may lower the incidence of this complication,[56] careful catheter manipulation, fluoroscopy, and minimizing catheterization time will obviate the need for lidocaine in most cases. Patients at highest risk for ventricular tachyarrhythmias are those with a prior history of ventricular tachycardia or fibrillation, pulmonary hypertension, congestive heart failure, and acute myocardial infarction. The incidence may be highest in patients with right ventricular infarction, in whom an irritable right ventricle may be more predisposed to ventricular tachyarrhythmias during bedside right heart catheterization. An occasional patient will develop ventricular ectopy some time following catheter placement. This may indicate catheter-tip migration or looping.

A new right bundle branch block, which can last up to 24 hours, may be seen in as many as 5% of patients undergoing right heart catheterization.[18,57] This block may occur because of the proximity of the conduction system to the ventricular septum, which may have been irritated by the catheter when it was placed. Up to 23% of patients with preexisting left bundle branch block,[57] will develop high-degree AV block at the time of right heart catheterization. This generally must be managed with a temporary pacemaker. At the time of right heart catheterization, a temporary pacemaker should be considered for any patient with a preexisting left bundle branch block, especially in the setting of acute myocardial infarction. Atropine, isoproteronol, or both should be available at the patient's bedside, even though they may prove ineffective. When heart block occurs in an unpaced patient during right heart catheterization, immediate attempts to sustain rhythm include: withdrawal of the offending catheter, external pacing, precordial thumping, or coughing.

Erroneous Data

Although not a complication in the usual sense, incorrect interpretation of data can lead to critical errors in patient management. Therefore, it is mandatory that at the time of catheter placement, transducers be correctly zeroed and calibrated at the mid chest in the supine patient. Dampened pressure tracings are not acceptable, particularly if the interpretation of pressure data is being used for "blind" catheter placement. In most cases, damping is due to a bubble in the catheter or transducer. This can be corrected by thoroughly flushing the catheter. Occasionally, damping is caused by a catheter-tip thrombus or a kinked catheter. Should damping occur, the catheter should be completely removed and replaced with another (kinking) or flushed and reused in the case of a thrombus at the tip. In patients with a low stroke volume, it may be difficult to distinguish pulmonary artery from pulmonary capillary wedge or right ventricular tracings, especially in patients with right ventricular infarction. In such cases, saturation data (abrupt increases in PO_2 in the wedge position), radiographic guidance, and timing pressure tracings with the electrocardiogram may be helpful. End diastole occurs at the onset of the R wave on the surface electrocardiogram. The upstroke of systolic pressures (e.g., right ventricular or pulmonary artery) is initiated after the R wave peaks but before the end of the T wave. With balloon inflation, the V wave in the pulmonary artery wedge position occurs at end systole, after the end of the T wave on the surface electrocardiogram (Fig. 6).

The measurement of thermodilution cardiac outputs, although simple to perform, must be carried out rigorously. Care must be taken to inject a fixed volume of 5% dextrose in water at a standardized temperature, with the computer constant properly adjusted for temperature, volume of injectate, and the catheter used. Generally, we obtain three readings over 2 to 3 minutes, with additional readings taken if the results do not agree. Severe tricuspid regurgitation or low output states may result in inaccurate values, caused by the loss or warming of the "cold" indicator prior to the appearance at the thermistor in the pulmonary artery. Shunts at the atrial, right ventricular, or pulmonary artery level also produce inaccurate output measurements. The indicator may be lost or diluted by right-to-left shunting or diluted by left-to-right shunting; the latter problem is further confounded by early recirculation of the indicator. The misinterpretation of spurious data may lead to the inappropriate management of such patients. The direct Fick method of output determination, utilizing blood oxygen content, should be used in the presence of shunt lesions.

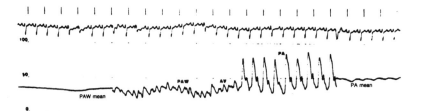

Figure 6. *Relationship of pulmonary artery and pulmonary artery wedge pressure waveforms to the surface electrocardiogram. The V wave in the pulmonary artery wedge tracing occurs after the T wave on the surface ECG. The upstroke of the pulmonary artery pressure occurs after the peak of the R wave, but prior to the end of the T wave. Note the marked difference between mean pulmonary artery and pulmonary artery wedge tracings. A = A wave; V = V wave; PA = pulmonary artery; PAW = pulmonary artery wedge pressure.*

In this discussion an attempt has been made to review the historic aspects, indications, and complications of central venous and right heart catheterization. Guidelines that can be used to minimize complications of central venous and right heart catheterization are given in Table 4.

Table 4

Guidelines to Minimize Complications of Central Venous and Right Heart Catheterization

---

General Considerations

1. Be certain that the indications for catheterization are firm. If the data can be reliably obtained by other means, catheterization should be avoided.
2. For catheterization of short duration, favor antecubital or external jugular routes over subclavian or internal jugular sites. Consider femoral route in patients with severe lung disease or coagulation abnormalities.
3. Avoid procedures in patients who are unable to cooperate.
4. If subclavian or internal jugular routes are taken, have patient in Trendelenburg position with attempt made to accentuate landmarks (e.g., towel between shoulder blades).
5. Use fluoroscopic guidance whenever possible. If catheter will not readily advance, consider use of dilute contrast material.
6. Perform catheterization with continuous electrocardiographic monitoring. Have defibrillation equipment in or near procedure room. Consider prophylactic temporary pacemaker placement in patients with underlying left bundle branch block.
7. Maintain strict sterility during catheter insertion and perform daily inspection of insertion site.
8. Inexperienced operators must be closely supervised throughout the procedure.

Optimal Performance of Percutaneous Puncture, Guidewire, and Catheter Placement

1. Advance a sharply beveled needle until blood is readily aspirated with a syringe. Drop the needle parallel to the axis of the vessel to facilitate guidewire passage.
2. If blood is not easily withdrawn, do not attempt to advance the guidewire.
3. If blood flow is pulsatile or the blood appears saturated, *do not place a sheath.* Venous or inadvertent arterial puncture can be

Table 4—(Cont'd)

Optimal Performance of Percutaneous Puncture, Guidewire, and Catheter Placement—(Cont'd)

confirmed by oximetry in most patients. Saturations less than 80% are usually venous blood.

4. If the guidewire does not advance readily, assess the wire's course with fluoroscopy. In some cases, a flexible J-tip will facilitate passage of wire. Use dilute contrast injections to identify anatomy. If the guidewire cannot be readily withdrawn through the needle, withdraw the wire and needle as a unit. Failure to do so may result in shearing of the wire and particulate embolus.

5. Following proper advancement of the guidewire, determine the wire's course if fluoroscopy is available (e.g., wire in RA or SVC and not heading cephalad in internal jugular vein or out contralateral subclavian vein with subclavian puncture).

6. Remove the needle over the guidewire while maintaining proximal pressure on the entry site to avoid blood loss. Make a nick with a #11 blade adjacent to the guidewire followed by initial dilation with a hemostat to facilitate dilation. Advance the dilator and sheath over the guidewire with gentle pressure and rotation at the skin. Never release the proximal end of the guidewire until it is visualized beyond the distal end of the dilator and sheath.

7. Have the patient stop breathing at end expiration during guidewire and sheath exchanges. Never allow the venous system to be open to air during normal respiration. Take care to avoid flushing air bubbles into the system following initial catheter placement.

8. Advance the catheter through the sheath to the desired anatomic location (e.g., SVC, RV, or pulmonary artery). If the catheter does not advance readily, confirm position under fluoroscopy.

Management of Patient Following Catheter Placement

1. Obtain a chest x-ray following the procedure to look for pneumothorax and to confirm proper catheter position. If multiple ipsilateral puncture attempts are unsuccessful (subclavian) never proceed to the contralateral side without first obtaining a chest x-ray to exclude pneumothorax.

2. Ensure proper transducer height and calibration to avoid erroneous data.

3. Change dressings daily. Never advance a catheter that has been in place more than a few hours.

Table 4—(Cont'd)

Management of Patient Following Catheter Placement—(Cont'd)

4. Do not infuse fluids through central venous catheters if blood cannot be readily withdrawn.
5. Never allow a pulmonary artery catheter to remain in "permanent wedge" position. Balloon inflation may result in pulmonary artery rupture or infarction. Carefully "trouble shoot" damped tracings.
6. Consider daily x-rays to confirm catheter position.
7. In most cases, pulmonary artery and central venous catheters should be changed to new site every 48 to 72 hours.

References

1. Forssman W: Die Sondierung des rechten Herzens. Klin Wochenschr 8:2085, 1929.
2. Cournand A: Cardiac catheterization. Development of the technique, its contributions to experimental medicine, and its initial application in man. Acta Med Scand (Suppl) 579:1, 1975.
3. Aubaniac R: Une nouvelle voie d'injection ou de ponction venneuse: la voie sous-claviculaire: veine soues claviere tronc brachiocephalique. Sem Hosp Paris 28:3445, 1952.
4. Keeri-Szanto M: The subclavian vein, a constant and convenient intravenous injection site. Arch Surg 72:179, 1956.
5. Borja AR: Current status of infraclavicular subclavian vein catheterization. Ann Thorac Surg 13:615, 1972.
6. Hermosura B, Vanagsland Dickey MW: Measurement of pressure during intravenous therapy. J Am Med Assoc 195:181, 1966.
7. Daily PO, Griepp RB, Shumway NE: Percutaneous internal jugular vein cannulization. Arch Surg 101:534, 1970.
8. McGoon MD, Benedetto PW, Greene BM: Complications of percutaneous venous catheterization: a report of two cases and review of the literature. Johns Hopkins Med J 145:1, 1979.
9. Furman S, Schweidel JB: An intracardiac pacemaker for Stokes-Adams seizures. N Engl J Med 261:943, 1959.
10. Swan JHC, Ganz W, Forrester J, et al: Catheterization of the heart in man with use of a flow-directed balloon-tipped catheter. N Engl J Med 283:447, 1970.
11. Foote GA, Schabel SI, Hodges M: Pulmonary complications of the flow-directed balloon-tipped catheter. N Engl J Med 290:927, 1974.

12. Gomez-Arnau J, Montero CG, Luengo C, et al: Retrograde dissection and rupture of pulmonary artery after catheter use in pulmonary hypertension. Crit Care Med 10:694, 1982.
13. McCloud TC, Putnam CE: Radiology of the Swan-Ganz catheter and associated pulmonary complications. Radiology 116:19, 1975.
14. Pape LA, Haffajee CI, Markis JE, et al: Fatal pulmonary hemorrhage after use of the flow-directed pulmonary artery catheter. Ann Intern Med 90:344, 1979.
15. Lipp H, O'Donoghue K, Resnekov L: Intracardiac knotting of a flow-directed balloon catheter. N Engl J Med 284:220, 1971.
16. Elliott CG, Zimmerman GA, Clemmer TP: Complications of pulmonary catheterization in the care of critically ill patients: a prospective study. Chest 76:647, 1979.
17. Boyd KD, Thomas SJ, Gold J et al: A prospective study of complications of pulmonary artery catheterizations in 500 consecutive patients. Chest 84:245, 1983.
18. Sprung CL, Pozen RG, Rozanski JJ, et al: Advanced ventricular arrhythmias during bedside pulmonary artery catheterization. Am J Med 72:203, 1982.
19. Rosenblum SE, Ratliff NB, Shirey EK, et al: Pulmonary artery dissection induced by a Swan-Ganz catheter. Cleveland Clin Q 51:671, 1984.
20. Rinaldo JE: Risks and benefits of pulmonary artery catheters. NY State J Med 84:484, 1984.
21. Brandstetter RD, Alarakhia N, Coli L, et al: Distal kinking of a pulmonary catheter as a cause of fatal hemoptysis. NY State J Med 84:521, 1984.
22. Willis C, Wight D, Zidulka A: Hypotension secondary to balloon inflation of a pulmonary artery catheter. Crit Care Med 12:915, 1984.
23. Myers ML, Austin TW, Sibbald WJ: Pulmonary artery catheter infections. A prospective study. Ann Surg 201:237, 1985.
24. Rowley KM, Chubb S, Walker Smith GJ, et al: Right-sided infective endocarditis as a consequence of flow-directed pulmonary catheterization. N Engl J Med 311:1152, 1984.
25. Shah KB, Rao TLK, Laughlin S, et al: A review of pulmonary artery catheterization in 6,245 patients. Anesthesiology 61:271, 1984.
26. Silver GM, Bogerty SA, Hayashi RM, et al: Arterial complications of attempted Swan-Ganz insertion. Am J Cardiol 53:340, 1984.
27. Ducatman BS, McMichan JC, Edwards WD: Catheter-induced lesions of the right side of the heart. J Am Med Assoc 253:791, 1985.
28. Teich SA, Halprin SL, Tay SB: Horner's syndrome secondary to Swan-Ganz catheterization. Am J Med 78:168, 1985.
29. Gore JM, Matsumoto AH, Layden JJ et al: Superior vena cava syndrome. Its association with indwelling balloon-tipped pulmonary artery catheters. Arch Intern Med 144:506, 1984.
30. Lois JF, Takiff H, Schecter MS, et al: Vessel rupture by balloon catheters complicating chronic steroid therapy. Am J Roentgenol 144:1073, 1985.

31. Iberti TJ, Benjamin E, Gruppi L, et al: Ventricular arrhythmias during pulmonary artery catheterization in the intensive care unit. Am J Med 78:451, 1985.
32. Falk RH, Zoll PM, Zoll RH: Safety and efficacy of noninvasive cardiac pacing. N Engl J Med 309:1166, 1983.
33. Lucas RV: Anamolous venous connections, pulmonary and systemic. In Adams FH, Emmanouilides GC (eds): Moss' Heart Disease in Infants, Children, and Adolescents. Baltimore, Williams and Wilkins, 1983, p 483.
34. Giesy J: External jugular vein access to the central venous system. J Am Med Assoc 9:1216, 1972.
35. Brandt RL, Foley WJ, Fink GH, et al: Mechanism of perforation of the heart with production of hydropericardium by a venous catheter and its prevention. Am J Surg 119:311, 1970.
36. Kron J, Sutherland D, Rösch J, et al: Arteriovenous fistula: a rare complication of arterial puncture of cardiac catheterization. Am J Cardiol 55:1445, 1985.
37. Bloch A: Murphy's Law and Other Reasons Why Things Go Wrong. Los Angeles, Price, Stern and Sloan, 1977.
38. Bernard RW, Stahl WM: Subclavian vein catheterization: a prospective study. Ann Surg 271:184, 1971.
39. Fein AM, Goldberg SK, Walkenstein MD, et al: Is pulmonary artery catheterization necessary for the diagnosis of pulmonary edema? Am Rev Respir Dis 129:1006, 1984.
40. Mostert JW, Kenny GM, Murphy GP: Safe placement of central venous catheter into internal jugular veins. Arch Surg 101:431, 1970.
41. Linos DA, Mucha P, Van Heerden JA: Subclavian vein. A golden route. Mayo Clin Proc 55:315, 1980.
42. Collier PE, Ryan JJ, Diamond DL: Cardiac tamponade from central venous catheters. Report of a case and review of the English Literature. Angiology 35:595,1984.
43. Maschke SP, Rogers HJ: Cardiac tamponade associated with a multi-lumen central venous catheter. Crit Care Med 12:611, 1984.
44. Krog M, Berggren L, Brodin M, et al: Pericardial tamponade caused by central venous catheters. Anesthesiology 48:445, 1978.
45. Hoar PF, Stone JG, Wicks AE, et al: Thrombogenesis associated with Swan-Ganz catheters. Anesthesiology 48:445, 1978.
46. Chastre J, Cornud F, Bouchama A, et al: Thrombosis as a complication of pulmonary-artery catheterization via the internal jugular vein: prospective evaluation by phlebography. N Engl J Med 306:278, 1982.
47. Mangaro DT: Heparin bonding and long-term protection against thrombogenesis. N Engl J Med 307:384, 1982.
48. Mathews RA, Park SC, Neches WH, et al: Iliac venous thrombosis in infants and children after cardiac catheterization. Cathet Cardiovasc Diagn 5:67, 1979.
49. Parish JM, Marschke RF, Dines DE, et al: Etiologic considerations in superior vena cava syndrome. Mayo Clinic Proc 56:407, 1981.

50. Warden GD, Wilmore DW, Pruit BA Jr: Central venous thrombosis. A hazard of medical progress. J Trauma 13:620, 1973.
51. Bradof J, Sands MJ Jr, Lahim PC: Symptomatic venous thrombosis of the upper extremity complicating permanent transvenous pacing. Reversal with streptokinase infusion. Am Heart J 104:1112, 1982.
52. Stone JG, Khambatta HJ, McDaniel DD: Catheter-induced pulmonary arterial trauma: can it always be averted? J Thorac Cardiovasc Surg 86:146,1983.
53. Goldenheim PD, Kazemi H: Cardiopulmonary monitoring of critically ill patients. N Engl J Med 311:717, 776, 1984.
54. Hendrick AM, Wilkinson A: Infectious complications of prolonged central venous (Hickman) catheterization. South Med J 67:639, 1978.
55. Applefield JJ, Caruthers TE, Reno DJ, et al: Assessment of the sterility of long-term cardiac catheterization using the thermodilution Swan-Ganz catheter. Chest 74:377, 1978.
56. Sprung CL, Marcial EH, Garcia AA, et al: Prophylactic use of lidocaine to prevent advanced ventricular arrhythmias during pulmonary artery catheterization: prospective double-blind study. Am J Med 75:906, 1983.
57. Akhtar M, Damato AN, Gilbert-Leeds CJ, et al: Induction of iatrogenic electrocardiographic pattern during electrophysiologic studies. Circulation 56:60, 1977.

Chapter 3

Complications of Retrograde Left Heart Catheterization and Interventional Angiography

Stephen A. Malone, Robert Palac, and Edward Murphy

Introduction

Despite its relatively short history, left heart catheterization with coronary arteriography has become one of the more common and routinely performed diagnostic procedures. In 1984, 570,000 cardiac catheterizations and 292,000 coronary arteriograms were performed.[1] In the last 10 years, interventional coronary arteriography in the form of intracoronary administration of thrombolytic agents, percutaneous transluminal angioplasty and, most recently, balloon valvuloplasty have further broadened the indications for imaging the coronary arteries and left ventricle. Despite the low incidence on a percent basis of major complications, the total number of patients suffering from adverse effects is sizable. This chapter reviews the indications, risks, and optimal technique of left heart catheterization. Major and vascular complications are defined and guidelines for management and prevention of these complications are presented.

From *Complications of Cardiac Catheterization and Angiography: Prevention and Management* edited by Jack Kron, M.D. and Mark J. Morton, M.D. © 1989, Futura Publishing Inc., Mount Kisco, NY.

History

The first attempts to visualize the coronary arteries were limited by difficulties both in selectively injecting the coronary arteries and the limited radiographic recording systems of the time. Initial studies involved nonselective catheter injections of the ascending aorta via direct puncture of the aortic arch.[2] In 1959, Sones and Shirey reported selective coronary arteriography by retrograde cannulation from the brachial artery.[3,4]

The combination of selective coronary cannulation from a peripheral artery with cinematographic recording provided easy access and high quality dynamic imaging. With the development of preshaped catheters, Judkins introduced the percutaneous femoral adaption which added speed, simplicity, and flexibility.[5] These developments, which facilitated the diagnosis and characterization of coronary artery disease, anticipated the advent of direct coronary revascularization, which began in the mid 1960s.[6,7]

During the past 10 years, three developments advanced left heart catheterization and coronary arteriography from a purely diagnostic procedure to a therapeutic modality. In 1977, Gruentzig demonstrated nonsurgical reduction in a coronary artery stenosis by percutaneous transluminal coronary angioplasty (PTCA).[8,9] In 1981, the first large clinical trial of the use of intracoronary streptokinase to reduce infarct size in acute coronary thrombosis was reported.[10] The percutaneous approach to treatment of valvular heart disease in the adult soon followed. In 1984 and 1985, Lababidi et al.[11] and Lock et al.[12] reported successful catheter balloon valvuloplasty (CBV) in young patients with congenital aortic stenosis and rheumatic mitral stenosis, respectively. Cribier et al.[13] followed, in 1986, with reports of successful percutaneous balloon valvuloplasty in elderly patients with acquired aortic stenosis. Thus, in less than 30 years, left heart catheterization and selective coronary arteriography have advanced to a high level, allowing precise anatomic and hemodynamic assessment of coronary and valvular heart disease, and have provided additional nonsurgical treatments for selected patients.

Indications

As the alternatives for the treatment of coronary artery disease and valvular heart disease expanded and the risks of catheterization

Table 1
Indications for Diagnostic Left Heart Catheterization and Coronary Arteriography

1. To establish or exclude the diagnosis of ischemic heart disease
   (a) chest pain of uncertain etiology
   (b) electrocardiographic evidence of myocardial ischemia without symptoms
   (c) critical occupations in relation to public safety
2. To direct management of patients with known ischemic heart disease (define operability or suitability for PTCA)
   (a) chest pain, congestive heart failure, arrhythmias, or mechanical complication following myocardial infarction
   (b) abnormal stress test following myocardial infarction
   (c) non Q-wave myocardial infarction
   (d) possible left main or three-vessel coronary artery disease by noninvasive testing
   (e) unstable angina
   (f) angina refractory to medical management
3. To direct management of patients with other cardiac symptoms
   (a) aborted sudden cardiac death
   (b) recurrent ventricular arrhythmias
   (c) preoperative evaluation for valvular or congenital heart disease
4. To assess left heart hemodynamics
   (a) valvular heart disease
   (b) congenital heart disease
   (c) cardiomyopathy
   (d) pericardial disease
5. To assess left ventricular global and regional systolic function by angiography
6. To quantify left side regurgitant lesions or left-to-right shunts by angiography

fell, the indications for left heart catheterization and coronary arteriography grew. A simplified outline of the general indications for left heart catheterization is given in Table 1.

Diagnostic Coronary Arteriography

The greatest percentage of left heart catheterizations are performed to determine the presence and extent of suspected coronary artery disease. Several authors have published lists of indications for coronary arteriography.[14-17] It should be remembered that although several guidelines exist, the chief indication for coronary arteriography is to define the coronary anatomy and associated left ventricular function in order to select appropriate therapy for ischemic heart disease.

Coronary arteriography is the only technique that provides a visual evaluation of the coronary anatomy. Therefore, it is the gold standard for the diagnosis of coronary artery disease, regardless of etiology. Thus, when the historic findings and noninvasive evaluations conflict or are equivocal, coronary angiography is the best examination for the confirmation or exclusion of coronary artery disease and its risks.

The most common reason for coronary arteriography is to direct the management of patients with known ischemic heart disease. It is used to assess risk for a future cardiac ischemic event in those with a history of unstable chest pain or in patients with a complicated course after myocardial infarction. Also, coronary arteriography defines the operability or suitability for PTCA in patients in whom angina is poorly controlled by medical therapy.

Left heart catheterization with coronary arteriography is indicated to assess possible ischemic myocardial disease in patients with recurrent ventricular arrhythmias or history of sudden cardiac death, or as part of the preoperative evaluation of patients with valvular or congenital heart disease. Less commonly, cardiac catheterization has been used to exclude coronary artery disease in patients who have evidence of silent myocardial ischemia. This is especially important in patients employed in occupations critical to public safety.

Diagnostic Left Heart Catheterization and Arteriography

Left heart catheterization is performed frequently in combination with right heart catheterization to evaluate valvular or congenital heart disease and to determine left ventricular function. Catheterization of the left ventricle allows one to measure left ventricular systolic and diastolic pressures and to inject contrast agents for left ventricular angiography. In addition, indicators can be injected for cardiac output measurements or shunt detection; also blood samples for oxygen content analyses can be obtained for shunt assessment.

The direct measurement of pressure gradients between the left atrium, left ventricle, and aorta remains the gold standard for the evaluation of stenotic mitral or aortic valves. Angiography of the left ventricle and aortic root is widely used to quantitate regurgitation through the mitral and aortic valves. Also, left ventriculography provides reliable, quantitative measurements of left ventricular size and global and regional systolic functions.

Thus, left heart catheterization remains the classic technique to define left heart hemodynamics and left ventricular function. However, recently improved noninvasive techniques may replace cardiac catheterization for some of the above purposes. Two-dimensional echocardiography provides good assessment of left ventricular wall motion and thickening in most but not all patients. From Doppler evaluations of stenotic and incompetent valves mean pressure gradients and the severity of regurgitation can be estimated, although volume flow measurements have been inadequate to date. Radionuclide ventriculography can provide high quality assessments of left ventricular volume, ejection fractions, and wall motions. The integration of noninvasive techniques with left heart catheterization is discussed further in Chapter 14.

Therapeutic Left Heart Catheterization

In contrast to diagnostic catheterization, the accepted indications for interventional left heart catheterization are still evolving. During the last decade, intracoronary administration of thrombolytic agents has been advanced for coronary reperfusion during the acute stages of transmural myocardial infarction. Administration of intracoronary streptokinase and recombinant tissue plasminogen activator during the first 3 to 6 hours of the onset of chest pain has produced small but sometimes significant improvements in early post myocardial infarction survival and myocardial function.[18,19] In a long-term follow-up of patients with acute myocardial infarction, early successful thrombolysis with intracoronary streptokinase improved the l-year survival rate, although nonfatal reinfarction rates were higher.[20]

Similarly, the indications for percutaneous transluminal coronary angioplasty (PTCA) are still evolving. The initial indication was anatomically suitable single-vessel coronary artery disease with demonstrable ischemia.[9,21] More recently, PTCA has been used to establish coronary artery reperfusion in patients during the early hours of myocardial infarction. The extent of myocardial salvage and the long-term patency results await confirmation by ongoing trials. The benefits versus risks of PTCA in patients who are mildly symptomatic or who have multivessel disease are presently being evaluated at a few medical centers.[22–24]

More recently, catheter balloon valvuloplasty (CBV) has been recommended as a palliative procedure for severe aortic stenosis and as a substitute for operative mitral commissurotomy in severe mitral stenosis.[25,26] Elderly patients with an increased surgical risk may be the most suitable candidates for this procedure. Application to other patients is likely as the technique improves, hemodynamic benefit is demonstrated, and long-term results are available to compare with surgery.

Technique

The goal of left heart catheterization and arteriography is to obtain a good quality, complete study with maximum patient safety. Many excellent descriptions of both the transfemoral and the brachial approach are available.[27–30] In any discussion of cardiac catheterization complications, several principles should be emphasized. Risks can be minimized by appropriate patient preparation, prompt attention to changes in the patient's condition, and tailoring the procedure to the individual.

Patient Preparation

This begins during the precatheterization evaluation and includes patient education. Patients with a history of known or suspected allergy to contrast media should be premedicated with antihistamines and steroids, as described in Chaper 9. Patients with ischemic heart disease should be stabilized on medical therapy prior to study. Pulmonary congestion in patients with congestive heart failure should be minimized without producing prerenal azotemia.

Patients with cardiogenic shock or hemodynamic instability should be stabilized with intravenous inotropic and vasoactive agents, and intra-aortic balloon pump counterpulsation should be considered. Nonionic contrast should be used for arteriography in individuals with unstable angina, congestive heart failure, or hemodynamic instability.

Patients with recurrent ventricular tachyarrhythmias should be stabilized with the best available medical therapy and direct current cardioversion must be readily available. Patients with monomorphic ventricular tachycardia may respond to overdrive pacing and a temporary pacemaker should be considered. The use of nonionic contrast may reduce the risk of arrhythmias; excessive contact with the endocardium should be avoided. During selective coronary arteriography, a temporary pacemaker (or central venous access with pacemaker available) and the use of nonionic contrast should also be considered for patients either with bradycardia or at high risk for bradycardia.

In the catheterization laboratory, intravenous atropine may be given before intracoronary injection to reduce the risk of prolonged asystole or severe bradycardia. In patients found to have high filling pressures, sublingual nitroglycerin or intravenous furosemide may be given prior to arteriography to reduce the possibility of sudden pulmonary edema. Conversely, patients with aortic stenosis or hypertrophic cardiomyopathy require elevated filling pressures to maintain stroke volume and must not be allowed to become dehydrated from overaggressive use of diuretics or the osmotic diuretic effect of contrast. Nonionic contrast agents are useful in minimizing blood volume changes in such patients.

Choice of Techniques

The current choice of brachial artery cutdown versus the percutaneous transfemoral approach should ultimately hinge on the operator's skill with either method and the patient's suitability. Although early studies of the hazards associated with left heart catheterization favored the brachial artery approach, later series have demonstrated that the transfemoral approach can be performed as safely.[31-34]

At times, the transfemoral approach may be more difficult or hazardous, as in patients with advanced aortoiliac disease or aortopelvic reconstructive surgery. Percutaneous brachial artery catheterization, using an arterial sheath, has been used in several centers as an alternative to brachial artery cutdown in patients with occlusive iliofemoral arterial disease. Although reported series are smaller in patient numbers, success rates of 95% to 97% are reported; local complication rates may be lower than with the cutdown approach.[35–38]

Attention to Details

Regardless of whether the brachial or transfemoral approach is chosen, certain subtleties in catheter technique are of paramount importance to reduce the risk of complications. The correct technique for guidewire and catheter manipulation includes the following:

1. During guidewire and catheter insertion and advancement, attention should be directed to the positions of the guidewire and catheter tip under fluoroscopy. The use of a safety J-wire often facilitates guidewire advancement in patients with extensive peripheral atherosclerosis or arterial tortuosity.
2. Care should be taken to prevent the passage of the advancing guidewire and catheter up the carotid arteries. The guidewire and catheter should not be advanced to the left ventricular apex if a mural thrombus is suspected.
3. Once the guidewire is removed and the catheter is connected to the manifold, the catheter tip pressure should be monitored continuously. A damped pressure indicates either thrombus formation or catheter tip impaction either against the vessel wall or in a small vessel and necessitates catheter withdrawal, aspiration, and flushing.
4. The coronary ostia should be entered carefully and with minimal catheter manipulation.
5. Meticulous attention must be paid to the guidewire; wiping it free of blood during catheter exchanges is imperative. Catheter exchanges and flushes should be performed as distally in the vascular tree as possible to avoid central embolization.
6. To further reduce the risk of thromboembolism, heparin should

be administered intravenously or intraarterially early in the catheterization procedure.

7. Several authors have suggested that the risk of thromboembolic complications rises as the duration of the procedure increases; thus, the briefer the procedure the shorter the time the patient is at risk.[39,40] However, sufficient time between coronary injections must be allowed for the systemic blood pressure, ST- and T-wave changes and QT interval, to return to normal to reduce the risk of ventricular fibrillation.

8. With the transfemoral approach, the pedal pulses and adequacy of distal flow should be checked immediately following catheterization and frequently thereafter for several hours. With the brachial approach, meticulous attention to the radial pulse is necessary following the catheterization.

Tailoring the Procedure

Throughout catheterization, the physician must integrate the returning anatomic and hemodynamic data with changes in the patient's condition and tailor the procedure to maximize patient safety without sacrificing diagnostic quality. Ischemic pain should be relieved before proceeding with the next injection of contrast. The volume of contrast should be minimized in patients with poor left ventricular function or with a pulmonary capillary wedge pressure greater than 30 mmHg. Pulmonary congestion, hypotension, and arrhythmias should be treated promptly. If a left main stenosis is suspected or discovered, the minimum number of left and right coronary injections required to assess the degree of stenosis and distal runoff should be performed.

Postcatheterization Care

Although left heart catheterization and coronary arteriography are now routinely performed in selected patients on an outpatient basis, meticulous postcatheterization care is still necessary for all patients. Vital signs, pulses, and the dressing and access site must be checked frequently for several hours following the procedure. Oral fluids are encouraged in patients without congestive heart failure to replace fluids lost in response to the osmotic diuresis from contrast. Adequate hydration is particularly important for patients with severe aortic stenosis who depend on higher filling pressures to sustain cardiac output. Patients with preceding renal insufficiency or diabetes are at higher risk for contrast-induced nephropathy and their urine output and renal function should be monitored carefully.

Some patients require intensive monitoring following catheterization. These include patients with unstable angina pectoris or myocardial infarction, or those receiving angioplasty, valvuloplasty, or intracoronary streptokinase. Depending on the various institutional protocols, these individuals may simply have electrocardiographic monitoring in the coronary care unit or may have retained arterial and venous access sheaths and right heart catheters. Intravenous anticoagulants and vasoactive agents may also be used.

Complications and Risk Factors

In the past 25 years, several large surveys have identified the risks of cardiac catheterization and angiography.[31-34,39,41-47] Judkins and Ganders have suggested that a 0.10% or less mortality rate is an acceptable risk.[48] The data available indicate that although complication rates have improved, this goal has been attained in only the more recent studies. Moreover, complication rates will increase because of the recent trend toward more aggressive management of acute myocardial infarction with diagnostic and interventional angiography[20].

Major Complications

The definitions of complications related to cardiac catheterization varies among the different surveys. However, the "major" complications, including mortality, myocardial infarction, and cerebrovascular accidents are the most easily quantified. For most surveys, mortality is defined as death occurring during the procedure or within the first 24 hours after the procedure. This time frame may be expanded if a later death is an identifiable consequence of an event in the laboratory. A myocardial infarction is defined as evidence of myocardial injury by ECG or cardiac enzyme analyses within 24 hours of the catheterization. In the Collaborative

Studies in Coronary Artery Surgery (CASS), mortality and myocardial infarction were assumed to be procedure-related up to 48 hours following catheterization.[45] A cerebrovascular accident is defined as any neurologic abnormality persisting for at least 24 hours after the study.

The incidences of major complications of left heart catheterization and coronary angiography in the largest surveys reported since 1973 are shown in Table 2. The vast majority of patients in these surveys had been evaluatied angiographically for coronary artery disease as opposed to earlier studies that evaluated a larger number of patients for valvular or congenital heart disease. The risk of death varied from 0.07% to 0.2% in the more recent prospective series to 0.45% in the earlier large study by Adams et al.[31] in 1973. A much higher mortality of 2.1% was reported by Takaro et al.[32] in 1973 from catheterizations performed as part of the VA Cooperative Study of Surgery for Coronary Arterial Occlusive Disease. This study included all fatalities within 10 days after arteriography, although 74% of deaths occurred within 24 hours of the procedure. Of the deaths in the VA Cooperative Study, 53% of the patients involved had an acute coronary occlusion based on evidence from angiography or histopathology. These data suggest a critical role for catheterization-induced coronary occlusion in catheterization related death. In the studies listed in Table 2, the overall incidence of myocardial infarction ranged from 0.07% to 0.6% and for cerebrovascular accidents from 0.03% to 0.23%.

Thromboembolism is believed to be the most frequent cause of the major complications.[32,33] A less frequent cause of myocardial infarction or death is coronary artery dissection from the injecion of contrast under an atherosclerotic plaque or catheter impingement with excessive force against the coronary artery intima. Catheter or guidewire manipulation in the arch or cranial vessels may also dislodge atherosclerotic debris, which may embolize to the brain with transient or permanent neurologic sequelae. Selective catheterization of aortocoronary bypass grafts or internal mammary artery to coronary grafts is likely to increase this complication because of increased catheter manipulation in the arch and subclavian arteries.

The variability in reported complication rates is the result of several factors: (1) Most reports are retrospective and suffer from incomplete accounting, most notable in surveys by Adams et al.,[31]

Table 2
Major Complications of Coronary Arteriography

Survey	Adams[31]		Tokaro[32]		Bourassa[33]	Adams[34]		Hansing[44]	Davis[45]		Kennedy[46]		Morton[47]	
Years of Study	1970–1		1968–72		1970–4	1973–4		1972–7	1975–6		1979–81		1977–82	
Technique	B	F	B	F	F	B	F	F	B	F	B	F	B	F
No. Patients	24124	22780	750	2300	5250	43080	45999	14050	1187	6328	23040	28934	183	7369
Death (%)	.13	.78	.3	2.2	.23	.12	.16	.19	.51	.14	.10	.12		.09
MI (%)	.22	1.01	—	—	.09	.15	.20	.13	.42	.22		.07		.11
CVA (%)	.03	.43	—	—	.13	.08	.09	.06	.08	.02		.07		.12
Total (%)	.38	2.22	—	—	.45	.35	.45	.38	1.01	.38		.28		.3

MI = Myocardial infarction; CVA = Cerebrovascular accident; B = Brachial technique; F = Percutaneous transfemoral technique.

Adams and Abrams,[34] and Takaro et al.[32] (2) Complication rates vary with the type and severity of underlying cardiac disease. More recent reports contain fewer cases of valvular heart disease and a predominance of coronary artery disease. The registry of the Society for Cardiac Angiography (SCA)[46] Study contained 77% coronary artery disease, 12% valvular disease, and 2.8% congenital heart disease, whereas the Collaborative Study of Coronary Artery Surgery (CASS)[45] was almost exclusively coronary artery disease. Laboratories with a higher prevalence of patients with normal coronary arteries had lower mortality rates. (3) Earlier studies[31,32] had reported higher major complication rates with the transfemoral approach than with the brachial technique, especially in institutions with yearly caseloads of less than 200. Local complications, especially arterial thrombosis, were more frequent with the brachial approach. One explanation offered was that since the transfemoral approach was easier to use, operators with less experience in coronary arteriography or its complications might be performing such examinations. However, in 1974 Adams and Abrams[34] repeated their survey of 475 institutions with open heart surgical teams. Analysis of the results of the 176 institutions responding revealed that the transfemoral approach can be performed with the same degree of safety as the brachial technique. In CASS, a higher morbidity was found with the brachial approach, especially for institutions where both approaches were used. The exception was institutions in which greater than 80% of the procedures were performed using the brachial approach. In these institutions complication rates were similar for brachial and transfemoral catheterization.

The risk directly attributable to coronary arteriography cannot always be assessed. In unstable patients at high risk for myocardial infarction, sudden death, or stroke, there is frequently no way to determine whether the event was due to the procedure or to the disease itself. CASS included deaths occurring the day after the procedure, even if the death was intraoperative and not clearly related to the catheterization. Hildner et al.[49] reported all complications associated with 1,606 diagnostic cardiac catheterizations from 24 hours before to 72 hours after the procedure. They found that spontaneous medical or surgical incidents were as common as procedure-related complications. Only vascular injury was clearly related to the procedure.

Despite the variations in reported mortality and morbidity rates, several patient characteristics have been repeatedly identified which predispose to major complications. In CASS,[45] these included left main coronary artery stenosis greater than 50%, triple vessel coronary artery disease, a left ventricular ejection fraction less than 0.30, congestive heart failure, hypertension, and multiple premature ventricular ectopic beats. In addition, the New York Heart Association functional class 4 angina was associated with an increased risk of death in the Society for Cardiac Angiography registry.[46]

Left main coronary artery disease has had the strongest association with increased risk for angiography, including a sevenfold increased risk of death.[45] Left main stenosis greater than 60% was found in 46%, 24%, 75%, and 47% of the deaths in the series reported by Adams et al.,[31] Takaro et al.,[32] Bourassa and Noble,[33] Davis et al.,[45] and Kennedy,[46] respectively. In CASS,[45] the mortality in patients with significant left main disease undergoing coronary angiography was 0.94%.

Patients with unstable angina are at increased risk for myocardial infarction during and following coronary angiography.[45] Critical aortic stenosis is associated with a higher incidence of sudden death following cardiac catheterization and angiography.[50] The Society for Cardiac Angiography registry identified ages less than 1 year or greater than 60 years as high-risk groups for procedure-related mortality.[50] However, CASS reported no increase in major complications in patients 65 years of age and older.[51]

Arrhythmias

The serious arrhythmias associated with coronary arteriography are ventricular fibrillation, ventricular tachycardia, and prolonged bradycardia. Of the three, ventricular fibrillation (Fig. 1) is the most common, with an incidence ranging from 0.32% to 1.28%.[33,34,45–47] Ventricular fibrillation, in the majority of cases, occurs after right coronary artery injection. It can occur in patients without significant atherosclerosis; in fact, in the series by Bourassa and Noble,[33] approximately one-half of the cases in which ventricular fibrillation was induced reportedly had normal coronary arteries. In the largest study addressing ventricular arrhythmias

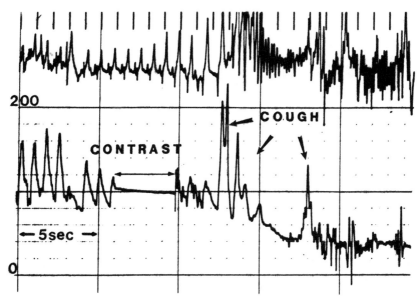

Figure 1. *Ventricular fibrillation following left coronary artery injection is shown. The upper tracing is the electrocardiogram and the lower is the catheter tip pressure. The patient was successfully defibrillated and suffered no long-term adverse effects.*

during coronary angiography, 67% of the episodes of ventricular tachycardia or ventricular fibrillation occurred after contrast injection into minimally diseased coronary arteries.[52] The electrocardiographic changes preceding these arrhythmias in patients with minimally diseased coronary arteries included prolonged bradycardia with a pause greater than 6 seconds or a large increase in T-wave amplitude and pronounced widening of the QRS and QT intervals. The arrhythmias occurred late in the procedure, i.e., after several previous injections.

The mechanism(s) behind ventricular fibrillation following coronary artery injection are unclear. Ischemia may play a role but most of the arrhythmogenic effects are believed due to the various components of the contrast agent. Contrast media has been shown to lower the ventricular fibrillation threshhold by altering myocardial metabolism.[53,54] Sodium iodide slows conduction by inactivating the fast sodium channel and thus may predispose to reentry

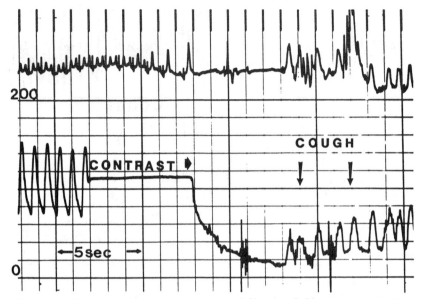

Figure 2. *Sinus arrest with hypotension following left coronary injection is shown. The upper tracing is the electrocardiogram and the lower is the catheter-tip pressure. Coughs aid the return to normal sinus rhythm.*

tachyarrhythmias.[55] The EDTA and sodium citrate in Renografin-76 are calcium sequestering agents and produce local hypocalcemia and prolong the QT interval.[56]

Bradycardia (Fig. 2) is a frequent consequence of intracoronary contrast injection. Mechanisms proposed include sinus node and atrioventricular node suppression by direct action of the hyperosmolar contrast, reflex vagal stimulation, and reflexes mediated by chemoreceptors located in the left ventricular myocardium.[57,58] The arrhythmias associated with angiography are further discussed in Chapter 9.

Vascular Complications

Taken collectively, local vascular complications are the most common significant risk of arterial catheterization. Potential peripheral vascular complications at the site of arterial puncture include arterial thrombosis, arterial laceration or dissection, pseudoaneurysm, hematoma, arteriovenous fistula, peripheral thromboembolism, and thrombophlebitis. The reported incidences of local vascular complications for several large series are shown in Table 3. The overall risks of vascular complications were 0.57% and 0.84%, in the SCA registry[46] and CASS[45] reports, respectively.

In early series, brachial artery catheterization was associated with marked reductions or loss of the radial pulse in 12.2% to 28% of cases.[59-62] Loss of pulse necessitated reopening the arteriotomy in 9.6% and 5.4% of cases in the surveys by Campion et al.[59] and Machleder et al.,[60] respectively. In the vast majority of cases, loss of pulse was associated with brachial artery thrombosis. Less common causes were arterial spasm, an obstructing intimal flap, or arterial stenosis.

Arterial thrombosis continues to be the most common complication after brachial arteriotomy. Brachial artery thrombosis occurred in 1.67% and 1.9% of the surveys by Adams et al.[31] and Davis et al.,[45] respectively. Predisposing factors to brachial artery thrombosis include small artery size, failure to remove a thrombus formed during catheterization, an initial flap retained at arterial repair, and arterial spasm following repair.[63] Other reported local complications of the brachial artery cutdown approach include peripheral thromboembolism, median nerve injury, either from laceration during dissection or from later bleeding with nerve compression by the hematoma, wound infection, or thrombophlebitis.

Percutaneous brachial artery catheterization using an arterial sheath is an alternative to brachial artery cutdown in patients with contraindications to the transfemoral technique. Fewer reports of complications are available. In the largest series, loss of radial pulse occurred in 2% and local hematomas in 4%.[35,37]

Local vascular complication rates for percutaneous transfemoral catheterization have fallen over the years. From different sources, the reported rates are 1.70% in 1968, 1.41% in 1973, 0.85% in 1976, 0.36% in 1979, and 0.40% in 1984.[62,31,34,45-47]

The most common local vascular complication of percutaneous transfemoral catheterization is intraluminal thrombus formation resulting in femoral artery occlusion (Fig. 3). A predisposition to femoral artery thrombosis was found in females with small femoral arteries by Bourassa and Noble[33] and Kloster et al.[64] Other risk

Table 3
Local Vascular Complications of Coronary Arteriography

Survey	Adams[31]		Bourassa[32]	Adams[34]		Davis[45]		Kennedy[46]		Morton[47]	
Years of study	1970-1		1970-4	1973-4		1975-6		1979-81		1977-82	
Technique	B	F	F	B	F	B	F	B	F	B	F
No. patients	24124	22780	5250	43080	45999	1187	6328	23040	28934	183	7369
Arterial Thrombosis, Dissection, or Rupture (%)	1.67	1.19	.68	1.13	.23	2.78	.37		.56	2.7	.4
Hematoma Requiring surgery (%)	.07	.16	—	.05	.14						—
Pseudoaneurysm (%)	.06	.06	.17	.04	.05						.08
Total (%)	1.80	1.41	.85	1.22	.42	2.78	.37		.57		.5

B = Brachial; F = Percutaneous transfemoral.

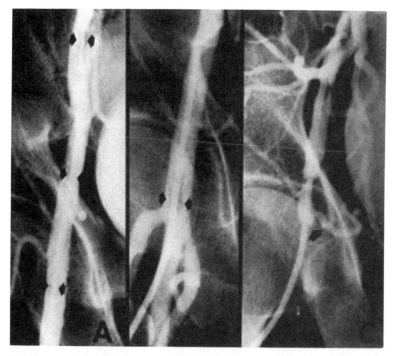

Figure 3. *Abnormal pullout iliofemoral arteriograms are shown for three patients who had left ventriculograms and coronary arteriograms. A. Fibrinous sheath around the catheter (arrows). B. Localized thrombus at catheter entry site (arrow). C. Occlusion of the femoral artery at the entry site (arrow). (Courtesy of Antonovic R, Rösch J, Dotter CT: The value of systemic heparinization in transfemoral angiography: a prospective study. Am J Roentgenol 127:223, 1976.)*

factors may include long procedures, excessive catheter manipulation, or frequent catheter changes. The improvement in femoral artery thrombosis rates in recent years is believed to be due to technical improvements and the use of heparin.[40]

Other local complications of the femoral artery approach include peripheral thromboembolism, pseudoaneurysm, arteriovenous fistula (Fig. 4), and large hematoma with vascular or nerve compromise. Retroperitoneal hemorrhage may occur following perforation of the iliac vessels. Local infection is uncommon with the

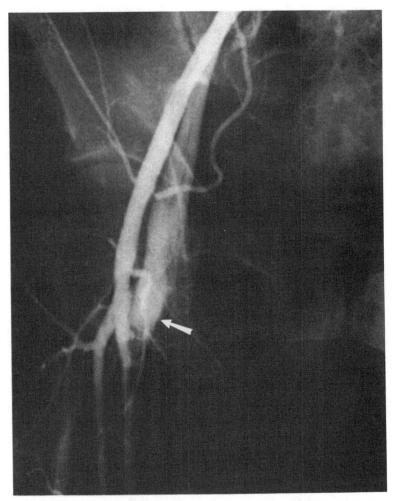

Figure 4. *An arteriovenous fistula (arrow) in a patient with a previous percutaneous transfemoral catheterization. The contrast dye was injected into the right iliac artery antegrade from a catheter placed via the left femoral artery. (Courtesy of J Rösch.)*

femoral technique, but rare cases of septic thrombophlebitis have occurred.

Complications related to femoral vein puncture occur even when catheterization is limited to the left heart. Inadvertent femoral vein puncture attends searching for the femoral artery, and the femoral vein may also be punctured when it lies posterior to the artery. The latter situation is perhaps the worst because the operator never knows that the vein was punctured.

The risk of peripheral vascular complications from PTCA in the absence of lytic therapy approximates that of the more recent surveys of diagnostic left heart catheterization.[65] Local vascular complication rates are higher with catheter balloon valvuloplasty.[13,66] The management of catheterization-related vascular injuries is discussed in Chapter 11.

Other Complications

Multiple other complications have been reported with left heart catheterization and coronary arteriography. Perforation of the heart or great vessels is uncommon and is usually associated with difficulty in catheter passage and excessive manipulation. Pulmonary edema may occur due to excess fluid administration, myocardial ischemia, or the bradycardia or negative inotropic effect of the contrast media. Hypotension may occur from the complications listed above, vasovagal reactions, anaphylactoid reactions, or contrast effects, including immediate vasodilation or late hypovolemia from osmotic diuresis. Fevers occur secondary to contrast reactions, local phlebitis or infection, or pyrogen reaction. Pyrogen reactions are caused by endotoxin contamination of resterilized catheters. Since disposable catheters are now used, pyrogen reactions occur much less frequently. Renal insufficiency can result from contrast nephrotoxicity or atheromatous emboli. Contrast nephropathy is further discussed in Chapter 10.

Additional Risks of Interventional Angiography

Systemic and selective administration of intracoronary thrombolytic agents has been advanced to reduce the size of a myocardial infarction.[10,67,68] The success of establishing coronary reperfusion has been found to decrease with the duration of chest pain or age of the thrombus. Early animal work indicates that salvage of myocardium is possible up to 6 hours after abrupt coronary occlusion.[69] However, while digestion of circulating fibrin and fibrinogen occurs within minutes of streptokinase infusion, clot lysis may take much longer, fail altogether, or result in rethrombosis in up to 30% of cases.[70,71]

The most comprehensive data regarding the results of streptokinase intracoronary infusion were reported from the Society for Cardiac Angiography registry.[72] The in-hospital mortality rate was 8.2%, although there was no control group.[66] Additional major complications included ventricular reperfusion arrhythmias in 4.9%, hypotension requiring therapy in 1.9%, dissection of the right coronary artery in 0.5% and hemorrhage in 1.3%. Other investigators have found a higher risk of hemorrhage, with 7% of patients requiring blood tranfusion after intracoronary streptokinase.[73,74] Other risks include anaphylaxis to streptokinase in 1.7% to 18% of cases and hemorrhage in the area of myocardial necrosis, which may predispose to fatal cardiac rupture.[75-77] The risk of bleeding from diagnostic or interventional catheterization early after the administration of thrombolytic agents is also increased.[78]

Percutaneous transluminal coronary angioplasty was first performed in 1977.[8] In 1983, the National Heart, Lung and Blood Institute reported the complication rates of its first 1,500 patients from its registry.[65] The major complication rate was 9.2%, which included in-hospital death (1.17%), nonfatal myocardial infarction (3.9%), or the need for emergency surgery (6.8%). The total major complication rate has fallen to 6% in the 1987 report despite inclusion of patients with more complex disease.[79]

Coronary artery occlusion was reported in 4.6% and coronary artery dissection or intimal tear distal or remote to the lesion was reported in 9.2%. Coronary dissection was associated with adverse effects in less than one-third of the cases. An additional 1.5% of cases sustained vascular complications, including arterial thrombosis (0.8%), pseudoaneurysm (0.13%), hematoma (0.33%), femoral arteriovenous fistula (0.07%), femoral artery aneurysm (0.07%), and arterial laceration (0.07%). Pericardial tamponade also has been reported as a complication of PTCA, from right ventricular perforation with the pacing wire, or as a rare complication of coronary artery perforation.[80,81]

Catheter balloon valvuloplasty was first performed in adults in 1986[13]; thus, the complication rates are not as well defined. In one series of 32 elderly patients undergoing aortic balloon valvuloplasty, the complications included in-hospital deaths (9.4%) and hemorrhage requiring transfusion (31.3%). One patient required surgical repair of a left ventricle perforation by the guidewire with cardiac tamponade and another received coronary artery bypass grafting and aortic valve replacement for continued angina after valvuloplasty. No embolic complications were reported. Aortic insufficiency was mildly increased in the majority of cases.

The largest series of patients receiving aortic balloon valvuloplasty is the French registry.[82] Of 607 patients receiving balloon dilatations, complications occurred in 23.5%. These included deaths during the procedure in 0.8%, in-hospital deaths in 8%, femoral artery complications in 13% (one-half of which required surgery), pulmonary edema and cardiogenic shock in 3.2%, stroke in 2%, and cardiac tamponade in 1%. Of note, in-hospital mortality was highest in patients over 70 years of age and in nonsurgical candidates. Furthermore, mortality declined with operator experience from 12% for the first 10 patients studied in each center to 4% for later patients.

Management and Prevention of Complications

Complication rates of left heart catheterization and arteriography have improved with the use of more adequate preventive measures. These preventive measures include anticipation of the high-risk patient; early recognition and stabilization of the patient with ongoing ischemia, pulmonary edema, or hemodynamic instability; adequate premedication, including that for contrast allergy; and the routine use of heparin.

Acute Coronary Artery Occlusion or Dissection

Coronary artery occlusion may occur during catheterization from thrombosis at the site of an atherosclerotic plaque, from catheter-induced thromboembolism (Fig. 5), or from subintimal coronary dissection (Fig. 6) produced by catheter trauma or PTCA. If coronary collaterals to the bed distal to the occlusion are inadequate, myocardial infarction will occur. In patients with embolic or spontaneous thrombotic occlusion, thrombolytic agents or PTCA may reestablish flow. Acute coronary occlusion following PTCA is caused

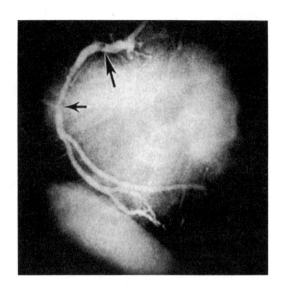

Figures 5A-C. *Acute right coronary artery occlusion from catheter-induced thromboembolism. A. A catheter tip thrombus (large arrow) and a severe mid-vessel stenosis (small arrow) are seen during the initial right coronary artery injection.*

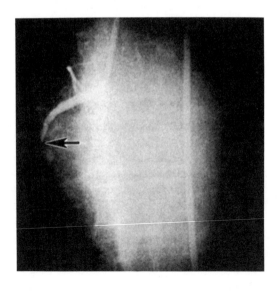

Figure 5B. *A second contrast injection reveals acute occlusion of the mid-right coronary artery (arrow) at the stenosis.*

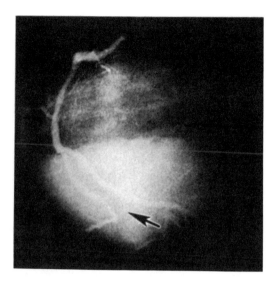

Figure 5C. *Percutaneous transluminal coronary angioplasty reestablishes mid-right coronary artery patency but distal thromboembolism occurs with occlusion of a posterior descending artery branch (arrow).*

by dissection or spasm, and less frequently by thrombosis or embolism. The retention of a guidewire across the lesion has allowed many of these occlusions to be successfully redilated or flow to be reestablished with intracoronary and systemic vasodilators. Intracoronary stents are now being investigated as a mechanism for maintaining patency in this setting. When mechanical or pharmacologic measures fail to reestablish flow, surgical revascularization may be necessary to prevent or minimize infarction. In this setting, systemic arterial to coronary shunt perfusion catheters may be useful to maintain myocardial viability prior to surgery and are currently being evaluated.

Subintimal coronary artery dissection has been reported in 0.05% of coronary angiograms.[32,83-86] Dissections of the right coronary artery are more common than of the left coronary artery[33]; however the majority of left coronary dissections result in myocardial damage, whereas only one-half of the right coronary artery dissections lead to myocardial infarction.[83] Predisposing factors for dissections include coronary artery medial degeneration, left main atherosclerosis, and excessive catheter manipulation, e.g., in the case of an unusual takeoff of the left main coronary artery from the aorta. The dissection is frequently caused or extended by the

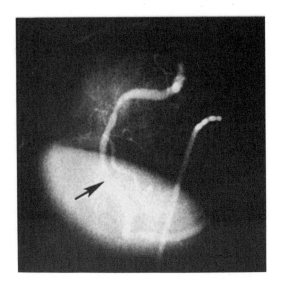

Figures 6A-C. *Right coronary artery dissection followed by acute coronary occlusion during percutaneous transluminal coronary angioplasty (PTCA) is shown. A. Before PTCA, there is a severe mid-right coronary narrowing (arrow).*

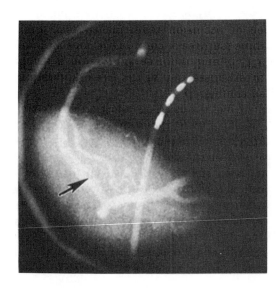

Figure 6B. *Following PTCA, coronary injection reveals a mid-vessel dissection (arrow).*

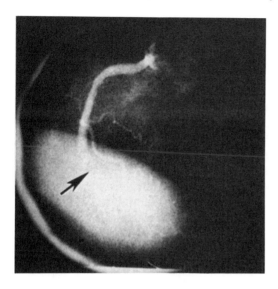

Figure 6C. *Coronary injection a few minutes later shows acute coronary occlusion (arrow).*

jet of contrast from the endhole of the coronary catheter, which is impacted on or in the intima. Many dissections are self-limiting and recanalization occurs frequently. If myocardium is jeopardized by the dissection, surgical revascularization is necessary.

The most important factor in preventing dissection is the use of pressure monitoring during selective coronary angiography. Contrast should never be injected into an artery with a damped pressure. Pressure damping indicates endhole impaction against or into the arterial wall. In this setting, contrast injection will force contrast under high pressure through the intima to produce dissection in the media. Some investigators have advocated the use of non-preformed catheters or blunt, soft-tipped catheters.[87] Regardless of the approach or the catheter used, the operator should refrain from manipulating the catheter within the coronary artery. After the coronary artery is cannulated, the catheter should be withdrawn a few millimeters from the vessel lumen. If the pressure tracing is normal, we advocate, at this time, a small test injection before the coronary artery is opacified completely.

Subintimal coronary artery dissection at the site of dilatation is a frequent sequela of PTCA and requires surgery in a small fraction of cases. Angiographic features of coronary lesions with an increased risk of dissection or occlusion requiring surgery after

PTCA include irregular borders, intraluminal lucency, and location of the stenosis at a bifurcation or in a curve.[88] Left main coronary artery dissection is a reported complication of PTCA, especially in patients with known left main coronary irregularity and may require emergency surgical revascularization.[65,89]

Catheter-induced (iatrogenic) coronary artery spasm occurs from mechanical irritation of the intima. The reported incidence varies from 0.26% to 2.9% and is believed to be highly related to the skill of the angiographer.[90,91] It is more frequent in the right coronary artery and with the Judkins' technique.[92] Iatrogenic spasm may be more resistant to reversal with nitroglycerin because of coexistent intimal injury. Multiple doses of sublingual or intracoronary nitroglycerin and sublingual calcium channel antagonists may be required. A case of refractory coronary artery spasm requiring emergency coronary bypass surgery has been reported.[93]

Arrhythmias

Intracoronary contrast injection has been shown to lower the ventricular fibrillation threshhold by multiple mechanisms, as described above and in Chapter 9. To minimize the cumulative toxic effects of intracoronary contrast injections, the operator should allow sufficient time between injections for systemic pressure, ST- and T-wave changes, and the QT interval to return to baseline. The incidence of ventricular fibrillation has been reduced by the use of sodium meglumine diatrizoate contrast in which EDTA and sodium citrate have been replaced by disodium calcium EDTA.[94] Recently, nonionic contrast has been shown to produce a much lower incidence of ventricular fibrillation and bradycardia than sodium meglumine diatrizoate.[95]

Bradycardia is a frequent consequence of intracoronary contrast injection. Atropine sulfate premedication has been shown to reduce the incidence of bradycardia.[96,97] Routine atropine sulfate administration for diagnostic coronary angiography is not without complications. The most important is tachycardia mediated increased myocardial oxygen demand. In addition, anticholinergic effects will produce a dry mouth and occasionally urinary retention. Atropine also renders subsequent ergonovine testing less reliable. We recommend the use of atropine before coronary arteriography, except in cases of unstable angina or if ergonovine testing is planned. For cases of unstable angina, vigorous cough or the use of nonionic contrast is an effective alternative.[98] In ergonovine testing, prophylactic right ventricular pacemaker placement is recommended.

Thromboembolic Complications

Fibrin and platelet adherance to guidewire and catheter surfaces soon after exposure to the bloodstream has been well demonstrated.[40,99,100] This layer of platelets is stripped from the guidewire and transferred to the catheter tip during guidewire withdrawal. Also, during catheter exchanges, platelet masses are deposited at the site of arterial puncture (Fig. 7) and adhere to the surface of the newly inserted catheter.

Meticulous attention to the details of guidewire and catheter insertion, removal, and flushing has reduced the thromboembolic complications of left heart catheterization and coronary angiography.[101] Double aspiration is performed each time a guidewire is used

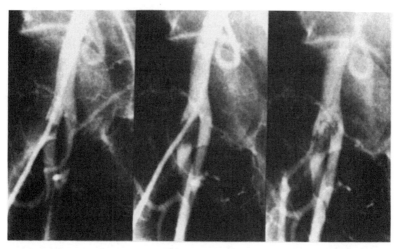

Figure 7. *Panels show progressively enlarging depositions of intraluminal thrombi at the catheter entry site during catheter withdrawal. (Courtesy of J Rösch.)*

or when a problem with aspiration occurs. The initial aspirate is vigorously withdrawn and discarded. A second aspiration is then performed, drawing a small amount of blood into the syringe and then injecting the catheter with heparinized (2,000–5,000 units/L of heparin) saline to clear the blood from the lumen. The operator should more forcibly flush catheters with sideholes, such as the pigtail catheter, because of their propensity for clot formation distal to the sideholes. Catheters are flushed every 2 minutes and guidewire manipulation time is limited to 2 minutes. The guidewire should be wiped free of blood before the catheter is inserted and the catheter aspirated and flushed before the guidewire is reinserted. The operator should avoid advancing the guidewire to the apex of the left ventricle if the possibility of a mural thrombus exists. Also, care should be taken to prevent the passage of the advancing guidewire or catheter up the carotid or subclavian arteries.

Left heart catheterization from a brachial artery cutdown has routinely been performed with systemic heparinization. In contrast, in the earlier years of the percutaneous transfemoral approach, heparin was not administered routinely. The catheter was simply flushed frequently with a dilute solution of heparin. After the demonstration of fibrin and platelet deposits on the outer surfaces of catheters, some investigators began injecting heparin boluses into the abdominal aorta as the catheter was introduced. It has been a matter of debate whether the decreased thromboembolic and major complication rates with the Judkins' method, in recent years, have been at least in part due to the adoption of systemic heparinization.

Several authors have advocated the routine use of initial bolus systemic heparin in doses varying from 2,000 units to 100 units/kg.[102–107] In one controlled study by Wallace et al. in 1973, a 45-unit/kg initial injection of heparin into the abdominal aorta was shown to statistically reduce catheterization-related thromboembolic complications and mortality.[103] In contrast, in the more recent CASS and SCA surveys, the use of heparin did not significantly influence the complication rates.[45,46] In the prospective study by Morton and Beanlands,[47] a small but statistically significant reduction in mortality was found in cases treated with systemic heparin.

We believe the potential benefits of heparin administration during left heart catheterization and coronary angiography outweigh any demonstrated risks of bleeding. Our protocol is to administer heparin in a dose of 10 units/lb at the time of arterial cannulation for routine left heart catheterization and coronary angiography. We give higher doses of heparin if nonionic contrast is used. Coaxial catheter systems and prolonged guidewire placement mandate the use of full systemic anticoagulation. Accordingly, we use 10,000 units of heparin for coronary angioplasty, and most centers utilize a similar amount. This larger dose of heparin is associated with bleeding, and a 0.7% incidence of excessive blood loss was reported in the NHLBI PTCA registry.[65] Due to its powerful effect on platelet aggregation, aspirin is routinely used in PTCA and may be of benefit in diagnostic coronary angiography as well. However, increased hematoma formation as well as frank bleeding will probably be more common in patients receiving antiplatelet therapy. We discourage the use of platelet-active medications in patients undergoing outpatient angiography.

Local Vascular Complications

The risk of local arterial complications can be reduced by careful operator technique and systemic heparinization. Also, a strictly followed postcatheterization regimen will recognize vascular complications earlier for prompt treatment to decrease long-term sequelae.

With the transfemoral approach, the pedal pulses and adequacy of distal flow should be checked immediately after catheterization and frequently for several hours. Immediate surgical embolectomy is indicated for femoral artery occlusion to relieve limb ischemia and to prevent propagation of the thrombus into more distal arterial branches.[108]

Evacuation of local hematomas is rarely required after diagnostic angiography utilizing the Judkins' technique. However, due to the lytic state after intracoronary streptokinase, hemorrhage from the arterial puncture site is common and the introducer sheath should remain in place until fibrinogen levels and the clotting cascade are repleted. Retroperitoneal bleeding may occur from inadvertent iliac vessel puncture and should be suspected if the patient complains of back pain or if bradycardia or hypotension occur. Retroperitoneal bleeding is usually self-limited following diagnostic arteriography. Evidence for continued bleeding should suggest arterial laceration and the need for surgical repair.

With the brachial cutdown approach, prevention of arterial thrombosis includes careful arteriotomy repair and routine administration of systemic heparin at the start of the procedure. Just prior to arteriotomy repair, the proximal and distal arterial segments should be checked for free bleeding. Immediately after arteriotomy closure, the radial artery should be palpated and the pulse amplitude should be the same as prior to arteriotomy. If the pulse is diminished or absent, the arteriotomy should be reopened. Thrombi should be removed from the distal arterial segment by inserting the Sones' catheter for aspiration or using a Fogarty embolectomy catheter; any intimal flaps should be resected. The radial pulse should be reexamined later the same day. If diminished or absent, arterial spasm or thrombosis has occurred. If no other signs of limb ischemia are present, the patient can be observed for return of the radial pulse on intravenous heparin with surgery consultation. In contrast to the transfemoral approach, arterial occlusion is more common with the brachial approach, but patients can be frequently observed for the development of limb ischemia and surgery is sometimes not required.

An uncommon local complication of transfemoral and brachial artery catheterizations is pseudoaneurysm (Fig. 8) formation from free communication between the artery and a liquifying hematoma. A pseudoaneurysm should be suspected if a pulsatile mass is detected on postcatheterization follow-up and should be surgically repaired because of the danger of continued enlargement and rupture.

The Incomplete Study

A "complication" not reported in series on left heart catheterization is the incomplete study. Studies may be incomplete because of a failure to adequately visualize all of the coronary artery branches due to poor framing, underfilling the arteries with contrast, or an insufficient number or poor choice of views. Alternatively, the procedure might be terminated early because of patient instability.

Newer data processing systems have made the incomplete study less common in recent years. Immediate video replay permits analyses of previously recorded coronary artery views during the procedure. Unfortunately, limits to video resolution, operator oversight, and patient instability or difficult anatomy have all resulted in incomplete studies from time to time.

High Risk Patients

Patient characteristics associated with an increased risk for major complications have been discussed above. These include left main coronary artery disease, severe triple vessel disease, congestive heart failure, unstable angina, and critical aortic stenosis. The high-risk patient with coronary artery disease should be stabilized on medical therapy, including beta-blockers, if tolerated, prior to study. Congestive heart failure should be controlled with diuretics, ni-

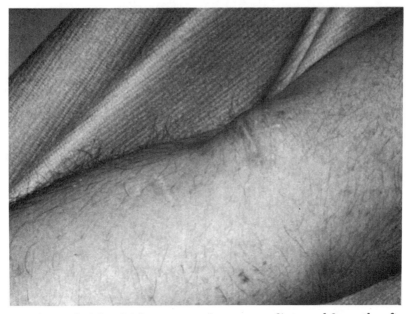

Figures 8A-C. *A brachial artery pseudoaneurysm diagnosed 6 months after left heart catheterization. A. The patient reported a gradually enlarging pulsatile mass at the previous arteriotomy site.*

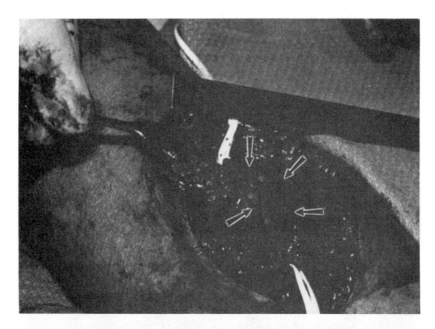

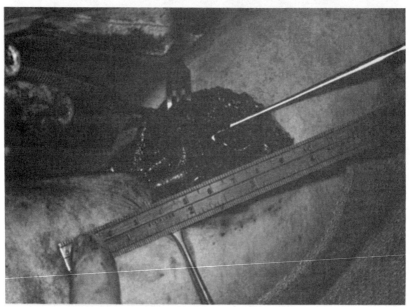

Figures 8B (top) and C (bottom). *At surgery, the overlying hematoma (arrows) and false lumen (held by forceps) are demonstrated.*

trates, and intravenous nitroprusside, if necessary. A temporary, prophylactic, pacemaker should be considered in patients with sick sinus syndrome, complete atrioventricular block or trifascicular conduction system disease, or evolving inferior wall myocardial infarction. Sublingual nitroglycerin or intravenous furosemide should be given prior to arteriography in patients with high preload conditions.

Coronary arteriography should be performed before ventriculography in patients with suspected multiple high-grade stenoses. If left main stenosis is suspected or discovered, the minimum number of left and right coronary artery injections required to assess the degree of stenosis and distal runoff should be performed. The volume of contrast should be minimized in patients with poor left ventricular function or pulmonary wedge pressure greater than 30 mmHg. Nonionic contrast media will lower the likelihood of ventricular fibrillation and minimize the hemodynamic changes that result from myocardial depression, peripheral vasodilatation, and volume loading.

Immediate attention should be given to changes in the patient's condition. Ischemia, pulmonary congestion, hypotension, and arrhythmias should be relieved promptly. Ischemic pain should be relieved before proceeding to the next injection of contrast. However, if acute coronary occlusion is suspected, reinjection of the suspected coronary artery is indicated. If angina cannot be controlled with medical therapy or hemodynamic stability cannot be maintained, intra-aortic balloon counterpulsation is useful. Emergency coronary bypass surgery is indicated for refractory ischemia or cardiogenic shock.

Future Directions

In less than 30 years, left heart catheterization with selective coronary arteriography has grown to become one of the most common diagnostic procedures performed today. Furthermore, it has advanced into interventional angiography with intracoronary thrombolysis and balloon angioplasty and valvuloplasty. The impact of these broadening applications is only now beginning to be realized.

As the techniques became more refined, complication rates fell, but collectively, major complications still occur in approximately one-third to 1% of diagnostic procedures and an even higher percentage of interventional procedures. Meticulous attention to details and changes in the patient's condition will minimize but will not eliminate risks entirely because acutely ill patients with advanced disease will continue to be studied and treated.

References

1. Dennison CF: National Center for Health Statistics Summary: National Hospital Discharge Survey. Washington, DC, 1984.
2. Dotter CT, Frische LH: Visualization of the coronary circulation by occlusion aortography: a practical method. Radiology 71:502, 1958.
3. Sones FM Jr., Shirey EK, Proudfit WL, et al: Cine-coronary arteriography. (abstract) Circulation 20:773, 1959.
4. Sones FM Jr., Shirey EK: Cine coronary arteriography. Mod Concepts Cardiovasc Dis 31:735, 1962.
5. Judkins MP: Selective coronary arteriography, part I: a percutaneous transfemoral technic. Radiology 89:815, 1967.
6. Favaloro R: Direct and indirect coronary surgery. Circulation 46:1197, 1972.
7. Garrett HE, Dennis EW, DeBakey ME: Aortocoronary bypass with saphenous vein graft: seven-year follow-up. J Am Med Assoc 223:792, 1973.
8. Gruntzig A: Transluminal dilatation of coronary-artery stenosis. Lancet 1:263, 1978.
9. Gruntzig AR, Senning A, Siegenthaler WE: Nonoperative dilatation of coronary-artery stenosis: percutaneous transluminal coronary angioplasty. N Engl J Med 301:61, 1979.
10. Rentrop P, Blanke H, Karsch KR, et al: Selective intracoronary thrombolysis in acute myocardial infarction and unstable angina pectoris. Circulation 63:307, 1981.
11. Lababidi Z, Wu J, Walls JT: Percutaneous balloon aortic valvuloplasty: results in 23 patients. Am J Cardiol 53:194, 1984.
12. Lock JE, Khalilullah M, Shrivastava S, et al: Percutaneous catheter commissurotomy in rheumatic mitral stenosis. N Engl J Med 313:1515, 1985.
13. Cribier A, Saoudi N, Berland J, et al: Percutaneous transluminal valvuloplasty of acquired aortic stenosis in elderly patients: an alternative to valve replacement? Lancet 1:63, 1986.
14. Bristow JD, Burchell HB, Campbell RW, et al: Report of the ad hoc committee on the indications for coronary arteriography. Circulation 55:969A, 1977.
15. Ambrose JA: Unsettled indications for coronary angiography. J Am Coll Cardiol 3:1575, 1984.

16. Grossman W: Cardiac catheterization: historical perspective and present practice. In W Grossman (ed): Cardiac Catheterization and Angiography. Philadelphia, Lea and Febiger, 1986, p 3.
17. King SB, Douglas JS: Indications, limitations, and risks of coronary arteriography and left ventriculography. In SB King, JS Douglas (eds): Coronary Arteriography and Angioplasty. New York, McGraw-Hill, 1985, p 122.
18. Raizner AE, Tortoledo FA, Verani MS, et al: Intracoronary thrombolytic therapy in acute myocardial infarction: a prospective randomized, controlled trial. Am J Cardiol 55:301, 1985.
19. Kennedy JW, Ritchie JL, David KB, et al: Western Washington randomized trial of intracoronary streptokinase in acute myocardial infarction. N Engl J Med 309:1477, 1983.
20. Simoons ML, Serruys PW, van den Brand M, et al: Early thrombolysis in acute myocardial infarction: limitations of infarct size and improved survival. J Am Coll Cardiol 7:717, 1986.
21. Hamby RI, Katz S: Percutaneous transluminal coronary angioplasty: its potential impact on surgery for coronary artery disease. Am J Cardiol 45:1161, 1980.
22. Vlietstra RE, Holmes DR, Reeder GS, et al: Balloon angioplasty in multivessel coronary artery disease. Mayo Clin Proc 58:563, 1983.
23. Dorros G, Stertzer SH, Cowley MJ, et al: Complex coronary angioplasty: multiple coronary dilatations. In Proceedings of the National Heart, Lung, and Blood Institute Workshop on the outcome of percutaneous transluminal coronary angioplasty. Am J Cardiol 53:126C, 1984.
24. Dorros G, Lewin RF, Janke L: Multiple lesion transluminal coronary angioplasty in single and multivessel coronary artery disease: acute outcome and long-term effect. J Am Coll Cardiol 10:1007, 1987.
25. McKay RG, Lock JE, Keane JF, et al: Percutaneous mitral valvuloplasty in an adult patient with calcific rheumatic mitral stenosis. J Am Coll Cardiol 7:1410, 1986.
26. McKay RG, Safian RD, Lock JE, et al: Balloon dilatation of calcific aortic stenosis in elderly patients: postmortem, intraoperative and percutaneous valvuloplasty studies. Circulation 74:119, 1986.
27. Tilkian AG, Daily EK: Cardiac catheterization and coronary arteriography. In AG Tilkian (ed): Cardiovascular Procedures: Diagnostic Techniques and Therapeutic Procedures. St Louis, CV Mosby, 1986, p 117.
28. Grossman W: Cardiac catheterization by direct exposure of artery and vein. In W Grossman (ed): Cardiac Catheterization and Angiography. Philadelphia, Lea and Febiger, 1986, p 45.
29. Judkins MP, Judkins E: Coronary arteriography and left ventriculography: Judkins technique: Part I: The Judkins technique. In SB King, JS Douglas (eds): Coronary Arteriography and Angioplasty. New York, McGraw-Hill, 1985, p 182.
30. Levin DC: Technique of coronary arteriography. In HL Abrams (ed):

Coronary Arteriography: A Practical Approach. Boston, Little, Brown, 1983, p 53.

31. Adams DF, Fraser DB, Abrams HL: The complications of coronary arteriography. Circulation 48:609, 1973.
32. Takaro T, Hultgren HN, Littmann D, et al: An analysis of deaths occurring in association with coronary arteriography. Am Heart J 86:587, 1973.
33. Bourassa MG, Noble J: Complication rate of coronary arteriography: a review of 5250 cases studied by a percutaneous femoral technique. Circulation 53:106, 1976.
34. Adams DF, Abrams HL: Complications of coronary arteriography: a follow-up report. Cardiovasc Radiol 2:89, 1979.
35. Fergusson DJG, Kamada RO: Percutaneous entry of the brachial artery for left heart catheterization using a sheath. Cathet Cardiovasc Diag 7:111, 1981.
36. Pepine CJ, Gunten CV, Hill JA, et al: Percutaneous brachial catheterization using a modified sheath and new catheter system. Cathet Cardiovasc Diag 10:637, 1984.
37. Campeau L: Percutaneous brachial catheterization. (letter) Cathet Cardiovasc Diag 11:443, 1985.
38. Eugster GS, Reisig AH, Ugaldea CT: Percutaneous left brachial catheterization using 5-French preformed (Judkins) catheters. Cathet Cardiovasc Diag 12:274, 1986.
39. Ross RS, Gorlin R: Cooperative study on cardiac catheterization: coronary arteriography. Circulation 37 and 38 (Suppl III):III-67, 1968.
40. Formanek G, Frech RS, Amplatz K: Arterial thrombus formation during clinical percutaneous catheterization. Circulation 41:833, 1970.
41. Sones FM: Cine coronary arteriography. Anesth Analg 46:499, 1967.
42. Selzer A, Anderson WL, March HW: Indications for coronary arteriography, risks vs benefits. Calif Med 115:1, 1971.
43. Green GS, McKinnon CM, Rosch J, et al: Complications of selective percutaneous transfemoral coronary arteriography and their prevention. Circulation 45:552, 1972.
44. Hansing CE: The risk and cost of coronary angiography: II. the risk of coronary angiography in Washington state. J Am Med Assoc 242:735, 1979.
45. Davis K, Kennedy JW, Kemp HG, et al: Complications of coronary arteriography from the Collaborative Study of Coronary Artery Surgery (CASS). Circulation 59:1105, 1979.
46. Kennedy JW: Complications associated with cardiac catheterization and angiography (from the Registry Committee of the Society for Cardiac Angiography). Cathet Cardiovasc Diagn 8:5, 1982.
47. Morton BC, Beanlands DS: Complications of cardiac catheterization: one centre's experience. Can Med Assoc J 131:889, 1984.
48. Judkins MP, Gander MP: Prevention of complications of coronary arteriography. Circulation 49:599, 1974.
49. Hildner FJ, Javier RP, Ramaswamy K, et al: Pseudocomplications of cardiac catheterization. Chest 63:15, 1973.

50. Kennedy JW and the Registry Committee of the Society for Cardiac Angiography: Mortality related to cardiac catheterization and angiography. Cathet Cardiovasc Diagn 8:323, 1982.
51. Gersh BJ, Kronmal RA, Frye RL, et al: Coronary arteriography and coronary artery bypass surgery: morbidity and mortality in patients ages 65 years or older: a report from the Coronary Artery Surgery Study. Circulation 67:483, 1983.
52. Nishimura RA, Holmes DR, McFarland TM, et al: Ventricular arrhythmias during coronary angiography in patients with angina pectoris or chest pain syndromes. Am J Cardiol 53:1496, 1984.
53. Wolf GL, Kroft L, Kilzer K: Contrast agents lower ventricular fibrillation threshhold. Radiology 129:215, 1978.
54. Lehman MH, Case RB: Reduced human ventricular fibrillation threshold associated with contrast-induced Q-T prolongation. J Electrocardiol 16:105, 1983.
55. Miller D, Lohse J, Wolf G: Slow response induced in canine Purkinje fiber by contrast medium. Invest Radiol 11:577, 1976.
56. Murdock DK, Euler DE, Scanlon PJ, et al: Electrophysiologic effects of intracoronary Renografin-76. (abstract) J Am Coll Cardiol 1:729, 1983.
57. Eckberg DL, White CW, Kioschos JM, et al: Mechanisms mediating bradycardia during coronary arteriography. J Clin Invest 54:1455, 1974.
58. Frink RJ, Merrick B, Lowe HM: Mechanism of the bradycardia during coronary angiography. Am J Cardiol 35:17, 1975.
59. Campion BC, Frye RL, Pluth JR, et al: Arterial complications of retrograde brachial arterial catheterization: a prospective study. Mayo Clin Proc 46:589, 1971.
60. Machleder HI, Sweeney JP, Barker WF: Pulseless arm after brachial artery catheterisation. Lancet 1:407, 1972.
61. Jeresaty RM, Liss JP: Effect of brachial artery catheterization on arterial pulse and blood pressure in 203 patients. Am Heart J 76:481, 1968.
62. Ross RS: Cooperative study on cardiac catheterizations: arterial complications. Circulation 37 and 38 (Suppl III):III-39, 1968.
63. Grossman W: Complications of cardiac catheterization: incidence, causes and prevention. In W Grossman (ed): Cardiac Catheterization and Angiography. Philadelphia, Lea and Febiger, 1986, p 30.
64. Kloster FE, Bristow JD, Griswold HE: Femoral artery occlusion following percutaneous catheterization. Am Heart J 79:175, 1970.
65. Dorros G, Cowley MJ, Simpson J, et al: Percutaneous transluminal coronary angioplasty: report of complications from the National Heart, Lung and Blood Institute PTCA registry. Circulation 67:723, 1983.
66. McKay RG, Safian RD, Lock JE, et al: Assessment of left ventricular and aortic valve function after aortic balloon valvuloplasty in adult patients with critical aortic stenosis. Circulation 75:192, 1987.
67. European Cooperative Study Group for Streptokinase Treatment in

Acute Myocardial Infarction: Streptokinase in acute myocardial infarction. N Engl J Med 301:797, 1979.

68. Timmis GC, Gangadharan V, Hauser AM, et al: Intracoronary streptokinase in clinical practice. Am Heart J 104:925, 1982.

69. Reimer KA, Lowe JE, Rasmussen MM, et al: The wavefront phenomenon of ischemic cell death: (I.) myocardial infarct size vs duration of coronary occlusion in dogs. Circulation 56:786, 1977.

70. Lee G, Amsterdam EA, Low R, et al: Efficacy of percutaneous transluminal coronary recanalization utilizing streptokinase thrombolysis in patients with acute myocardial infarction. Am Heart J 102, 1159, 1981.

71. Harrison DG, Ferguson DW, Collins SM, et al: Rethrombosis after reperfusion with streptokinase: importance of geometry of residual lesions. Circulation 69:991, 1984.

72. Kennedy JW, Gensini GG, Timmis GC: Acute myocardial infarction treated with intracoronary streptokinase: a report of the Society for Cardiac Angiography. Am J Cardiol 55:871, 1985.

73. Merx W, Dorr R, Rentrop P, et al: Evaluation of the effectiveness of intracoronary streptokinase infusion in acute myocardial infarction: postprocedure management and hospital course in 204 patients. Am Heart J 102:1181, 1981.

74. Timmis GC, Gangadharan V, Ramos RG, et al: Hemorrhage and the products of fibrinogen digestion after intracoronary administration of streptokinase. Circulation 69:1146, 1984.

75. McGrath KG, Patterson R: Anaphylactic reactivity to streptokinase. J Am Med Assoc 252:1314, 1984.

76. Sharma GVRK, Cella G, Parisi AF, et al: Thrombolytic therapy. N Engl J Med 306:1268, 1982.

77. Little WC, Rogers EW: Angiographic evidence of hemorrhagic myocardial infarction after intracoronary thrombolysis with streptokinase. Am J Cardiol 51:906, 1983.

78. Topol EJ, Califf RM, George BS, et al: A randomized trial of immediate versus delayed elective angioplasty after intravenous tissue plasminogen activator in acute myocardial infarction. N Engl J Med 317:581, 1987.

79. Holmes DR, Vlietstra RE, Kelsey S, et al: Comparison of current and earlier complications of angioplasty: NHLBI PTCA registry. (abstract) J Am Coll Cardiol 9:19A, 1987.

80. Goldbaum TS, Jacob AS, Smith DF, et al: Cardiac tamponade following percutaneous transluminal coronary angioplasty: four case reports. Cathet Cardiovasc Diagn 11:413, 1985.

81. Kimbiris D, Iskandrian AS, Goel I, et al: Transluminal coronary angioplasty complicated by coronary artery perforation. Cathet Cardiovasc Diagn 8:481, 1982.

82. Berland J, Cribier A, Guermonprez J, et al: Complications of aortic balloon valvuloplasty: the French registry. (abstract) Circulation 76 (Supp IV):IV-495, 1987.

83. Morise AP, Hardin NJ, Bovill EG, et al: Coronary artery dissection secondary to coronary arteriography: presentation of three cases and review of the literature. Cathet Cardiovasc Diagn 7:283, 1981.
84. Feit A, Kahn R, Chowdhry I, et al: Coronary artery dissection secondary to coronary arteriography: case report and review. Cathet Cardiovasc Diagn 10:177, 1984.
85. Weiner RD, Boston BA, Mintz GS, et al: Catheter-induced coronary artery dissection. (abstract) Circulation 64 (Suppl IV):IV-108, 1981.
86. Haas JM, Peterson CR, Jones RC: Subintimal dissection of the coronary arteries: a complication of selective coronary arteriography and the transfemoral percutaneous approach. Circulation 38:678, 1968.
87. Van Tassel RA, Gobel FL, Rydell MA, et al: A less traumatic catheter for coronary arteriography. Cathet Cardiovasc Diagn 11:187, 1985.
88. Ischinger T, Gruentzig AR, Meier B, et al: Coronary dissection and total coronary occlusion associated with percutaneous transluminal coronary angioplasty: significance of initial angiographic morphology of coronary stenoses. Circulation 74:1371, 1986.
89. Slack JD, Pinkerton CA, Van Tassel JW, et al: Left main coronary artery dissection during percutaneous transluminal coronary angioplasty. Cathet Cardiovasc Diagn 12:255, 1986.
90. Lavine P, Kimbiris D, Linhart JW: Coronary artery spasm during selective coronary arteriography: a review of 8 years experience. (abstract) Circulation 48 (Suppl IV):IV-89, 1973.
91. Chahine RA, Raizner AE, Ishimori T, et al: The incidence and clinical implications of coronary artery spasm. Circulation 52:972, 1975.
92. O'Reilly RJ, Spellberg RD, King TW: Recognition of proximal right coronary artery spasm during coronary arteriography. Radiology 95:305, 1970.
93. Lafia P, Dincer B: Coronary artery catheter-induced spasm. Cathet Cardiovasc Diagn 8:607, 1982.
94. Murdock DK, Johnson SA, Loeb HS, et al: Ventricular fibrillation during coronary angiography: reduced incidence in man with contrast media lacking calcium binding additives. Cathet Cardiovasc Diagn 11:153, 1985.
95. Gertz EW, Wisneski JA, Chiu D, et al: Clinical superiority of a new nonionic contrast agent (Iopamidol) for cardiac angiography. J Am Coll Cardiol 5:250, 1985.
96. Glassman E, Roberts G: Prevention of arrhythmias during coronary arteriography by prophylactic atropine. (abstract) Circulation 39 and 40 (Suppl III):III-90, 1969.
97. Richards KL, Browning JD, Hoekenga DE: Prevention of contrast-induced bradycardia during coronary angiography. Cathet Cardiovasc Diagn 7:185, 1981.
98. Cheng TO: Against routine use of atropine during coronary arteriography. (letter) Cathet Cardiovasc Diagn 7:459, 1981.
99. Talano JV, Tonaki H, Meadows WR, et al: Platelet aggregates in preformed polyurethane catheters following coronary arteriography:

an electron microscopy study. (abstract) Circulation 45 and 46 (Suppl II):II-32, 1972.

100. Wilner GD, Casarella WJ, Baier R, et al: Thrombogenicity of angiographic catheters. Circ Res 43:424, 1978.

101. Page HL, Campbell WB: Percutaneous transfemoral coronary arteriography: prevention of morbid complications. Chest 67:221, 1975.

102. Nelson RM, Osborn AG: Systemic heparinization for percutaneous catheter arteriography. (abstract) Circulation 43 and 44 (Suppl II):II-205, 1971.

103. Wallace S, Medellin H, De Jongh D, et al: Systemic heparinization for angiography. Am J Roentgenol Rad Ther Nucl Med 116:204, 1972.

104. Walker WJ, Mundall SL, Broderick HG, et al: Systemic heparinization for femoral percutaneous coronary arteriography. N Engl J Med 288:826, 1973.

105. Eyer KM: Complications of transfemoral coronary arteriography and their prevention using heparin. Am Heart J 86:428, 1973.

106. Luepker RV, Bouchard RJ, Burns R, et al: Systemic heparinization during percutaneous femoral artery cathetrization. (abstract) Circulation 48 (Suppl IV):IV-89, 1973.

107. Antonovic R, Rösch J, Dotter CT: The value of systemic arterial heparinization in transfemoral angiography: a prospective study. Am J Roentgenol 127:223, 1976.

108. Yellin AE, Shore EH: Surgical management of arterial occlusion following percutaneous femoral angiography. Surgery 73:772, 1973.

Chapter 4

Complications of Transseptal Catheterization and Transthoracic Left Ventricular Puncture

Mark J. Morton and Henry L. DeMots

Transseptal Left Heart Catheterization

History

Ross and Cope separately reported techniques for left heart catheterization by atrial septal puncture in 1959.[1,2] At that time, left heart catheterization was in its infancy. Retrograde catheterization was 9 years old and other techniques, left ventricular puncture, left atrial puncture, and transbronchial left atrial puncture were available but were too cumbersome or dangerous for routine application. Pulmonary capillary wedge estimation of left atrial pressures[3] were available and some of the limitations of this technique were understood[4] but would need to be relearned.[5,6] Most importantly, this was the dawn of surgical management of valvular heart disease with the successful replacement of mitral and aortic valves occurring 1 and 2 years later, respectively. Thus, much like coronary angiography, this diagnostic technique evolved just prior to meaningful surgical therapy.

The technique, modified by Brockenbrough in 1960 to include a catheter suitable for angiography, was popular for left heart catheterization and angiography in the 1960s.[7,8] The catheter and needle combination could be used to rapidly catheterize the right ventricle, right atrium, left atrium, and left ventricle in sequence. The 8.5 French catheter has excellent fidelity and provides good angio-

From *Complications of Cardiac Catheterization and Angiography: Prevention and Management* edited by Jack Kron, M.D. and Mark J. Morton, M.D. © 1989, Futura Publishing Inc., Mount Kisco, NY.

graphic images of the left atrium or left ventricle. The cooperative study of cardiac catheterization in the late 1960s revealed that transseptal left atrial puncture comprised 14.3% of 12,367 procedures.[9] Complications related to transseptal catheterization were reported in 4%. Cardiac perforation occurred in 2.4%, with tamponade resulting in about one-half of these procedures. Two patients died as a consequence of tamponade (0.1%). One patient died from pulmonary embolism (0.05%). Systemic embolism occurred in 0.3% of patients. These relatively low complication rates remain the bench mark and probably have not been improved upon despite vastly improved fluoroscopy and new techniques.

Perhaps one reason that transseptal catheterization complications have not declined is that the use of the procedure has.[10] Thus, trainees learn on fewer cases and practitioners have fewer to do to maintain their skills. Two factors have contributed to the decline of catheterization by the transseptal technique: (1) the decline of rheumatic heart disease and (2) the further development of rapid, safe, and successful retrograde techniques.[11]

Several important additions to Brockenbrough's equipment and technique have been made in the last decade. The first was the introduction, by Mullins,[12] of the dilator sheath system to transseptal catheterization in children. This technique was extended to adults in 1982 by Laskey and his colleagues who used a preshaped pigtail catheter to enter the left atrium and ventricle.[13] This advance permitted the simultaneous assessment of left atrial pressure through the sheath, and the left ventricle through the pigtail. In addition, the preshaped pigtail catheter theoretically reduced the chance of left atrial or left ventricular perforation or of myocardial stain during contrast angiography.[14] Balloon-tipped, flow-directed catheters have also been used for antegrade left ventricular and aortic catheterization for pressure measurements, contrast injections, or to facilitate guidewire placement for balloon valvuloplasty.[15-18]

Indications for the Procedure

The simplest way to reduce procedure-related complications is to not use the procedure, unless it is absolutely indicated. Our indications for the procedure are listed in Table 1. As confidence

Table 1
Indications for Transseptal Left Heart Catheterization

I. Measurement of transvalvular pressure gradients
Mitral valve
1. Doppler gradient inconclusive or unreliable
2. PCW tracing unreliable
3. Prosthetic mitral valve

Aortic valve
1. Doppler gradient inconclusive or unreliable
2. Retrograde catheterization not possible
3. Prosthetic aortic valve

II. Left ventricular angiography
Assessment of mitral regurgitation
1. Doppler inconclusive or unreliable
2. Retrograde catheterization not possible

III. Valvuloplasty
Mitral or aortic valve antegrade

IV. Septostomy

V. Pulmonary vein wedge angiography

VI. Measurement of pulmonary venous pressure gradients

in the use of noninvasive techniques to select therapy for native valvular heart disease increases, the need for diagnostic transseptal left heart catheterization will continue to decline. Therapeutic catheterizations probably will continue to increase, and the major need for this procedure in the future may be in valvuloplasty and septostomy. At present, we are not convinced that noninvasive techniques can adequately assess the function of mechanical prostheses. Therefore, at our institution, transvalvular gradients in patients with suspected prosthetic dysfunction are measured with catheters on both sides of the valve and valvular competence is assessed by contrast angiography.

We agree with Schoenfeld et al.[16] and with Dunn[19] that transseptal catheterization should be performed to evaluate prosthetic mitral valve stenosis and failure to do so, may result in unnecessary valve rereplacement. However, we do not agree with Karsh et al.[20] that aortic mechanical prostheses may be crossed safely without disturbing hemodynamics, and therefore, transseptal catheterization can be performed to evaluate mechanical aortic prostheses for possible stenosis. Furthermore, we do not cross bioprostheses retrograde, although other institutions do.[21-23] Our reasons for not crossing these prostheses retrograde relate to concerns for leaflet fracture and debris embolization balanced against the relative safety of transseptal left heart catheterization in operated patients. For these reasons, most adult patients at our institution undergo diagnostic transseptal left heart catheterization for the evaluation of prosthetic valve dysfunction.

Complications

Table 2 lists the complications of eight relatively contemporary series of transseptal left heart catheterizations.[10,13,14,16,17,24-26] Although prospectively maintained registries provide a more accurate and representative view of complication rates than do reported series, the results are surprisingly similar to those of the cooperative study reported two decades ago. The procedure shares risks common to all catheterization and angiography, e.g., access vessel injury, embolism, contrast reaction, and arrhythmia. There are, however, risks peculiar to transseptal left heart catheterization, which must be recognized and for which effective contingency plans must be available. The major risk is cardiac perforation by the transseptal needle, catheter, or both. Perforation can occur in the right atrium, posterior left atrium, pulmonary vein, left atrial appendage, and left ventricle as well as from the right atrium into the aorta. Any of these structures can bleed into the pericardium and cause tamponade. Almost all deaths related to this procedure are caused by tamponade. For this reason, anyone who lacks the ability to recognize and treat tamponade should never perform transseptal left heart catheterization, which in our laboratory, includes the rapid availability of subxyphoid pericardiocentesis. In addition, a thoracotomy tray ready for use is present in the laboratory and, if necessary the cardiology faculty will perform a thoracotomy and pericardiotomy. Fortunately, most patients for whom this procedure is indicated for diagnostic purposes will have had prior cardiac

Table 2
Contemporary Transseptal Catheterization

Author	Dates	Patients	Complications	Success %
Kawachi[14]	?-'81	32	0	LV 97
Lew[24]	'79-'82	207	1 perforation 1 tamponade	LA 90 LV 92
Laskey[13]	?-'82	56	3 perforations 2 tamponade	
Lam[17]	'80-'82	47	2 perforations	LA 77 LV 97
Bagger[16]	'72-'83	178	2 embolus	LA 97 LV 100
Lundqvist[25]	'72-'84	278	8 perforations 0 tamponade 3 embolus	LA 91 LV 96
O'Keefe[26]	'80-'85	141	5 perforations 0 tamponade 1 embolus 1 femoral v hemotoma	?
Schoonmaker[10]	'78-'86	250	6 perforations 1 tamponade with death 1 broken needle	LA 99
	Total	1,189	34 (2.8%) 1 death (0.08%)	LA 77%-99% LV 92%-100%

surgery. Because the pericardial space usually is obliterated by adhesions, cardiac perforation with tamponade does not occur in patients with prior valve replacement.

Vascular complications are probably lower for transseptal left heart catheterization than for retrograde left heart catheterization because the vein rather than the artery is used. Nevertheless, both excessive bleeding from femoral vein laceration[26] and femoral vein thrombosis with pulmonary embolus[19] have been reported, although the incidence is very small. Furthermore, these complications are not unique to transseptal left heart catheterization but may occur with any right heart catheterization from the femoral vein. We have also reported inadvertent bladder puncture during transseptal left heart catheterization which occurred during attempts to puncture the femoral vein.[27] Iliac or inferior vena cava venous perforation may also occur as the stiff Brockenbrough catheter and needle are being passed through these structures.

Systemic embolus is a disastrous complication that may result in a stroke. Embolus occurred in 0.3% of transseptal left heart catheterizations in the cooperative study and in 0.6% of catheterizations reported in Table 2. These data suggest that the risk of embolus has not decreased despite improvements in technique. Unfortunately, many patients who undergo transseptal left heart catheterization are at risk for left atrial thrombi and embolus by the nature of their disease processes. Many will have associated atrial fibrillation and prosthetic heart valves. Several factors appear to be related to embolus and may be avoided. Foremost, no patient with a left atrial thrombus or myxoma should have transseptal left heart catheterization. Thus, two-dimensional echocardiography should be performed before catheterization in these patients to exclude these findings where possible. The catheter must be kept out of the left atrial appendage, a common source for emboli particularly in patients with atrial fibrillation. Lastly, left atrial angiography should probably not be performed in patients at risk for embolus. Left ventricular size and function can be measured by noninvasive techniques; left atrial angiography cannot exclude mitral valve incompetence.

The incomplete study is infrequent with transseptal left heart catheterization but occurs as indicated in Table 2. Difficulty engaging and puncturing the interatrial septum accounts for most of these difficulties. The study reported by Lam et al. reveals a high failure rate of left atrial catheterization.[17] It should be noted that this consecutive series was their first experience with the Mullins sheath, and septal puncture was not even obtained in 6 of the 47 patients. Once in the left atrium, a sheath system coupled with a balloon floatation catheter, if necessary, should eliminate all failures to enter the left ventricle. Even when inadvertent perforation occurs, the majority of diagnostic studies can be completed. Infrequently, an interrupted inferior vena cava will be encountered during transseptal left heart catheterization. To avoid potential disaster, the operator must be aware of this congenital anomaly. The catheter will proceed to the right atrium SVC junction, through the azygous extension. Attempts to puncture the interatrial septum will result in azygous laceration. Although transseptal puncture has been performed from the superior vena cava, we recommend that the operator who lacks experience with this approach terminate the procedure if inferior vena cava interruption is present.

Equipment failures may produce complications, including incomplete study. Fracture of the distal transseptal needle has been reported infrequently.[9,10] More commonly, the needle may perforate the distal catheter or, less often, a dilator-sheath system. This complication, if unrecognized, will result in the inability of the operator to advance the catheter or sheath through the septum following needle puncture.

Factors associated with complications include several that may be considered contraindications for the procedure (see Table 3). Anticoagulation with coumadin is prevalent in patients undergoing transseptal left heart catheterization. Considering the possibility of cardiac perforation in unoperated patients, we are reluctant to perform transseptal left heart catheterizations when the prothrombin time is prolonged in these patients. Transseptal left heart catheterization in patients who have had previous cardiac surgery and are receiving anticoagulation therapy has been reported from our institution and no complications related to cardiac perforation or tamponade were noted in 117 patients.[27,28] We are, accordingly, less rigorous regarding the coagulation status of operated patients.

Anatomic abnormalities may make transseptal left heart catheterization difficult or, as indicated above, with interrupted inferior vena cava, impossible. Giant left or right atrium may make finding the fossa ovalis extremely difficult and firm impingement impossible. Thoracic skeletal abnormalities may severely distort the re-

Table 3
Contraindications To Transseptal Left Heart Catheterization

Anticoagulation (especially unoperated patient)
Severe aortic root dilation
Severely enlarged right or left atrium
Severe thoracoskeletal abnormality
Recent systemic embolus
Left atrial clot or myxoma (absolute)
Interrupted IVC (absolute)
Congenital heart disease with disturbance of the normal landmarks

lationships of the interatrial septum and other landmarks. Aortic root dilatation from aneurysm or dissection pushes the right atrium posterior and narrows the small window of interatrial septum available for puncture, increasing the likelihood of aortic puncture. The juxtaposition of the aorta and the medial wall of the right atrium are illustrated in Figure 1. Lastly, it is our experience that pericardial effusion increases the likelihood of cardiac perforation during transseptal left heart catheterization. Although we have no data to support this notion, it is conceivable that without the support of the tough pericardium, the thin friable atrium can be perforated by a stiff catheter or a transseptal needle.

Optimum Performance of Transseptal Left Heart Catheterization to Avoid Complications

As stated earlier, the easiest way to avoid complications is to not perform the procedure unless it is absolutely indicated. As the indications for transseptal left heart catheterization decline, fewer people will be performing these procedures and therefore, fewer should be trained to perform them. Many descriptions of the technique[13,26,29,30] as well as reviews of the anatomic considerations[31,32] are available. The procedure should not be attempted without first carefully studying this important information. Since failure to accomplish retrograde catheterization is a frequent indication for transseptal left heart catheterization, knowledge re-

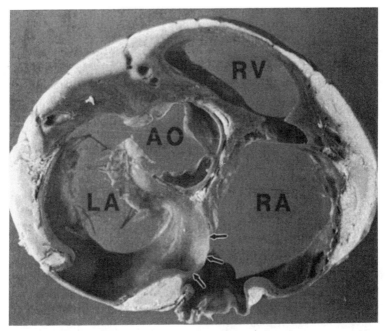

Figure 1. *Coronal section of a heart fixed at physiologic pressure. The section is 1-cm thick and passes through the aortic sinuses of valsalva. The specimen is viewed from the cephalic aspect. The relationships of the right atrium (RA), left atrium (LA), aorta (AO), and right ventricular outflow tract (RV) are shown. The thin fossa ovalis is identified in the posterior interatrial septum by arrows. The key finding is that the medial wall of the RA is equally composed of AO and LA. Thus, the transseptal needle must be directed posteromedially to avoid aortic puncture during transseptal left atrial catheterization.*

garding the several highly successful methods for retrograde catheterization of the aortic valve should be mastered by all who perform left heart catheterization.[11]

Selection and Preparation of Equipment

At the present time we are using either the USCI 8.5 French Brockenbrough catheter or an 8 French USCI Mullins sheath system over the Brockenbrough needle for adult transseptal catheterization (C.R. Bard, Billerica, MA.) Pediatric catheterization techniques are elaborated in Chapter 7. The advantage of the stiff Teflon Brockenbrough catheter is that it provides excellent stabilization for impingement and puncture of thick or distorted atrial septums. The disadvantages are (1) difficulty passing the catheter over the needle through the septum and (2) the catheter's stiffness and lack of maneuverability in the left atrium. Both of these drawbacks decrease the likelihood of entering the left ventricle and promote left atrial perforation as the stiff catheter is clumsily maneuvered around the left atrium. The Teflon Brockenbrough catheter can best be used for left atrial catheterization in patients with mitral valve prostheses in whom left ventricular catheterization is not anticipated and in whom difficult atrial septal puncture can be anticipated.

The advantages of the Mullins sheath are that a sheath-dilator system is more tapered than the Brockenbrough catheter and allows a wide choice of catheters for pressure measurements and for angiography of the left ventricle. The sheath also facilitates the placement of wires and catheters for balloon valvuloplasty. The sideport on the sheath permits simultaneous left atrial and left ventricular pressure measurements when the left ventricle is catheterized. Mitral valve disease occasionally prevents left ventricular catheterization with the Brockenbrough catheter, but it should never be a problem with the sheath system and a more maneuverable preshaped pigtail or a balloon-floatation catheter.[13–15,17] The disadvantages of the sheath are its flexibility, which may increase the difficulty of septal puncture, and the long coaxial sheath-catheter system, which invites clot formation in unanticoagulated patients. The sideport of the sheath must be filled with heparinized saline and meticulously flushed every few minutes while it remains within the patient. Thus, the sheath system may be best suited for use in unoperated patients with aortic valve disease, especially those with native combined aortic and mitral valve disease.

After selecting the equipment, the operator must measure the Brockenbrough needle against the length of the catheter or sheath. Although the position of the needle can be seen within the catheter on fluoroscopy, the needle point can be kept in the catheter by placing one or two fingers between the needle pointer and the hub of the catheter or sheath. The relationship between the pointer and the curved tip of the needle must be determined precisely. Treating the needle roughly can result in torsional bending and a wide angle between the pointer and tip. Failure to note this or to observe the orientation of the needle tip prior to puncture may lead to aortic or posterior left atrial puncture (see Fig.1). Especially with the stiff preformed Brockenbrough catheter, the needle must not be inserted without straightening the catheter. If the catheter is not straightened, the needle will gouge the outside curve of the lumen, filling its tip with Teflon shavings. The use of a stylet will reduce this hazard,[30] and is used routinely in some laboratories. The needle, catheter, or sheath sideport are all flushed and filled with heparinized saline. If a Brockenbrough catheter is to be used to catheterize the left ventricle, we size and shape a tip occluder at this time. This device, introduced by Dr. J. Michael Criley, allows the operator to pull the catheter tip down and anteriorly across the mitral valve, into the left ventricle, avoiding manipulation of the catheter.[29] The occlusive tip also reduces the likelihood of contrast extravasation from the endhole into the myocardium.

The right femoral vein is used for access. The left femoral vein can be used but is very awkward and may require repositioning of the patient's hip and chest to obtain impingement. The skin and soft tissue are incised and dissected to provide free movement of the catheter. The sheath or catheter is then passed over a guidewire into the superior vena cava. The catheter or sheath system is then aspirated and flushed with heparinized saline. The saline-filled needle is then passed through the catheter or sheath to lie just inside the tip. During passage, the needle must negotiate substantial tortuosity in the pelvis. The curved tip should be allowed to rotate and follow the path of least resistance. The needle must never be pushed. It will perforate the catheter if excessive force is applied. The needle is aspirated and flushed with heparinized saline and connected to a pressure transducer. Pressure is measured and compared with previous capillary wedge pressure measurements if available. The landmarks are identified fluoroscopically. The left atrial shadow, bronchi, aortic and mitral valve calcification, or prostheses are noted. A catheter placed in the ascending aorta may be used to identify this structure. This technqiue should be considered in patients with a dilated aortic root. Other operators have used two-dimensional echocardiography to avoid aortic root puncture.[33] Biplane fluoroscopy is also helpful when available.[26]

The needle and catheter are pointed medially and drawn down

across the aorta. The needle is then turned posteriorly to about 5:00 and the limbic edge is crossed. The tip may then move medially and slight advancement of the catheter will produce secure impingement. The catheter or sheath must not be permitted to flex with the impingement move because the needle may be forced through the side of the catheter during the process. If the position appears to be correct, impingement is secure, and the needle tip pressure is recording right atrial pressure, the septum is then punctured with a swift firm movement. We stabilize the catheter or sheath with the left hand at the groin and pop the needle forward with the right hand. At this time, the patient may experience upper chest or neck discomfort.

Several pressure waveforms may be observed after attempted puncture. The most likely is left atrial pressure, which usually will be higher than right atrial pressure. However, even if the two pressures are similar, left atrial pressure can be differentiated by the more clearly defined A and V waves in the left atrial tracing. If the needle does not enter the left atrium, it will be in the right atrium, embedded in the septal wall, in the pericardial space or in the aorta. If the needle fails to puncture the septum, it will usually be observed to slide up the septum. Its right atrial location will be confirmed by the pressure waveform. A second attempt can be made by repeating the entire procedure, except that the catheter should be more securely impinged against the septal wall. If the needle is embedded in the septal wall, the waveform will be a randomly moving smooth line bearing no relationship to cardiac activity. The needle may be withdrawn, flushed, and another attempt made. Puncture of the aorta is diagnosed by recognizing the arterial pressure waveform recorded through the needle. Intrapericardial pressure waveform usually reflects cardiac activity but is distinguished from intracavitary pressures because it usually is negative. Aspiration of serous fliud through the needle confirms that it has entered the pericardial space. Successful septal puncture can be confirmed by the pressure waveforms and, if desired, by measuring the saturation of a small amount of blood aspirated through the needle or by contrast injection.

When the needle has been advanced successfully to the left atrium, the needle catheter combination should be rotated so that the tip is oriented horizontally at 3:00. The needle-catheter combination is then advanced. If only the catheter is advanced, it may push the septal wall off the end of the needle. After an initial period of resistance, the catheter will advance abruptly. As this abrupt advance occurs, the needle should be withdrawn because a protruding needle may puncture the opposite wall of the left atrium and the catheter may follow it. When the catheter has been advanced successfully to the left atrium, the needle is removed, the catheter aspirated and flushed, and pressure is recorded. It is good practice to note atrial and arterial pressures at this time.

The left ventricle can be entered by several techniques. The Brockenbrough catheter usually is placed posteriorly and must be rotated counterclockwise (anteriorly) and withdrawn to bring it across the mitral valve. The tip occluder may facilitate this process. A variety of catheters may be used through a sheath. Regardless of technique utilized, the operator must avoid manipulating stiff catheters or wires in the left atrial appendage, which is easily perforated. Finally, the position of the Brockenbrough catheter tip in the left ventricle should be confirmed soon after placement as it may burrow into the posterior wall, producing ectopy, perforation, or myocardial extravasation of contrast during angiography. With all catheters placed, the operator should consider using heparin. If no difficulties have been encountered and particularly if coronary angiography is to be performed subsequently, we would administer heparin, 10 units/lb intravenously, at this time; others use 5,000 units.[13] The larger dose may be more important with the coaxial sheath system.

Management of Complications

Perforation

Cardiac Perforation will occur despite the best technique; therefore, all operators must be able to recognize and plan to deal with this complication and its sequelae. We inform all patients who are undergoing this procedure that pericardiocentesis or thoracotomy and pericardiotomy may be necessary to manage perforation. The catheterization laboratory is equipped to perform pericardiocentesis and thoracotomy rapidly. Emergency echocardiography is available to help diagnose and follow tamponade. Needle perforation is usually recognized by recording aortic or extracardiac pressure, as noted previously. In either case, the needle should be withdrawn promptly and the catheter pulled back. If the catheter also was inserted into the aorta, we recommend it be removed in the operating room so that thoracotomy and suture closure of the perforation may be performed rapidly, if necessary. If the catheter has perforated the atrium, the two approaches advocated have been (1) to remove the catheter and observe for signs of tamponade in the catheterization laboratory and (2) to remove the catheter in the operating room. We prefer the former approach for most patients. If no signs of tamponade develop, the diagnostic catheterization is completed. It is important to recognize that rapid increases in right atrial pressure may not occur in these patients and that cardiac output and arterial pressure must be monitored closely. We do not administer heparin to these patients.

Difficult Septal Puncture

A tough septum with a poorly defined limbic ledge is the usual finding in patients with mitral valve replacement. Furthermore the interatrial septum will frequently bulge into the right atrium in the presence of left atrial hypertension. This smooth convex surface makes impingement difficult and maintenance of the 5:00 position of the needle tip during puncture, challenging. Fortunately, the left atrium in these patients is large and can be entered safely by experienced operators without first identifying the usual tactile landmarks. The needle frequently will skid up the septum in this setting. When this happens, the best attempt should be made to impinge the catheter before the needle is brought into contact with the septum to secure the impingement. The needle is then popped forward briskly. Frequently, when the left atrium is large and bulging, the best place to obtain impingement is slightly lower than usual on the septum. As noted previously, the stiff Brockenbrough catheter may offer some advantages over the sheath system for difficult septal puncture. Occasionally, septal puncture may be aided by altering the curvature of the Brockenbrough needle.[29] This must be done with care to prevent breakage. Increasing the curve may be helpful if the needle skids up the septum repeatedly. Alternatively, if the septum is to be punctured low and bulges into the right atrium, a straighter tip may be advantageous.

Once in the left atrium, the catheter must be advanced over the needle. With a tough, thick septum, this may be difficult to do with the Brockenbrough catheter, but firm steady pressure usually resolves the issue. Occasionally, time passes and the operator must choose between the need to flush the catheter or sheath and the desire not to withdraw the needle and repuncture the septum. Occasionally, a second septal puncture in a more favorable location is the right choice. Alternatively, if only left atrial pressure is needed, the needle connected to stiff tubing and a low displacement transducer, carefully cleared of bubbles, produces adequate pressure records. Left atrial and left ventricular pressure can be recorded simultaneously, the needle withdrawn, and output measured. This contingency plan suggests the need to formulate the catheterization in advance in order that the most difficult procedure is performed last. As noted previously, difficulty passing the catheter or sheath over the needle should suggest the possibility of catheter or sheath perforation. The operator should inspect the fluoroscopic image carefully for evidence that the needle is indeed passing through the endhole.

Difficulty Entering the Left Ventricle

The two major problems related to entering the left ventricle from the left atrium with transseptal left heart catheterization are (1) knowing where the catheter is and (2) the ability to direct the catheter where the operator wants it to go. The first problem is solved by understanding the anatomy, the expected course of the catheter, and the use of biplane fluoroscopy or a C-arm to observe both AP and lateral catheter tip positions. Usually, the catheter or sheath is directed posteriorly and may actually be in the left upper or left lower pulmonary vein after its initial passage across the septum. Attempts to pass the catheter into the left ventricle from this position will obviously be unsuccessful and may result in pulmonary vein perforation. The catheter must be withdrawn and rotated anteriorly (counterclockwise) in order to pass through the mitral valve. This movement is best appreciated on lateral fluoroscopy. Now, when the catheter is advanced, it will enter the left ventricle or left atrial appendage, depending on how tight the catheter curve is relative to the position of the mitral valve and interatrial septum. This relationship is most readily appreciated on AP fluoroscopy, although the left atrial appendage can also be seen to lie just anterior to the mitral valve on lateral fluoroscopy. Attempts to advance the catheter in the left atrial appendage in unoperated patients will almost always result in perforation. Thus, manipulation of the stiff Brockenbrough catheter alone, except as described above, may result in left atrial or pulmonary vein perforation and is not recommended. To bring the catheter tip down across the mitral valve, we use a tip occluder wound into a tight spiral. If rotated anteriorly, the tip frequently will fall into the left ventricle, without manipulation, as the tip occluder is inserted. This is fortunate, because the catheter is even stiffer with the tip occluder in place, and the tip is sharper.

Alternatively, the sheath system allows the use of a preshaped pigtail catheter, as described elsewhere.[13,14] The rounded tip is unlikely to produce perforation, but forays into the left atrial appendage may still promote embolization and should be avoided. Finally, a balloon-floatation catheter is relatively atraumatic and will cross almost all mitral valves with minimal manipulation. Utilizing all of these techniques and avoiding the anatomic problems that are relative contraindications to the procedure, the incomplete procedure should be prevented in 99% of the patients studied.

Transthoracic Left Ventricular Puncture

History

Direct puncture of the left ventricle was introduced over 35 years ago by Pondomenech[34] and was brought into routine clinical use by Brock a few years later.[35] It is not surprising that surgeons were frequently responsible for the early series reported on this dramatic procedure.[36,37] Clearly other methods of left heart catheterization have relegated left ventricular puncture to infrequent use and for good reason. Either transseptal or retrograde left heart catheterization is safer, although left ventricular puncture is probably less technically demanding and certainly faster. While 260 procedures were reported in the cooperative study in 1968,[38] the frequency with which this procedure is performed at our institution has fallen to less than one per year. In the mid 1970s, in contrast, we performed 22 left ventricular puncture procedures over a 3-year period.[27]

Indications for Left Ventricular Puncture

The only indications for this procedure are the need to measure left ventricular pressure or to perform left ventricular angiography when no other means of obtaining these aims are available or are more dangerous than left ventricular puncture. For most patients, the clinical setting will be combined mitral and aortic valve replacement with mechanical prostheses. Double valve replacement with bioprostheses can be studied adequately by antegrade catheterization of the left atrium and left ventricle using the sheath and catheter techniques described above to provide simultaneous left atrial and left ventricular pressure measurements. Alternatively, the aortic valve can be crossed retrograde, but we believe the transseptal approach is easier and safer in operated patients. Several investigators have reported techniques for crossing aortic mechanical valves (tilting disk, ball valve) retrograde.[20,39] However, other investigators have reported important disturbances in hemodynamics during crossing of ball valves[40] and tilting disk valves.[41] Furthermore, the product engineering division of Shiley does not recommend retrograde crossing of their tilting disk prostheses.[42] For these reasons, when left ventricular pressure measurement and angiography are required following double valve replacement with mechanical prostheses, we will perform left ventricular puncture. Because other techniques can be used to assess patients with native valve disease, we have not studied this type of patient in over 15 years. In addition, transthoracic left ventricular puncture in unoperated patients carries the additional risk of tamponade and we view the unoperated state as a relative contraindication to this procedure.

Complications

The complication rates with this procedure, as reported from three small series in the past decade, are shown in Table 4.[27,43,44] The complication rate of 15% is greater than the 3.1% reported in the 1968 cooperative study.[38] This form of left heart catheterization shares with all left heart catheterizations the problems of emboli, arrhythmia, and contrast reaction. The unique feature of this procedure is the need to puncture the left ventricular apex. Obviously,

Table 4
Recent Studies of Complications of Transthoracic Left Ventricular Puncture

Author	Dates	Patients	Complications
Morton[27]	'73-'76	22	2 hemothorax 1 TIA
Baxley[43]	'72-'79	17	2 hemothorax 1 postop bleeding 1 TIA
Vignola[44]	'77-'79	7	0
		46	7 (15%)

some bleeding will occur. In patients with prior surgery, the bleeding will be into the left pleural space. In unoperated patients, the bleeding will be into the pericardium and tamponade may result. The bleeding is somewhat unpredictable but probably is related to needle size and anticoagulation status. These biases not withstanding, operators have performed guidewire exchanges to place 7 French catheters into the left ventricle and ultimately catheterize the aorta antegrade.[45] In addition, patients on anticoagulants have been studied at our institution[27,28] and in the cooperative study.[38] We now insist on a normal prothrombin time before performing left ventricular puncture. Bleeding may result in minimal pleural discomfort or hemothorax requiring thoracostomy, drainage, and transfusion. In one reported instance, the left ventricular puncture hole bled after open heart surgery and had to be sutured.[43] Since many of these patients return for prosthetic valve rereplacement, surgeons need to be alerted to this possible complication. Other problems specific to this procedure are inadvertent puncture of the right ventricle, coronary laceration, pulmonary puncture resulting in pneumothorax, and postpericardiotomy syndrome, which may occur late after the procedure. In our experience, contrast extravasation is more prevalent with this procedure because once the needle is placed, it cannot be maneuvered. The operator is frequently faced with the dilemma of proceeding with borderline needle placement or pulling back and making another puncture

(Fig. 2). Contrast irritation of the ventricle may also produce unwanted ventricular ectopy, making it difficult or impossible to interpret the left ventriculogram. Except for difficulties with the left ventriculogram, however, incomplete procedure is rarely a complication of transthoracic left ventricular puncture.

Factors Associated with Complications

Anticoagulation, unoperated state, and needle size all appear to influence bleeding. Embolism may occur if a clot is dislodged from the ventricular apex.

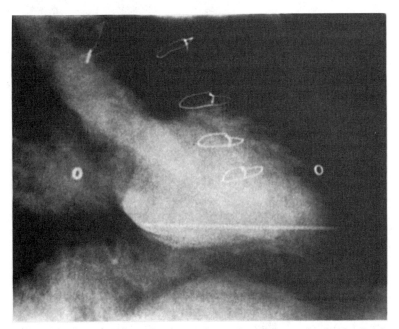

Figure 2A. *An end-diastolic frame from cineangiography in the RAO projection showing placement of the 18-gauge thin-wall transthoracic needle. Unfortunately, the needle was positioned more caudally than ideal. However, the injection of contrast medium through this needle, which has only sideholes, was without incident.*

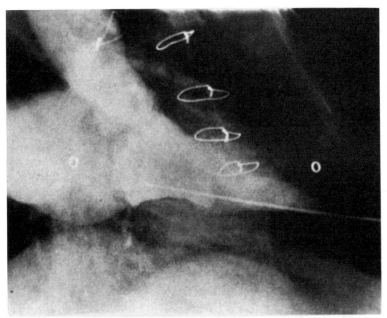

Figure 2B. *An end-systolic frame from the same patient shows severe mitral regurgitation with aortic and mitral valve replacement with St. Jude prostheses, which are only faintly radioopaque. The mechanism of regurgitation was found to be paravalvular at surgery.*

Optimal Performance to Avoid Complications

This procedure should only be performed by a few experienced operators and only when other alternatives have been exhausted or are not appropriate. In addition, the operator should be comfortable with transseptal left heart catheterization if simultaneous left atrial, left ventricular and aortic pressures are to be recorded during left ventricular puncture (Fig. 3). Coumadin is discontinued an adequate time before the procedure to allow prothrombin time to fall to normal. If there is grave concern regarding embolism, the patient can be maintained on heparin until 6 hours before the procedure. We routinely consult our cardiothoracic surgeons to let them know what we plan to do and to enlist their support for dealing with complications. An echocardiogram is performed to exclude left ventricular and left atrial thrombi. Right heart, transseptal left atrial, and retrograde aortic catheterizations are performed. Cardiac output is measured by direct Fick and by indicator-dilution techniques. The patient is then rotated into the 30° RAO position even though we have a C-arm imaging system. This maneuver tips the apex upward against the chest wall, making it easier to identify the apical impulse. Using this approach, we have not had problems with pneumothorax. Vignola and colleagues have used echocardiography to localize the apex in seven patients and successfully performed left ventricular puncture.[44] This approach is interesting but we have not used it because we have found that the left ventricular apex is obvious in lateral recumbancy.

The arms are then raised above the head to spread the ribs and

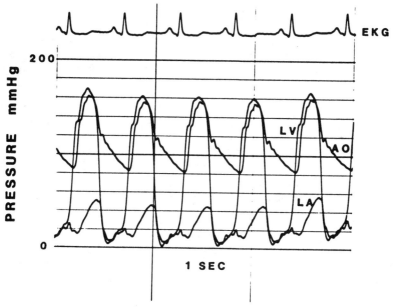

Figure 3. *Left ventricular (LV), aortic (AO), and left atrial (LA) pressures are recorded on equisensitive transducers as soon as the transthoracic needle enters the left ventricle. The good hydraulic characteristics of the St. Jude prostheses are evident despite severe mitral regurgitation by the low transvalvular gradient, both during systole and diastole.*

facilitate fluoroscopy and angiography. The apex is identified by palpation and its position, under fluoroscopy, is marked on the skin with a clamp. Usually, we prefer to enter at the most caudal interspace of the impulse. As always, the intercostal space is traversed over the cephalic aspect of the rib. The skin, intercostal space and pleura are anesthetized with lidocaine. A narcotic analgesic may be administered now, or if necessary during or after left ventricular puncture. The patient is cautioned not to cough or take deep breaths during the puncture. The breath is then held in mid-expiration as the needle is directed over the rib on a line midway between the aortic and mitral valves, in a plane horizontal to the table. We use an 18-gauge thin-wall needle with multiple sideholes and a closed beveled tip. The needle is connected directly to a stopcock and pressure tubing, and the system flushed with heparinized saline prior to puncture. Pressure is monitored during the puncture to confirm proper tip position. Once the needle is in the left ventricle, it is aspirated, flushed, and pressure recorded simultaneously on equisensitive left atrial, left ventricular, and aortic transducers (Fig. 3). If the needle bends markedly during systole, its shaft may be traversing the septum or free wall. While this may allow adequate pressure measurements, angiography can result in extravasation. Cardiac output is measured by an indicator-dilution technique for valve area calculations. If angiography is to be performed, the needle is connected to a prefilled injector and connecting tubing. The needle is carefully filled with contrast, and a test injection is performed to ensure that the sideholes are free in the left ventricular cavity. Left ventriculography is then recorded in the RAO projection in mid-expiration. We have not been able to incorporate our lateral camera into this procedure successfully. The technician must remain alerted to stop the injection should extravasation occur. The needle is then removed, a finger is held over the puncture site for several minutes, and a bandage applied. To detect evidence of pneumo- or hemothorax, fluoroscopy is performed. If coronary angiography is to be done subsequently, it is performed without heparin anticoagulation. Following catheterization, the patient is returned to the Coronary Care Unit for careful monitoring; an upright chest x-ray film is taken immediately to once again look for evidence of pneumo- or hemothorax. The chest x-ray is repeated if the patient becomes dyspneic or evidence of left pleural liquid appears.

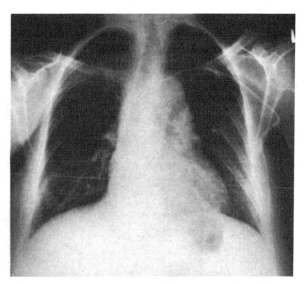

Figure 4A. *The chest roetgenogram prior to catheterization of the same patient as shown in Figures 2 and 3, reveals cardiomegaly and congestive heart failure. The St. Jude prostheses are not visible.*

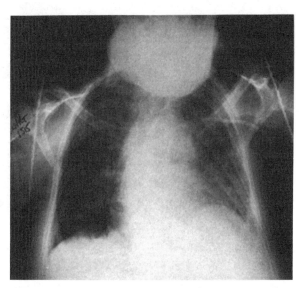

Figure 4B. *Immediately after catheterization, volume loss and a small amount of pleural fluid are noted in response to transthoracic left ventricular puncture.*

99

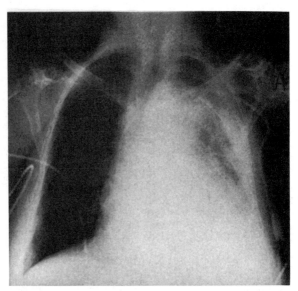

Figure 4C. *Six hours later, the patient was short of breath and had auscultatory evidence for hemothorax, confirmed by this film.*

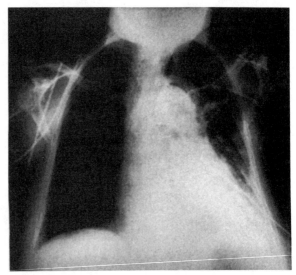

Figure 4D. *Tube thoroacostomy drainage resulted in prompt resolution of symptoms and bleeding stopped spontaneously.*

100

Management of Complications

Pneumo- or hemothorax are treated conservatively, if possible, and in consultation with the cardiothoracic surgeon. Tube thoracostomy may be necessary for extensive pleural blood or air (Fig. 4). Continued bleeding suggests coronary artery laceration and the need for open thoracotomy.

References

1. Ross J Jr: Transseptal left heart catheterization: a new method of left atrial puncture. Ann Surg 149:395, 1959.
2. Cope C: Technique for transseptal catheterization of the left atrium: preliminary report. J Thorac Cardiovasc Surg 37:482, 1959.
3. Hellems HK, Haynes FW, Dexter L: Pulmonary "capillary" pressure in man. J Appl Physiol 2:24, 1949.
4. Editorial: Pulmonary wedged catheter pressures. Circ Res 1:371, 1953.
5. Hosenpud JD, McAnulty JH, Morton MJ: Overestimation of mitral valve gradients obtained by phasic pulmonary capillary wedge pressure. Cathet Cardiovasc Diagn 9:283, 1983.
6. Schoenfeld MH, Palacios IF, Hutter AM, et al: Underestimation of prosthetic mitral valve areas: role of transseptal catheterization in avoiding unnecessary repeat mital valve surgery. J Am Coll Cardiol 5:1387, 1985.
7. Brockenbrough EC, Braunwald E: A new technique for left ventricular angiocardiography and transseptal left heart catheterization. Am J Cardiol 6:1062, 1960.
8. Brockenbrough EC, Braunwald E, Ross J Jr: Transseptal left heart catheterization: a review of 450 studies and description of an improved technique. Circulation 25:15, 1962.
9. Braunwald E: Transseptal left heart catheterization. Circulation 37 and 38(Suppl III):III-74, 1968.
10. Schoonmaker FW, Vijay NK, Jantz RD: Left atrial and ventricular transseptal catheterization review: losing skills? Cathet Cardiovasc Diagn 13:233, 1987.
11. Laskey WK: (Percutaneous) Retrograde left ventricular catheterization in aortic valve stenosis. Cathet Cardiovasc Diagn 12:75, 1986.
12. Mullins CE: New catheter and technique for transseptal left heart catheterization in infants and children. Circulation 59-60(Suppl II):II-251, 1979.
13. Laskey WK, Kusiak V, Untereker WJ, et al: Transseptal left heart catheterization: utility of a sheath technique. Cathet Cardiovasc Diagn 8:535, 1982.
14. Kawachi K, Kitamura S, Oyama C, et al: An improved method for

transseptal left heart catheterization. Cathet Cardiovasc Diagn 9:303, 1983.

15. Kotoda K, Hasegawa T, Mizuno A, et al: Transseptal left heart catheterization with Swan-Ganz flow-directed catheter. Am Heart J 105:436, 1983.

16. Bagger JP, Sennels F, Vejby-Christensen H, et al: Transseptal left heart catheterization with a Swan-Ganz flow-directed catheter: reviewed 173 studies. Am Heart J 109:332, 1985.

17. Lam W, Juska J, Pietras R: Transseptal balloon catheterization of the left ventricle in adult valvular heart disease. Am Heart J 107:147, 1984.

18. Palacios I, Block PC, Brandi S, et al: Percutaneous balloon valvotomy for patients with severe mitral stenosis. Circulation 75:778, 1987.

19. Dunn M: Is transseptal catheterization necessary? J Am Coll Cardiol 5:1393, 1985.

20. Karsh DL, Michaelson SP, Langou RA, et al: Retrograde left ventricular catheterization in patients with an aortic valve prosthesis. Am J Cardiol 41:893, 1978.

21. Handler JB, Thompson SI, Viewig WVR, et al: Transseptal and retrograde left ventricular catheterization in patients with the stent-mounted xenograft valve prosthesis in the aortic position. Cathet Cardiovasc Diagn 5:411, 1979.

22. Morris DC, King SB, Douglas JS, et al: Hemodynamic results of aortic aortic valvular replacement with porcine xenograft valve. Circulation 56:841, 1977.

23. Johnson A, Thompson S, Viewig WVR, et al: Evaluation of the in vivo function of the Hancock porcine xenograft in the aortic position. J Thorac Cardiovasc Surg 75:599, 1979.

24. Lew AS, Harper RW, Federman J, et al: Recent experience with transseptal catheterization. Cathet Cardiovasc Diagn 9:601, 1983.

25. Lundqvist C, Olsson SB, Varnaukas E: Transseptal left heart catheterization: a review of 278 studies. Clin Cardiol 9:21, 1986.

26. O'Keefe JH, Vliestra RE, Hanley PC, et al: Revival of the transseptal approach for catheterization of the left atrium and ventricle. Mayo Clin Proc 60:790, 1985.

27. Morton MJ, McAnulty JH, Rahimtoola SH, et al: Risks and benefits of postoperative cardiac catheterization in patients with ball valve prostheses. Am J Cardiol 40:870, 1977.

28. Kloster FE, Bristow JD, Seaman AJ: Cardiac catheterization during anticoagulant therapy. Am J Cardiol 28:675, 1971.

29. Ross J Jr: Considerations regarding the technique for transseptal left heart catheterization. Circulation 34:391, 1966.

30. Baim DS, Grossman W: Percutaneous approach and transseptal catheterization. In Grossman W (ed): Cardiac Catheterization and Angiography. Philadelphia, Lea and Febiger, 1986, pp 71–75.

31. Walmsley R, Watson H: The medial wall of the right atrium. Circulation 34:400, 1966.

32. Bloomfield DA, Sinclair-Smith BC: The limbic ledge: a landmark for transseptal left heart catheterization. Circulation 31:103, 1965.

33. Itzhak K, Glassman E, Cohen M, et al: Use of two-dimensional echocardiography during transseptal cardiac catheterization. J Am Coll Cardiol 4:425, 1984.
34. Ponsdomenech ER, Nunez VB: Heart puncture in man for Diodrast visualization of ventricular chambers and great arteries: its experimental and anatomophysiological bases and technique. Am Heart J 41:643, 1951.
35. Brock R, Milstein BB, Ross DN: Percutaneous left ventricular puncture in assessment of aortic stenosis. Thorax 11:163, 1956.
36. Bjork VO, Cullhed I, Hallen A, et al: Sequelae of left ventricular puncture with angiocardiography. Circulation 24:204, 1961.
37. Levy MJ, Lillehei CW: Percutaneous direct cardiac catheterization: a new method, with results in 122 patients. N Engl J Med 271:273, 1964.
38. Braunwald E: Percutaneous left ventricular puncture. Circulation 37–38(Suppl III):III-80, 1968.
39. MacDonald RG, Feldman RL, Pepine CJ: Retrograde catheterization of left ventricle through tilting disc valves using a modified catheter system. Am J Cardiol 54:1372, 1984.
40. Shabetai R, Krotkiewski A, Reeves JT: A pitfall in the postoperative evaluation of aortic Starr-Edwards valves. J Thorac Cardiovasc Surg 53:288, 1967.
41. Falicov RE, Walsh WF: Retrograde crossing of aortic Bjork-Shiley prosthesis. Am J Cardiol 43:1062, 1979.
42. Morris PE: Retrograde left ventricular catheterization in patients with a Bjork-Shiley valve prosthesis. Am J Cardiol 44:578, 1979.
43. Baxley WA, Soto B: Hemodynamic evaluation of patients with combined mitral and aortic prostheses. Am J Cardiol 45:42, 1980.
44. Vignola PA, Swaye PS, Gosselin AJ: Safe transthoracic left ventricular puncture with echocardiographic guidance. Cathet Cardiovasc Diagn 6:317, 1980.
45. Wong PHC, Chow JSF, Chen WWC, et al: Aortic catheterization via percutaneous left ventricular puncture. Cathet Cardiovasc Diagn 9:421, 1983.

Chapter 5

Complications of Temporary Pacing and Electrophysiologic Studies

Peter J. Kudenchuk and Jack Kron

Therapeutic Temporary Pacing

History

"When sudden death happens without any manifest cause, then it is owing to a palsy of the heart." Herophilus first noted this association between sudden death and apparent cardiac standstill in 300 B.C. Some 18 centuries later, currents from voltaic pile or a Leyden jar were used to stimulate cardiac nerves and muscle in hope of reviving dead animals.[1]

Cardiac pacemakers were first used for the treatment of Stokes-Adams attacks due to advanced atrioventricular block. The earliest efforts at temporary cardiac pacing, reported in 1952, consisted of needle electrodes placed subcutaneously on the chest wall, and attached to a pacemaker generator.[2] This relatively noninvasive form of external cardiac pacing was employed primarily in the emergency treatment of ventricular standstill. While successful, external cardiac stimulation techniques were shortlived because they frequently induced painful thoracic and diaphragmatic muscle contractions, and, on occasion, even skin burns.

From *Complications of Cardiac Catheterization and Angiography: Prevention and Management* edited by Jack Kron, M.D. and Mark J. Morton, M.D. © 1989, Futura Publishing Inc., Mount Kisco, NY.

Although cardiac catheterization by transvenous or arterial routes had been performed in animals since 1844,[3] the first successful human heart catheterization did not occur until 1929.[4] Techniques of intracardiac pacing awaited clinical introduction for nearly 30 more years. In 1958 Thevenet described a method of invasive transthoracic pacing which he accomplished by implanting a pacing wire percutaneously through the thorax and directly into the myocardial wall of the right ventricle.[5] Two years later, Bellet reported the limited success of such pacing among 9 patients suffering cardiac collapse.[6] In 1958, transvenous endocardial pacing was also successfully performed.[7] In large measure, the transvenous approach has subsequently displaced other modalities for temporary intracardiac pacing. However, transthoracic pacing still remains an alternative therapy in the cardiac arrest setting where time and ease of placement are critical factors.

Recently, external cardiac pacing has reemerged as a low risk means of providing emergency cardiac stimulation in cases of symptomatic bradycardia or asystole.[8] Modification of the electrodes has largely eliminated the stinging and burning sensations previously experienced by most patients. Furthermore, changes in the duration and shape of the delivered stimulus have reduced the current amplitude necessary to externally pace the heart. This has largely eliminated the painful muscular contractions associated with the earlier version of the external pacemaker.

Indications For Temporary Pacing

Indications for temporary cardiac pacing can be divided into three categories: definite indications, definite nonindications, and the controversial "middle ground" (Table 1).[9] Pacing is definitely indicated for any symptomatic bradyarrhythmia that cannot be readily revised pharmacologically. Pacing is not indicated for asymptomatic conduction disturbances having a low probability of becoming symptomatic or life-threatening. Between these extremes, however, lies a host of asymptomatic conduction abnormalities whose treatment relies principally upon clinical judgment and where there is often disagreement about the necessity of pacing.

Table 1
Indications for Temporary Cardiac Pacing

Circumstance	Definitely Indicated	Probably Indicated	Not Indicated
Complete AV block			
congenital (AV node)			
Asymptomatic			X
Symptomatic	T, P		
Acquired (HIS-P)			
Asymptomatic		T, P	
Symptomatic	T, P		
Surgical (persistent)			
Asymptomatic	T	P	
Symptomatic	T, P		
Second degree HB			
Type I (AV nodal)			
Asymptomatic			X
Symptomatic	T, P		
Type II (HIS-P)			
Asymptomatic		T, P	
Symptomatic	T, P		
First degree AVB			
AV Nodal			
Asymptomatic			X
Symptomatic			X
HIS-Purkinje			
Asymptomatic			X
Symptomatic			X
Bundle branch block			
Asymptomatic			X
Symptomatic			X
Sick sinus syndrome			
Symptomatic	T, P		
Asymptomatic			X
Hypersensitive carotid sinus syndrome			
Symptomatic	T, P		
Asymptomatic			X

Table 1 (Cont'd)
Indications for Temporary Cardiac Pacing

Circumstance	Definitely Indicated	Probably Indicated	Not Indicated
Tachycardia prevention*			
Associated with bradycardia	T, P		
Associated with QT prolongation	T	P	
Atrial flutter	T, P		
Atrial fibrillation			X
AV nodal reentry	T, P		
WPW with recip. tachy	T, P		
VT	T	P	

Adapted from: Zipes DP, Duffin EG: Cardiac pacemakers. In Braunwald E, (ed): Heart Disease: A Textbook of Cardiovascular Medicine. Philadelphia, W.B. Saunders Co, 1984, p 746, with permission.

T = temporary pacing; P = permanent pacing; X = pacing not indicated; * = the primary role of temporary and permanent pacing in tachycardia prevention is controversial, but may be appropriate in selected patients.

Complications of Temporary Pacing

Noninvasive External Pacing

Complications stemming from newer modes of external noninvasive cardiac stimulation principally relate to patient discomfort. Such discomfort is generally caused by muscle contraction. Subjectively, it may be described as a "twitch" to an intense "stinging," and is a function of the intensity of stimulus amplitude, and perhaps of the integrity of the skin underlying the pacing electrodes.

Transthoracic Pacing

Transthoracic pacing is a dangerous procedure which should only be used when other pacing modalities cannot be employed.

Potential risks include: pneumothorax, hemopericardium with tamponade, coronary artery laceration, and major organ or vessel injury. Roberts and Greenberg ,in their literature review of 44 human cases of successful transthoracic pacing, found no instance of fatality attributable to the procedure, and only 2 cases of nonlethal pericardial hemorrhage.[10] However, in a recent autopsy series of 20 patients receiving either transthoracic pacing wires or intracardiac injections via a variety of approaches, complications occurred in all patients and included: inferior vena cava puncture, right atrial puncture, pulmonary artery puncture, lung or liver puncture, internal mammary artery puncture, and right or left coronary artery laceration.[11] The incidence of complications appeared to be least with a percutaneous approach, entering the heart from the 5th intercostal space along the parasternal line. But even with this approach, three instances of pulmonary artery puncture were reported. Active cardiopulmonary resuscitation during pacemaker introduction is particularly likely to aggravate the incidence of such complications.

Transvenous Temporary Pacing

Complications due to the transvenous placement of temporary pacemakers may be related to access site, design of the pacing catheter, the pacing procedure itself, and the duration of pacing.[12]

Access Site

Choice of a particular venous access site for temporary pacemaker placement hinges on several concerns: hemostasis, thrombosis or thromboembolism, lead stability, infection, and the suitability of the selected site to the patient. In general, the choice of access route is governed by similar considerations to those of central venous and right heart catheterization (Chapter 2). Bleeding, thrombosis, and thromboembolism are problems not infrequently encountered during transvenous pacemaker placement. Anticoagulated patients are particularly prone to local bleeding complications. Superficial veins not juxtaposed to arteries, such as the cephalic or basilic veins in the arm, or the external jugular vein offer safety in this setting. If punctured below the inguinal ligament to avoid the risk of retroperitoneal hemorrhage, the femoral vein is a good alternative for some patients. Direct pressure to control bleeding can be readily applied to this site. The internal jugular and subclavian veins should only be used in emergency situations for reasons discussed in detail in Chapter 2.

Inadvertent arterial puncture may occur from attempts to percutaneously cannulate a vein in almost any location and has been reported to occur in as many as 10% of subclavian catheterization attempts.[13] When there is doubt about the identity of the vessel cannulated, measurement of oxygen saturation from an extracted blood sample can discriminate between venous and arterial vessels. We also recommend that whenever possible, fluoroscopic visualization of an initially placed small guidewire be obtained prior to placement of a larger cannula or introducer sheath. On occasion, a pacing catheter intended for the right ventricle has been inadvertently placed within the left ventricle because of unrecognized arterial puncture.

Thromboembolic Complications

Thrombosis following transvenous placement of pacesmaker electrodes is often associated with infection and may result in venous obstruction (Fig.1).[14,15] However, much of the data regarding this complication stems from studies of permanent pacemaker systems, and thus may be due to the chronic indwelling nature of the leads. Brachial phlebographies performed in 100 consecutive patients 44 months following placement of permanent pacemakers found a 39% incidence of thrombotic lesions in veins used to pass the pacemaker lead into the right ventricle.[16] However, only 12% of these 39 patients had clinical symptoms or signs of impaired venous return. Other reports have noted thrombosis of axillary, subclavian and innominate veins,[17-19] superior vena cava syndrome,[20-22] and even thrombotic occlusion of major dura mater sinuses.[23] It is uncertain whether similar problems can develop in vessels retaining pacemaker electrodes for shorter spans of time. The actual incidence of subclavian thrombosis in these such patients is probably closer to 2% to 3%.[24] The treatment of these complications also remains speculative. Although use of anticoagulants is appealing and successful in small groups of patients, no controlled trial using thrombolytic agents or anticoagulants has been per-

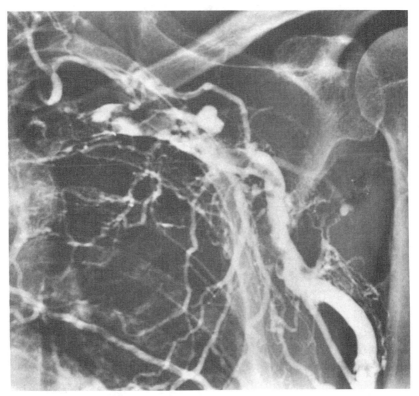

Figure 1. *Phlebogram demonstrating recent subclavian thrombosis in a patient who had undergone placement of a temporary transvenous pacemaker. Note extensive collateralization and intaluminal filling defects representing clot in the subclavian and axillary veins.*

formed.[25] At present, removal of the temporary pacing catheter (with culture of the catheter tip) as soon as possible appears to be the most prudent initial recommendation. A short course of intravenous anticoagulation should be considered for upper extremity sites, however, a prolonged course of warfarin therapy may be required for femoral vein thrombosis.

Other thromboembolic complications, specifically pulmonary embolism, have also been linked to indwelling pacing catheters.[26] In a recent study of 100 patients undergoing temporary transvenous pacing, this complication occurred in 2.7% of insertions and was seen exclusively when a femoral vein was selected as the placement site.[12] Phlebitis attributable to the pacing catheter was also observed in 5% of the 100 patients. However, there was no statistically significant difference in the frequency of phlebitis between upper or lower extremity cannulation sites.

Catheter Migration

Complications stemming from the instability of a pacing catheter may also be related to its site of placement. Pacemaker malfunction (defined as a failure to sense and/or capture) occurs in up to 37% of temporary transvenous pacemaker placements.[12] Such problems are more frequently seen when an arm vein is chosen as the site of cannulation, and are probably related to shifts in catheter position with arm motion. In one recent study, 37% of brachial venous pacemakers, as opposed to only 9% of femoral venous catheters (P = .005) required repositioning or replacement because of malfunction.[12]

Complications Related to Access Site

Certain central venous sites harbor unique potential complications. Internal jugular and subclavian vein cannulations have been associated with air aspiration and air embolization, a complication whose incidence is estimated at 1% to 10%. This complication can be minimized by placing the patient in the Trendelenburg position at the time of venipuncture, and having the patient maintain end-expiratory apnea at the time the venous cannula is transiently open to the atmosphere.[24]

Pneumothorax is a reported complication with either subclavian or internal jugular approaches and may occur in 0.25% to 2.3% of patients, depending upon the experience of the operator.[13,27] Rarely, left subclavian vein puncture has also been associated with chylothorax due to perforation of the thoracic duct[28,29] or with osteomyelitis of the first rib.[30]

Overall complications, including malfunction, bleeding, infection, thromboembolism, or arrhythmia are more common from the femoral site. Local infections at the site of insertion as well as sepsis are also more frequently seen in patients having femoral venous catheters. Three large reported surveys of temporary pacing have supported use of the subclavian or internal jugular veins for temporary pacing. The incidence of complications from such sites has ranged from 4% to 18%, with no pacing-related complication having resulted in patient death.[31–33] Based on available data, the internal jugular and subclavian veins would appear to be the most ideal locations from which to place a temporary pacemaker, whereas the basilic, cephalic, external jugular, or femoral veins may be more suitable in anticoagulated patients.

Pacing Catheter Complications

The temporary transvenous pacing catheter may perforate any vascular structure enroute to the heart, and may induce cardiac arrhythmias via local mechanical irritation. Ventricular tachycardia during pacemaker insertion may occur in up to 6% of patients; and cardiac perforation (with and without tamponade) in 4% of patients.[12] Both the right atrium and right ventricle are relatively thin-walled structures and thus susceptible to perforation, although puncture of the interventricular septum has also been known to occur.[34] We believe the incidence of right ventricular perforation during temporary pacing to be much higher than reported. Right ventricular perforation is recognized by: a sudden increase in threshold, a change from endocardial to epicardial electrogram from the distal electrode, pleural or pericardial pain, or a pericardial friction rub. Our practice is to confirm the presence of perforation by recording from the distal electrode (Fig. 2) and then to withdraw the catheter and reposition it if necessary to obtain a good pacing threshold. If tamponade is suspected, echocardiography should be performed to demonstrate pericardial fluid and evidence of abnormal right atrial or right ventricular filling.[35,36] One might expect larger, stiffer pacing catheters to produce a higher incidence of complications and a lower incidence of malfunction once placed. However, the choice of a smaller (5 or 6 French), as opposed to a larger (7 French), pacing catheter appears to have no significant bearing on either the incidence of pacemaker complications (29% vs 16%, respectively) or malfunction (46% vs 32%, respectively).[12]

Transient right bundle branch block has been reported to occur in 2% to 10% of patients undergoing right heart catheterization for pacemaker placement or for hemodynamic monitoring purposes, and is probably due to focal trauma to the right bundle in its superficial course near the tricuspid valve. Transient complete in-

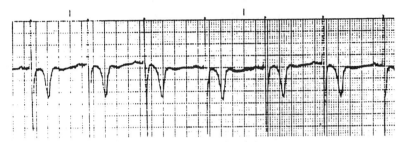

Figure 2. *Unipolar recording from distal electrode demonstrating epicardial electrogram in a patient whose temporary pacemaker lost caputre. Withdrawal of electrode demonstrated reemergence of ventricular capture and an intracavitary ventricular electrogram similar to that of Figure 11.*

terruption of atrioventricular conduction has been reported to occur in patients with preexisting left bundle branch block. Such block usually resolves within 24 hours.

Finally, because of their design and usual short duration of placement, temporary pacing wires, unlike their permanent pacing wire counterparts, are usually easily removed by simple withdrawal of the catheter. Retention of a temporary electrode is a reported, but rare, phenomenon.[37]

Hemodynamic and Electrophysiologic Complications

In the process of pacing the heart, patients may develop additional complications: induced pacemaker dependence, induced ventricular tachyarrhythmias, and hemodynamic deterioration. Pacemaker dependence is an incompletely understood phenomenon whereby a previously present escape focus either fails to reassert control over heart rhythm or only does so following a prolonged period of asystole when temporary pacing is abruptly terminated. This phenomenon has been observed in studies of sinus node function during electrophysiologic testing, and may occur at other pacemaker sites by similar mechanisms.[38,39] Because the appearance of this phenomenon is unpredictable, one is advised to avoid the abrupt termination of temporary pacing. A preferred method of assessing the presence or absence of an underlying rhythm is to gradually slow the paced heart rate until it falls below the rate of the patient's intrinsic rhythm, at which time the pacer generator can be turned off.

The mechanical induction of transient ventricular tachyarrhythmias during pacemaker placement is far more common than the electrical induction of such arrhythmias during ventricular pacing. The risk of mechanically induced ventricular fibrillation is particularly high among younger patients suffering an acute inferior myocardial infarction, among whom the incidence of ventricular fibrillation at the time of catheter manipulation can be as high as 14%.[40] During pacing, patients without a clinical history of ventricular tachyarrhythmias are at minimal risk of developing such arrhythmias, even with multiple paced beats delivered at "vulnerable periods" of the cardiac cycle.[41,42] However, patients with a history of ventricular tachycardia or fibrillation or with recent acute myocardial infarction, may be at higher risk for developing ventricular tachyarrhythmias.[43-45] Pacing during the vulnerable period of the cardiac cycle may occur as a consequence of pacemaker-sensing failure or nondemand pacing (Fig. 3). Based on data from intracardiac electrophysiologic studies, a single inappropriately placed ventricular paced stimulus may induce a sustained ventricular tachyarrhythmia in up to 16% of patients having a clinical history of ventricular tachyarrhythmias.[42] For these reasons, all patients undergoing temporary pacemeaker placement should be electrocardiographically monitored and defibrillation equipment should be readily available. This is particularly applicable to situations where rapid or "burst" pacing is used to overdrive and terminate a tachyarrhythmia. Such rapid pacing has been reported to not infrequently result in acceleration of ventricular tachycardia, necessitating electrical cardioversion.[46] Finally, because the transvenous pacing catheter provides a relatively low resistance electrical pathway from the external environment to the heart, inadvertent application of an alternating form of current (AC) to the proximal poles of the pacemaker electrode could result in disastrous ventricular fibrillation. Therefore, if not connected to a temporary pacemaker generator, any exposed metal leads extending from the pacemaker catheter should be wrapped with insulating material (most commonly a rubber examination glove).

Hemodynamic deterioration in patients undergoing temporary ventricular pacing has been attributed to inappropriate pacing rates and the loss of atrial augmentation of ventricular filling, or "atrial

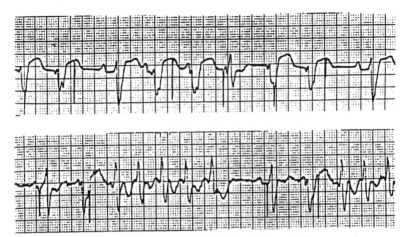

Figure 3. *Pacemaker with frequent sensing failure. In lower strip, pacemaker spike falls on beginning of T wave followed by a run of nonsustained ventricular tachycardia.*

kick." It is a more common occurrence in patients with impaired left ventricular function, in whom atrial transport may contribute up to 40% of cardiac output. During phasic shifts from a sinus rhythm to a ventricular paced rhythm, when ventricular systole is not preceded by an appropriately timed atrial contraction, systolic blood pressure may decrease by 20–40 mmHg, and cardiac output may decline by up to 1.5–2.0 L/min (Fig. 4).[47] Another potential cause of hemodynamic deterioration is failure to recognize noncapture during pacing. During the decay of a pacer spike of high amplitude, an ECG artifact simulating a QRS complex may be observed despite cardiac asystole (Fig. 5). This artifact can be differentiated from true ventricular capture by obtaining an ECG in multiple leads, at least one of which should demonstrate an unequivocal QRS-T complex if pacer capture is occurring, and by confirming the presence of a palpable arterial pulse with each paced beat.

Time Related Complications

Sepsis, phlebitis, and pulmonary embolism during temporary pacing are related to the duration of lead placement. Although

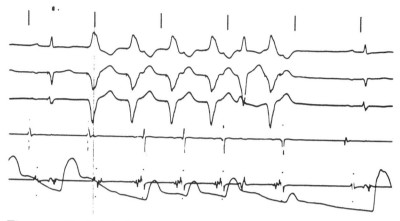

Figure 4. *Marked decline in systemic blood pressure in patient undergoing ventricular pacing during programmed electrical stimulation. Systolic blood pressure may fall by 20 to 40 mmHg in some patients undergoing ventricular pacing.*

temporary pacemakers can remain in position for days to weeks, the longer the catheter is in place, the greater the risk of problems.[48] The overall incidence of sepsis, phlebitis, or pulmonary embolus in 113 patients undergoing transvenous temporary pacing was 7%.[12]. When the duration of implantation in these patients was investi-

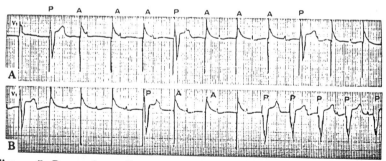

Figure 5. *Pacemaker spike with failure to pace. Only beats marked "P" are paced beats. During decay of a pacer spike of high voltage, an artifact may be produced that can stimulate a QRS complex (A). (From Roberts JR, Greenberg MI: Emergency transthoracic pacing. Ann Emerg Med 10:600, 1981, with permission.)*

gated, it was found that the complication rate was only 2% in those patients who were paced less than 72 hours, but rose to 12% after 72 hours. Most complications were limited to the femoral site of cannulation. There is scant data available regarding pacers retained in subclavian or internal jugular sites for prolonged periods, although reports of alimentation catheters placed in the subclavian vein state an incidence of sepsis in 7.5% of patients.[13]

Intracardiac Electrophysiologic Studies

History

The intracardiac electrophysiologic study is a systematic approach to cardiac arrhythmias, which is performed by recording and measuring a variety of electrophysiologic events within the heart, both in the native state and in response to programmed stimulation. Initially, electrophysiologic studies principally observed the presence and timing of atrial, His bundle, and ventricular activation. In the early 1970s, programmed stimulation was applied to these studies, allowing one to determine sinus node function, the refractory periods of various components of the AV conduction system, and the induction of arrhythmias. Currently, electrophysiologic cardiac stimulation forms a cornerstone for the diagnosis, evaluation, and treatment of otherwise sporadic life-threatening cardiac arrhythmias.[38] More recently, the technique of catheter ablation of the bundle of His, accessory pathways, and foci of tachyarrhythmias has been applied to selected patients with refractory tachyarrhythmias.[49] Once identified, such pathways or foci have been successfully ablated by delivering electric shocks through transvenous pacing catheters.

Indications and Technique

Intracardiac electrophysiologic studies are performed to evaluate suspected abnormalities of atrioventricular conduction, sinus node dysfunction, life-threatening tachyarrhythmias, and recurrent syncope of unknown etiology but in which an arrhythmia is strongly suspected. A variety of techniques and stimulation protocols are employed during electrophysiologic studies (Figs. 6 and 7). Programmed stimulation for drug testing and anatomic determination uses one to four extrastimuli delivered to one or more sites in the right ventricle, right or left atria (the latter via the coronary sinus), and occasionally to the left ventricle. Isoproterenol infusion is sometimes used during programmed stimulation to enhance the induction of ventricular or supraventricular arrhythmias. Detailed discussion of the variety of techniques employed in patients undergoing electrophysiologic study is beyond the scope of this chapter, and the reader is referred to a text detailing this information.[38]

Closed-chest catheter ablation of cardiac tissue has been used to treat refractory cardiac arrhythmias stemming from an identified arrhythmia focus, an accessory pathway, or arrhythmias due to rapid conduction through the atrioventricular junction. The technique involves meticulous attention to detail, first and foremost of which is proper positioning of the catheter at the site of intended ablation. In the region of the AV junction, this site is identified by a location evidencing maximum deflection of the His bundle electrogram ($\geq$ 150 mV). In the case of an accessory pathway(s) previously mapped to a septal position, the catheter should be positioned within the os of the coronary sinus, in proximity to the earliest retrograde activity of the accessory pathway. While left free-wall accessory pathways may be altered by direct-current shocks delivered from a distal position within the coronary sinus, many investigators prefer a surgical approach in such situations, limiting closed chest techniques primarily to posterior septal accessory pathways. This is because electrical discharge within the coronary sinus may result in coronary sinus rupture and cardiac tamponade. Catheter ablation of ventricular tachycardia foci re-

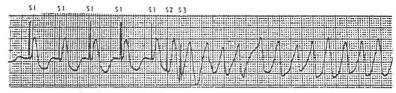

Figure 6. *Technique of programmed stimulation. Note five ventricular paced beats labeled S1 followed by two extrastimulated beats labeled S2 and S3 delivered during diastole at shorter coupling intervals. S3 is followed by the induction of ventricular tachycardia.*

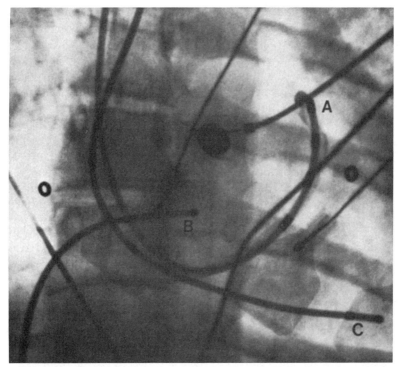

Figure 7. *Catheter placement during electrophysiologic study. A. Catheter with four electrodes placed in the coronary sinus from the left antecubital vein. Pacing and recording of electrical activity from the left atrium can be performed from this site. B. Tripolar catheter for recording of HIS Bundle electrogram is placed across the tricuspid valve from right femoral vein access site. C. Hexapolar catheter is placed via right subclavian vein to pace right ventricle. Proximal electrodes may be used to pace or record from right atrium. Note that the apical position of the distal electrodes demonstrates proper radiographic appearance of the temporary transvenous ventriuclar pacemaker.*

quires detailed endocardial mapping in order to identify the earliest site of endocardial activation preceding the surface ventricular tachycardia QRS complex. This site is interpreted to be the exit point of the ventricular tachycardia focus, and is the location to which the ablation catheter must be directed. Any potential site of ablation must take the proximity of coronary vessels into account, lest these be damaged by the energies used during such procedures.

Following proper positioning of the ablation catheter (cathode), and placement of a patch electrode (anode) adjacent to the left scapula, one or more direct-current shocks are applied to the catheter thru a cardioverter. The amount of electrical energy employed for each shock may vary from 35 to 500 J, usually 200 J. For shocks delivered from the coronary sinus, immediate surgical standby is mandatory in the event of coronary sinus perforation.

Complications

Complications inherent to the placement of any transvenous pacemaker catheter apply equally to those placed during the course of an electrophysiologic study. In a recently assembled registry from six university centers with active electrophysiology laboratories, major complications of 8,545 electrophysiologic studies performed in 4,015 patients were reported.[27] The reported incidence of cardiac perforation, major hemorrhage, arterial injury, or major venous thrombosis ranged from 0.1% to 0.5% of patients (.05% to .23% of studies). Cardiac perforation and major venous thrombosis were the most frequent complications encountered. The incidence of cardiac perforation is much higher in laboratories where the stimulating electrode is left in place for several days. Several complications are unique to the electrophysiologic study. These are principally due to induction of malignant arrhythmias during programmed stimulation, and the risks entailed in closed-chest catheter arrhythmia ablation techniques (Table 2).

Table 2
Major Complications of Clinical Cardiac Electrophysiologic Studies
(n = 8,545 studies in 4,015 patients)

Complication	n	% of studies	% of patients
Death	5	.06	.12
Cardiac perforation	19	.22	.5
Major hemorrhage	4	.05	.1
Arterial injury	8	.1	.2
Major venous thrombosis	20	.23	.5

From Horowitz LN: Safety of electrophysiologic studies. *Circulation* 73: II28, 1986, with permission.

Programmed Stimulation

Patients undergoing programmed stimulation of the heart frequently develop symptomatic arrhythmias. Cardioversion is required in 30% to 60% of such patients who develop ventricular arrhythmias, and 1% to 2% of patients in whom supraventricular tachycardias are induced.[50] Myocardial infarction, cerebrovascular events, or systemic arterial embolization are infrequent sequelae to arrhythmia induction and cardioversion.

The mortality rate from electrophysiologic studies is reported to be 0.12%.[27] Of 5 such deaths reported among a total of 4,015 patients in a recent survey, the cause of death in 2 patients was refractory ventricular tachycardia-fibrillation or electromechanical dissociation during electrophysiologic testing; 1 patient died of incessant ventricular tachycardia shortly after study, and 2 patients who died within 24 hours of study were in extremis and probably would have expired irrespective of electrophysiologic testing. This mortality rate of 0.12% is comparable to that reported during coronary angiography (0.10%). In 565 patients undergoing serial electrophysiologic studies at the Oregon Health Sciences University there have been two deaths. Both were related to the hemodynamic and electrophysiologic effects of rapidly administered antiarrhythmic drugs used during serial testing.

Catheter Ablation

The delivery of 50–400 J of energy thru an electrode catheter during closed-chest arrhythmia ablation procedures, delivers explosive concussion waves to the heart, which may exceed 1–2 atmospheres of pressure. Such concussive energy has been reported to rupture the thin-walled coronary sinus and result in acute cardiac tamponade.[51] The incidence of this complication has been as high as 27% among coronary sinus ablative procedures reported by the Percutaneous Mapping and Ablation Registry.[52] The local injury sustained from delivery of such shocks to the myocardium has been observed on a cellular level as disruption of membrane integrity with necrosis of myocytes and later replacement of these cells by fibrocytes, histiocytes, and round cells[53] compatible with focal sub-endocardial infarction.

Catheter ablation procedures frequently cause tachy- and bradyarrhythmias that may occur immediately or up to 48 hours following shock. These usually resolve within 2–3 days. Other acute complications have included transient hypotension and coronary artery spasm.[54] Acute coronary occlusion with myocardial infarction is as yet an unreported event during catheter ablation, but nonetheless of concern during such procedures. Later complications have included development of complete heart block, endocardial thrombi, large atrial thrombus,[55] damage to the support structures of the tricuspid and aortic valves, and sudden death.[56]

Guidelines For the Optimal Performance of Temporary Pacing

External Noninvasive Pacing

External noninvasive pacing is performed by first cleansing the skin of salt and natural oils. Two high impedance, large stimulating electrode patches are then placed. The posterior electrode patch is attached over the left subscapular area at the cardiac level; the anterior patch is placed over the left precordium, close to the lower left sternal edge, thus minimizing possible pectoralis muscle contraction during pacing. These leads are then attached to the external pacemaker, whose output is lowered to 0. An appropriate pacemaker rate is chosen. The pacemaker output current may then be adjusted at 10 mA increments (up to the device's maximum output of 140 mA) until a stimulated QRS-T complex closely and reliably follows each pacing artifact. Stimulation thresholds have been reported to usually range between 40–70 mA.

Transthoracic Pacing

Transthoracic pacing is indicated in unstable, unawake patients in whom time and circumstances do not permit use of fluoroscopy or flow-directed pacing catheters, and where external noninvasive pacing has failed.[10] The vast majority of such pacemakers are introduced during the course of cardiopulmonary resuscitation, where cardiac output is generally insufficient to direct a catheter into the ventricle, and use of fluoroscopy is out of the question because of ongoing chest compression. Transthoracic pacing kits are available (Elecath 11-KTM1, Electro-Catheter Corporation, Rahway, New Jersey) and include a blunt cannula with sharp inner trocar, J-shaped bipolar pacing wire, and electrical connector (Fig. 8).

We prefer percutaneous puncture of the heart from the subxyphoid approach despite reports of higher complication rates from this site.[11] We are concerned that left parasternal cardiac puncture too frequently may produce lung laceration and pneumothorax in mechanically ventilated patients. The cannula with trocar are inserted in the left xyphocostal notch and then directed either toward the sternal notch, or toward the right or left shoulder at an angle (between skin and needle) of 30°. The needle is advanced approximately three-quarters of its total length after which the trocar is withdrawn and a syringe attached (Fig. 9). Aspiration of blood con-

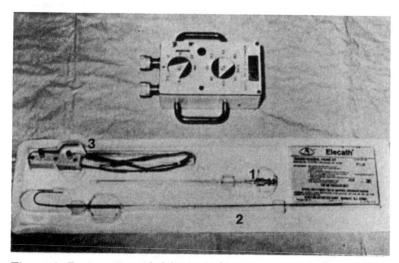

Figure 8. *Equipment needed for transthoracic pacing: 1. blunt steel cannula with inner trocar point; 2. bipolar pacing wire with sleeve; 3. electrical connector. (From Roberts JR, Greenberg MI: Emergency transthoracic pacing. Ann Emerg Med 10:600, 1981, with permission.)*

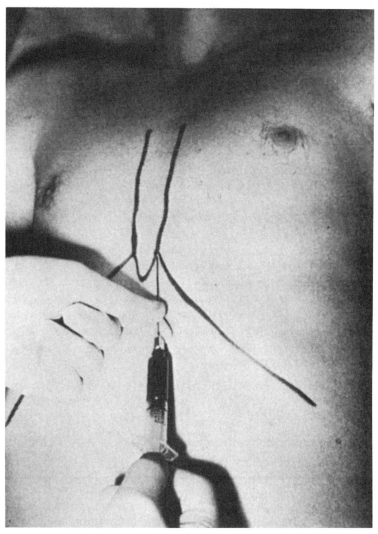

Figure 9. *Proper position and angle for successful placement of pacing wire into right ventricle. The cannula with trocar are inserted in the left xyphosternal notch at an angle of 30° and directed toward the sternal notch (or alternatively, toward the right or left shoulder). The cannula with trocar is advanced three-quarters of its length, after which the trocar is removed and a syringe attached to the cannula. Aspiration of intraventricular blood confirms proper position of the cannula. (From Roberts JR, Greenberg MI: Emergency transthoracic pacing. Ann Emerg Med 10:600, 1981, with permission.)*

firms proper positioning of the cannula. Failure to aspirate blood should prompt needle withdrawal and reapproach to the heart. When it is certain that the needle lies within a cardiac chamber (either the right or left ventricle), the pacing wire is placed through the cannula and advanced as far as possible without losing control of its distal end. Passage of the pacing sytlet should be easy, if the cannula lies within the heart cavity. Once the pacing stylet advances past the distal tip of the cannula, it spontaneously resumes its J-shape. The cannula is then carefully withdrawn over the pacing wire. The wire is inserted into its connector and to an external pacemaker generator adjusted initially to maximum output. If pacing is unsuccessful, the pacing wire may be rotated and gradually withdrawn until appropriate ventricular capture is achieved. The pacemaker generator output may then be briefly decreased to determine pacing threshold, and then returned to an output representing three to five times this value. Although pacing thresholds of no greater than 1–1.5 mA are preferred during placement of transvenous endocardial pacing electrodes, with emergent transthoracic pacing any current strength necessary to produce ventricular capture may be employed. Proper placement of the pacemaker should be verified and pneumothorax excluded by chest x-ray (Fig. 10). Immediate steps should then be taken to place a more stable transvenous pacing catheter.

Transvenous Temporary Pacing

Transvenous pacing can be accomplished from several venous venous access sites: internal or external jugular, subclavian, antecubital, or femoral veins. Jugular, subclavian, and femoral veins are approached percutaneously, whereas antecubital veins may be entered either percutaneously or by cutdown venotomy. The choice of venous access site is directed by clinical circumstances. Both internal jugular and subclavian approaches offer rapid approach to the right heart, with relatively good catheter stability and sterility. The femoral approach is hampered by the increasing risk of infection from an indwelling catheter from the groin and risk of thrombophlebitis from lower extremity immobilization. The antecubital, external jugular, or femoral veins are the sites of choice in anti-coagulated patients in whom control of bleeding from any access

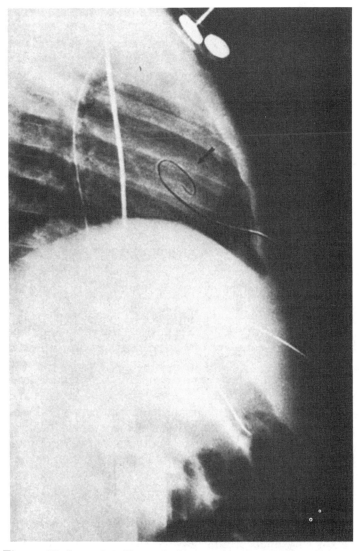

Figure 10. *Lateral radiograph demonstrates transthoracic pacing wire (arrow) in the right ventricle. (From Roberts JR, Greenberg MI: Emergency transthoracic pacing. Ann Emerg Med 10:600, 1981, with permission.)*

location must be considered. However, the incidence of venospasm, phlebitis, and catheter instability due to limb motion are disadvantages to the use of an arm vein.

A variety of transvenous pacing catheters are currently available. These range from 4–6 French floating bipolar catheters with inflatable balloon tips and 4 French semifloater catheters, both of whose lightweight design allows for flow direction into the right ventricle; pulmonary artery catheters with a right ventricular pacing port; and a variety of 5–8 French nonflow directed woven Dacron catheters (e.g., USCI, Billerica, MA). Transvenous pacing catheters, regardless of design, ideally should be directed into position under x-ray visualization.[48] Fluoroscopic guidance is mandatory for placement of stiff woven Dacron catheters to avoid mechanical injury to vascular structures. The right ventricular apex is the preferred destination for pacing catheters because of the greater lead stability achieved in that location.

When fluoroscopy is not readily available, a floating or semifloating pacing catheter may also be directed into proper position by electrocardiographic guidance. The approximate length of catheter needed to reach the right ventricular apex from a venous entrance site should always be initially estimated. The distal electrode of the pacing wire is then connected via a sterile alligator clip to lead V1 of a standard electrocardiograph. An intracardiac recording is made as the catheter is advanced (Fig. 11).[57] Achievement of proper position is determined both by a dramatic increase in QRS voltage as the catheter enters the right ventricle and by ST-segment elevation suggesting catheter contact with the endocardium. Under desperate circumstances, transvenous pacing can be achieved by attaching the catheter to an active external generator and advancing the catheter until "blind" ventricular capture is achieved.

Proper placement of the transvenous pacing catheter should be confirmed by chest radiography (Fig. 7). In addition, a pacing threshold of no more than 1–1.5 mA confirms proper contact of the pacemaker with endocardium. Pacing threshold should be verified daily to confirm proper catheter positioning and pacemaker function. However, the pacemaker generator output should be set at three to five times threshold in order to ensure consistent ventricular capture during pacing.

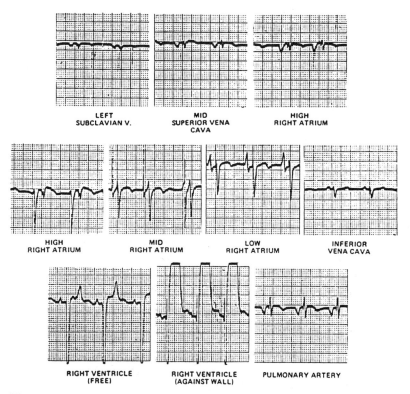

Figure 11. *As the pacemaker approaches the right atrium, the amplitude of the P waves increases progressively. Since atrial depolarization is inferiorly directed in this patient, P waves recorded above the atria have a negative deflection, whereas those low in the atria and in the inferior vena cava are positive. As the catheter enters the ventricle, the QRS amplitude increases markedly and a QS complex is inscribed. When the catheter tip touches the endocardial surface, marked ST-segment elevation is seen. As the electrode passes into the pulmonary artery, the QRS amplitude diminishes, and a negative P wave is inscribed since the catheter tip is again above the level of the atria. (From Bing OHL, McDowell JW, Hantman J, et al: Pacemaker placement by electrocardiographic monitoring. N Engl J Med 287:247, 1971, with permission.)*

Success of Temporary Pacing

Temporary cardiac pacing, by whatever means, is most likely to be successful when employed in metabolically stable patients for the treatment of cardiac conduction disturbances. Pacing by any modality, is less likely to be successful in the setting of severe hyperkalemia, hypoxia, acidosis, or severe cardiotoxic drug intoxication; in asystolic cardiac arrest; and following a prolonged period of cardiac arrest. Transthoracic pacing, in particular, has been used with the greatest frequency in such situations.

Ornato and colleagues reported a retrospective analysis of 54 adult patients treated with either transvenous or transthoracic pacemakers following prehospital bradysystolic cardiac arrest. Time between cardiac arrest and institution of cardiopulmonary resuscitation was 4.8 ± 4.3 minutes, and time from the onset of arrest to temporary pacemaker placement was 56.2 ± 20.4 minutes. Pacing achieved electrical capture in 38 of 60 pacemaker placements (63%). Three patients (5%) developed a pulse with pacing, one patient (1.6%) survived to be admitted to the hospital, but none survived to be discharged from the hospital. The authors concluded that "even with pacing, bradyasystolic-arrest victims appear to be irretrievable. Early pacemaker insertion after emergency department arrival did not affect the electrical capture rate nor did it influence survival."[58] Among a smaller series of 21 unsuccessfully resuscitated patients reported by Tintinalli and White in 1981, electrical capture occurred in only 8 patients (38%), only 2 of whom achieved even a transient blood pressure with pacing.[59]

Similar results occur with noninvasive external pacing. Among 29 patients in whom external noninvasive pacing was recently reported to be ineffective, 25 patients (86%) were unconscious and in cardiac arrest.[8] The reason for this high incidence of electrical noncapture, electromechanical dissociation, profound power failure, and dismal outlook for patients in cardiac arrest even with pacing, is probably due to the uncorrectable severity of their metabolic status and underlying ventricular dysfunction.

When used under less tenuous circumstances and among relatively more stable patients, temporary pacing is considerably more successful in achieving and maintaining electromechanical stability. Transvenous pacing, in particular, is almost universally successful among such individuals, although in some circumstances abnormalities in underlying cardiac tissue may require higher pacing currents in order to achieve consistent capture.[31]

External pacing is also more successful when performed under nondesperate circumstances. In a recent study of 134 patients receiving external pacing for a variety of brady- and tachyarrhythmias, electrical ventricular responses were produced in 105 patients (78%).[8] In another study of external pacing among 16 normal male subjects and 15 patients with a variety of bradyarrhythmias, only 1 patient could not be successfully paced even at maximum generator output.[60]

Summary

Cardiac pacing is indicated in the prophylactic, therapeutic, diagnostic, or ablative management of certain cardiac arrhythmias. The particular form of pacing used in a given situation depends upon the level of urgency. For most patients, transvenous pacing is the modality of choice. Electrophysiologic studies make use of more specialized equipment and catheters, usually placed from multiple access sites and should be performed only by individuals specifically trained and skilled in this area. Complications of intracardiac pacing are related to the type of pacemaker selected for placement, the site from which the pacer is placed, the process of pacing itself, and the length of time over which pacing is required. These problems can be minimized through the proper identification of patients most likely to benefit or incur harm from cardiac pacing procedures, the proper selection and tailoring of available modalities of pacing to the specific clinical situation, and a readiness to treat ensuing complications.

References

1. Registers of the Royal Humane Society of London, Nichols and Sons, 1774–1785.
2. Zoll PM: Resuscitation of the heart in ventricular standstill by external electrical stimulation. N Engl J Med 247:768, 1952.
3. Cournand AF: Nobel Lecture, December 11, 1956. In Nobel: Lectures, Physiology and Medicine 1942–1962. Amsterdam, Elsevier Publishing Co., 1964, p. 529.
4. Forssman MW: Die Sondierung des rechten herzens. Klin Wochenschr 8:2085, 1930.
5. Thevenet A, Hodges PC, Lillehei CW: The use of myocardial electrode

inserted percutaneously for control of complete atrioventricular block by an artificial pacemaker. Dis Chest 34:621, 1958.

6. Bellet S, Muller OF, DeLeon AC, et al:The use of an external pacemaker in the treatment of cardiac arrest and slow heart rates. Arch Intern Med 105:361, 1960.

7. Furman S, Robinson G: Use of an intracardiac pacemaker in the correction of total heart block. Surg Forum 9:245, 1958.

8. Zoll PM, Zoll RH, Falk RH, et al: External noninvasive temporary cardiac pacing: clinical trials. Circulation 71:937, 1985.

9. Zipes DP, Duffin EG: Cardiac pacemakers. In Braunwald E (ed): Heart Disease: A Textbook of Cardiovascular Medicine. Philadelphia, W.B. Saunders Co, 1984, p 746.

10. Roberts JR, Greenberg MI: Emergency transthoracic pacemaker. Ann Emerg Med 10:600, 1981.

11. Brown CG, Gurley HT, Hutchins BM, et al: Injuries associated with percutaneous placement of transthoracic pacemakers. Ann Emerg Med 14:223, 1985.

12. Austin JL, Preis LK, Crampton RS, et al: Analysis of pacemaker malfunction and complications of temporary pacing in the coronary care unit. Am J Cardiol 49:301, 1982.

13. Sitzmann JV, Townsend TR, Siler MC, et al: Septic and technical complications of central venous catheterization. Ann Surg 202:766, 1985.

14. Sidd JJ, Stellar LI, Gryska PF, et al: Thrombus formation on a transvenous pacemaker electrode. N Engl J Med 280:887, 1969.

15. Robboy SJ, Harthorne JW, Leinbach RC, et al: Autopsy findings with permanent pervenous pacemakers. Circulation 26:205, 1969.

16. Mitrovic V, Thormann J, Schlepper M, et al: Thrombotic complications with pacemakers. Int J Cardiol 2:363, 1983.

17. Sethi GK, Bhayana JN, Scott SM: Innominate venous thrombosis: a rare complication of transvenous pacemaker electrodes. Am Heart J 87:770, 1974.

18. Griepp RB, Daily PO, Shumway NE: Subclavian-axillary vein thrombosis following implantation of a pacemaker catheter in the internal jugular vein. J Thorac Cardiovasc Surg 60:889, 1970.

19. Swinton NW, Edgett JW, Hall RJ: Primary subclavian-axillary vein thrombosis. Circulation 38:737, 1968.

20. Williams DR, Demos NJ: Thrombosis of superior vena cava caused by pacemaker wire and managed with streptokinase. Thorac Cardiovasc Surg 68:134, 1974.

21. Matthews DM, Forfar JC: Superior vena caval stenosis: a complication of transvenous endocardial pacing. Thorax 34:412, 1979.

22. Kaulbach MG, Krukonis EE: Pacemaker electrode-induced thrombosis in the superior vena cava with pulmonary embolism. Am J Cardiol 26:205, 1970.

23. Floyd WL, Mahaley MS: Cerebral dural venous sinus thrombosis following cardiac pacemaker implantation. Arch Intern Med 124:368, 1969.

24. Bernard R, Stahl W: Subclavian vein catheterizations: a prospective

study I: noninfectious complications, II: infectious complications. Ann Surg 173:184, 1971.

25. Fritz T, Richeson JF, Fitzpatrick P, et al: Venous obstruction: a potential complication of transvenous pacemaker electrodes. Chest 83:534, 1983.
26. Prozan GB, Shipley RE, Madding GF, et al: Pulmonary thromboembolism in the presence of an endocardial pacing catheter. J Am Med Assoc 206:1564, 1968.
27. Horowitz LN: Safety of electrophysiologic studies. Circulation 73(II):II28, 1986.
28. Marsac J, Frija G, Bismuth V: Chylothorax et pathologie lymphatique de la pleure. Rev Fr Mal Respir 10:227, 1982.
29. Polla B: Contralateral chylothorax: one more complication of subclavian venous puncture. Chest 87:271, 1985.
30. Rosenfeld LE: Osteomyelitis of the first rib presenting as a cold abscess nine months after subclavian venous catheterization. PACE 8:897, 1985.
31. Donovan KD, Lee KY: Indications for and complications of temporary transvenous cardiac pacing. Anaesth Inten Care 13:63, 1985.
32. Krueger SK, Rakes S, Wilkerson J, et al: Temporary pacemaking by general internists. Arch Intern Med 143:1531, 1983.
33. Hynes JK, Holmes DR, Harrison CE: Five-year experience with temporary pacemaker therapy in the coronary care unit. Mayo Clin Proc 58:122, 1983.
34. Harris JP, Nanda NC, Moxley R, et al: Myocardial perforation due to temporary transvenous pacing catheters in pediatric patients. Cathet Cardiovasc Diagn 10:329, 1984.
35. Iliceto S, Antonelli G, Sorino M, et al: Two-dimensional echocardiographic recognition of complications of cardiac invasive procedures. Am J Cardiol 53:846, 1984.
36. Gondi B, Nanda NC: Real-time, two-dimensional echocardiographic features of pacemaker perforation. Circulation 64:97, 1981.
37. Antonelli D, Grinberg C, Barzilay J: Retention of a semifloating electrode catheter. Int J Cardiol 9:105, 1985.
38. Josephson ME, Seides SF: Clinical cardiac electrophysiology: techniques and interpretations. Philadelphia, Lea and Febiger, 1979.
39. Ward RW, Waxman MB: Depression of distal AV conduction following ventricular pacing. PACE 4:84, 1981.
40. Mooss AN, Ross WB, Esterbrooks DJ, et al: Ventricular fibrillation complicating pacemaker insertion in acute myocardial infarction. Cathet Cardiovasc Diagn 8:253, 1982.
41. Vandepol CJ, Farshidi A, Speilman SR, et al: Incidence and clinical significance of induced ventricular tachycardia. Am J Cardiol 45:725, 1980.
42. Kudenchuk PJ, Kron J, Walance CG, et al: Reproducibility of arrhythmia induction with intracardiac electrophysiology testing: patients with clinical sustained ventricular tachyarrhythmias. J Am Coll Cardiol 7:819, 1986.
43. Cueni TA, White RA, Burkart F: Pacemaker-induced ventricular tachy-

cardia in patients with acute inferior myocardial infarction. Int J Cardiol 1:93, 1981.

44. Tommaso C, Belic N, Brandronbrener M: Asynchronous ventricular pacing: a rare cause of ventricular tachycardia. PACE 5:561, 1982.

45. Ridgeway NA, Alison HW, Isham CA: Ventricular tachycardia due to a transvenous catheter pacemaker. South Med J 78:219, 1985.

46. Peters RW, Scheinman MM, Morady F, et al: Long-term management of recurrent paroxysmal tachycardia by cardiac burst pacing. PACE 8:35, 1985.

47. Escher DW: The use of cardiac pacemakers. In Braunwald E (ed): Heart Disease: A Textbook of Cardiovascular Medicine. Philadelphia, WB Saunders Co., 1980, p 757.

48. Cohen SL: Temporary and permanent pacemakers. In Grossman W (ed): Cardiac Catheterization and Angiography. Philadelphia, Lea and Febiger, 1985, pp 517–535.

49. Scheinman MM, Morady F, Hess DS, et al: Catheter induced ablation of the atrioventricular junction to control refractory supraventricular arrhythmias. J Am Med Assoc 248:851, 1982.

50. DiMarco JP, Garan H, Ruskin JN: Complications in patients undergoing cardiac electrophysiologic procedures. Ann Intern Med 97:490, 1982.

51. Fisher JD, Brodman R, Kim SG, et al: Attempted nonsurgical electrical ablation of accessory pathways via the coronary sinus in the Wolff-Parkinson-White syndrome. J Am Coll Cardiol 4:685, 1984.

52. Scheinmann MM: Catheter ablation for patients with cardiac arryhthmias. PACE 9:551, 1986.

53. Lerman BB, Weiss JL, Buckley BH, et al: Myocardial injury and induction of arrhythmia by direct current shock delivered via endocardial catheters in dogs. Circulation 69:1006, 1984.

54. Hartzler GO, Giorgi LV, Diehl AM, et al: Right coronary spasm complicating electrode catheter ablation of a right lateral accessory pathway. J Am Coll Cardiol 6:250, 1985.

55. Kunze KP, Schluter M, Costard A, et al: Right atrial thrombus formation after transvenous catheter ablation of the atrioventricular node. J Am Coll Cardiol 6:1428, 1985.

56. Bharati S, Scheinmann MM, Morady F, et al: Sudden death after catheter-induced atrioventricular junctional ablation. Chest 88:883, 1985.

57. Bing OHL, McDowell JW, Hantman, et al: Pacemaker placement by electrocardiographic monitoring. N Engl J Med 287:247, 1971.

58. Ornato JP, Carveth WL, Windle RJ. Pacemaker insertion for prehospital bradysystolic cardiac arrest. Ann Emerg Med 13:101, 1984.

59. Tintinalli JE, White BC: Transthoracic pacing during CPR. Ann Emerg Med 10:113, 1981.

60. Falk RH, Zoll PM, Zoll RH: Safety and efficacy of noninvasive cardiac pacing. N Engl J Med 309:1166, 1983.

Chapter 6

Complications of Endomyocardial Biopsy

Jeffrey D. Hosenpud

Historical Perspectives

Biopsy of the human heart during life was an uncommon event and performed only during thoracotomy, until the early 1950s. Sutton and colleagues[1] first reported percutaneous needle biopsy of the left ventricle in 1956. Bercu et al.[2] further developed the technique and in 1964 reported results from animal and human myocardial biopsies. Their technique utilized a modified Menghini renal biopsy needle which was inserted percutaneously in the fifth intercostal space and directed toward the interventricular septum. Tissue adequate for histologic examination was obtained from all 10 patients. Two patients had presumed intrapericardial bleeding that was manifest by new pericardial friction rubs.

The earliest experience with the transvascular approach for cardiac biopsy was reported by Konno and Sakakibara in 1962.[3] The cardiac bioptome was a modified cardiac catheter containing a small jaw at the tip linked by a wire running through the catheter and connected to a moveable handle that opened and closed the jaws. Because of its simplicity and relative safety, catheter biopsy of the heart became the technique of choice. Subsequent to the initial report, a variety of minor modifications of the basic technique have been described.[4-9] Currently the most common technique used in the United States, developed at Stanford University and reported by Caves et al.,[5] employs a modification of the Konno bioptome (Fig. 1). The bioptome is inserted percutaneously into the right internal jugular vein, directed through the right atrium, across the tricuspid

From *Complications of Cardiac Catheterization and Angiography: Prevention and Management* edited by Jack Kron, M.D. and Mark J. Morton, M.D. © 1989, Futura Publishing Inc., Mount Kisco, NY.

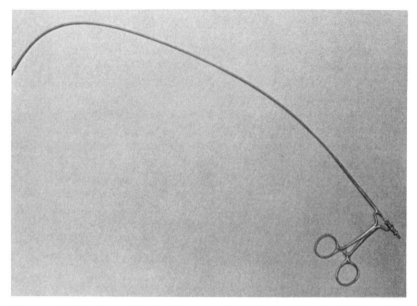

Figure 1. *The Caves-Schulz Bioptome developed at Stanford University.*

valve, and to the right ventricular septum near the apex. The King's bioptome is a smaller diameter, Teflon-coated modification of the Konno bioptome and is the most commonly used biopsy catheter in Europe. A final major modification of the cardiac biopsy technique is a long sheath that is placed in the specific chamber to be biopsied. This was originally described by Brooksby and colleagues,[10] and has had its major application in left ventricular biopsy and right ventricular biopsy from the femoral vein approach.[8,9]

Indications for the Procedure

Evaluation of Myocardial Disease

Endomyocardial biopsy has been performed in several groups of patients at the Oregon Health Sciences University. These have included patients with unexplained myocardial dysfunction, either those without valvular or coronary disease or those whose myocardial dysfunction is out of proportion to their underlying disease.

The majority of these patients will have nonspecific histologic findings on biopsy consistent with cardiomyopathy[11,12] or biopsies without diagnostic abnormalities. However, a variety of diseases can be diagnosed by endomyocardial biopsy—specifically, allergic, infectious, or idiopathic lymphocytic myocarditis,[13,14] granulomatous diseases of the heart, such as sarcoidosis or giant cell myocarditis,[15,16] amyloidosis, hemochromatosis, and some storage diseases[17-19] (Table 1).

Another group of patients who routinely undergo endomyocardial biopsy at the Oregon Health Sciences University are those with unexplained serious cardiac arrhythmias, whether or not myocardial dysfunction is present. Typically, these are young, otherwise healthy patients who present with ventricular tachycardia or high-degree atrioventricular block. Several recent reports, including one from this institution, demonstrate that myocardial abnormalities are common in this group of patients, even in the absence of overt cardiac dysfunction.[20-22] Figure 2 demonstrates histopathology consistent with giant cell myocarditis in a young patient who presented with ventricular tachycardia and normal ventricular function.

Table 1
Indications to Endomyocardial Biopsy

Dilated cardiomyopathy
  r / o myocarditis
Restrictive cardiomyopathy
  r / o amyloid
  r / o hemochromatosis
  r / o sarcoidosis
  Restriction vs. constriction
Endocardial fibrosis /
  fibroelastosis
Anthracycline cardiac
  toxicity
Cardiac allograft
  rejection
Unexplained ventricular arrhythmias or conduction disease

---

r / o = rule out.

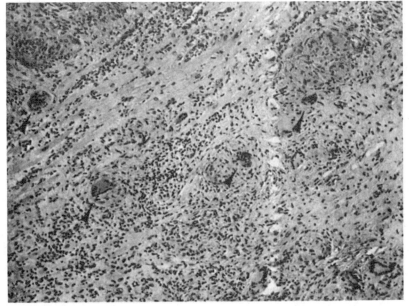

Figure 2. *Multiple giant cells with granuloma formation (arrow) are scattered throughout the myocardium (190X).*

Monitoring Cardiotoxic Drugs

The most active and widely used used antineoplastic agents are the anthracyclines (doxorubicin, daunorubicin). Myocardial toxicity is their primary side effect, limiting their usefulness and, not infrequently, effective antitumor therapy must be discontinued because of impaired systolic function and congestive heart failure. Toxicity appears to be enhanced by prior mediastinal irradiation, underlying cardiac disease, and increasing age. Bristow and colleagues have demonstrated that assessments of cardiac systolic function may underestimate the degree of anthracycline cardiac toxicity.[23] Serial endomyocardial biopsies studied by electron microscopy, which show the characteristic changes of intracellular vacuolization and myofibrillar loss, are more predictive of subsequent myocardial dysfunction than is current ejection fraction.[23]

Monitoring Cardiac Allograft Rejection

Survival following cardiac transplantation has steadily improved over the past decade. Although improved immunosuppressive agents have played a role in increased survival, another major factor has been surveillance endomyocardial biopsies for the diagnosis of rejection. Typically, endomyocardial biopsies are performed weekly for the first month following transplantation; their frequency is then reduced over subsequent months to a baseline frequency of three to four times a year. The diagnosis of rejection is based on lymphocyte infiltration and myocyte necrosis (Fig. 3), and is graded based on severity.

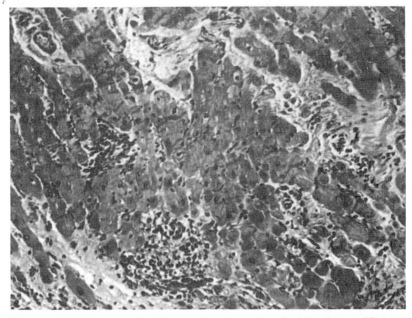

Figure 3. *Endomyocardial biopsy demonstrating lymphocytic infiltration and necrosis consistent with moderate acute rejection of a cardiac allograft (190X).*

Complications

Procedural Complications

Based on experiences from a single large center[24] and collated from several centers,[25] the overall incidence of complications associated with the endomyocardial biopsy procedure is between 1% and 2% (Table 2). As with most catheterization complications, the incidence declines with operator and institutional experience. At the Oregon Health Sciences University, the complication rate for the first 50 biopsies was 14% and for the subsequent 250 biopsies, 0.8%.

The most frequent problem with endomyocardial biopsy is not reflected in these statistics; it is the inability to gain access to the internal jugular vein. This can occur in as many as 10% of procedures. Reasons for failure to cannulate the internal jugular vein include: (1) the inability to find the appropriate landmarks in a given patient (large neck, obesity); (2) volume depletion with very

---

Table 2
Complications of Endomyocardial Biopsy

Cardiac perforation
  Tamponade
Arrhythmias
Conduction abnormalities
Air embolism
Pneumothorax
Vascular trauma
Nerve palsy
  recurrent laryngeal
  Horner's syndrome
Arterial complications
  with LV Biopsy
  vascular trauma
  emboli
Inadequate or inappropriate sampling, handling, or interpretation

low systemic venous pressure; (3) tamponade of the internal jugular vein caused by bleeding into the carotid sheath from unsuccessful cannulation of the jugular vein or inadvertent puncture of the carotid artery, or overzealous infiltration of a local anesthetic into the carotid sheath.

Cardiac perforation is the most serious complication associated with heart biopsy. Perforation occurs exclusively with right ventricular biopsy because the right ventricular free wall is so much thinner than the left ventricular wall. In patients with dilated cardiomyopathy, the right ventricular free wall may be thinned further. Perforation occurs because the biopsy forceps can cut transmural specimens from the free wall of the right ventricle. Accordingly, biopsy specimens must be taken from the interventricular septum. Improper placement of the bioptome is caused by technical considerations discussed below. The Caves-Schulz bioptome has a bend aligning the tip with the bioptome handle. The orientation of the bioptome tip is then directed by the position of the handle and, with the patient supine, should be directed completely posterior (towards the floor) to ensure that the tip is pointed at the interventricular septum. Both operator error and patient anatomy can result in misplacement of the bioptome tip and thus, the sampling site. The operator must be sure, before inserting the bioptome, that the bend and tip are in line with the bioptome handle. Because of the delicate shaft, this orientation can be disrupted by rough handling. The proper insertion technique is to cross the tricuspid valve with the bioptome directed anteriorly and to then rotate it posteriorly. For this reason, the bioptome tip can become caught in coarse trabeculations. When the handle is rotated posteriorly, the flexible shaft is twisted, leaving the bioptome tip in an anterior orientation. This is avoided by withdrawing the bioptome tip 1 to 2 cm away from the ventricular wall following the posterior rotation, to ensure that the tip is free. The bioptome is then again advanced with the jaws open, impinged on the endocardium, and the biopsy taken. In patients with severe right ventricular enlargement, rotation of the entire heart occurs in the chest, with a portion of the right ventricular free wall wrapping around posteriorly. Even though the bioptome tip is properly positioned in a posterior orientation, the biopsy can taken from the free wall.

In the Stanford series, ventricular perforation occurred in four patients for an overall incidence of 0.14%. Three of the four patients required needle or catheter evacuation of hemopericardium, the remaining patient required no intervention.[24] In the multicenter series, the incidence of perforation was 0.59% (14 of 2,337 patients) with thoracotomy, and pericardial drainage was required in 6 patients.[25]

A second group of complications includes the induction of arrhythmia and conduction abnormalities. Premature ventricular contractions are frequently produced when the tip of the bioptome is placed against the endocardium. Sustained ventricular tachycardia or fibrillation are unusual, but have been reported.[24] Supraventricular arrhythmias also occur, and at this institution transient and spontaneously resolving atrial fibrillation has been induced in two patients and junctional bradycardia in one. The overall incidence of dysrhythmias in a large survey was 0.81%.[25]

Conduction abnormalities, specifically right bundle branch block and occasionally left fascicular block, can occur with endomyocardial biopsy as with any other right heart catheterization procedure.[26] The right bundle branch block is usually transient and is presumed to be secondary to trauma to the right bundle due to its location in the subendocardial tissue (Fig. 4). As can be seen in Figure 4, permanent damage to the right bundle could potentially occur if a biopsy sample is taken high on the interventricular septum.

A variety of other complications related to the insertion site has been reported and covered in detail in Chapters 2 and 3. These complications include traumatic dysfunction and/or anesthesia of the vagus branch, which carries the recurrent laryngeal nerve, causing hoarseness and trauma to the sympathetic trunk and producing a Horner's syndrome. Pneumothorax is an infrequent complication of internal jugular venous cannulation, as is air embolism, bleeding or thrombosis of the vein, and the introduction of infection. Finally, an entire group of complications related to arterial catheterization have to be considered with the left ventricular biopsy procedure. These include systemic embolization, arterial trauma with either bleeding or thrombosis, arteriovenous fistula formation, and infection.

Complications Related to Tissue Handling and Interpretation

Complications related to the interpretation of the pathologic specimen can be divided into those related to adequacy of the sam-

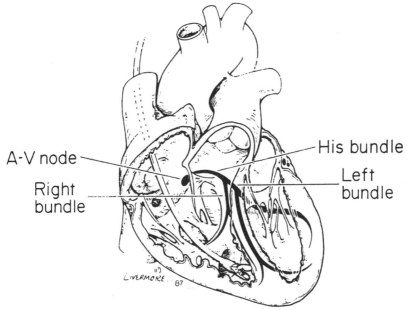

A-V node

Right
bundle

His bundle

Left
bundle

Figure 4. *The cardiac conduction system. Note damage to right bundle branch, which can occur if the biopsy is obtained high on the right side of the interventricular septum.*

ple, those related to handling and fixation, and those related to interpretation. These constitute, possibly, the most serious complications associated with endomyocardial biopsy because they threaten to render the entire procedure invalid.

The amount of total tissue available is of critical importance if several studies requiring different fixation techniques are used. For instance, tissue for standard light microscopy is usually fixed in 10% formalin, tissue for electron microscopy in glutaraldehyde, and tissue for immunofluorescence is rapidly frozen in liquid nitrogen. Assuming each of these studies are required, a minimum of five to six biopsy specimens should be obtained to allow for adequate analysis by each technique and to minimize sampling error. Sampling error can be an important factor in the diagnosis of certain disease states such as inflammatory myocarditis, granulomatous disease of the heart, anthracycline cardiac toxicity, and cardiac allograft rejection. Finally, it should be noted that the flexible biopsy forceps available for use with a long sheath (Cordis Co.)

have much smaller sampling jaws, and the biopsies obtained are approximately one-fourth to one-third the size of tissue samples obtained by the Caves-Schulz bioptome. If the smaller jaws are used, two to three times the number of samples otherwise indicated should be obtained.

As with any tissue, traumatic handling of myocardium can produce artifacts that may prevent the correct diagnosis from being made. If the bioptome is not sharp, the tissue can be torn, causing separation of the myofibers and distortion at the borders of the sample. Some authors recommend leaving the biopsy specimens out of fixative for 1 to 2 minutes to reduce contraction band artifacts. The experience at this institution has shown that fixation at room temperature rather than in cold solutions minimizes contraction artifacts. Furthermore, leaving the tissue exposed produces some loss of cellular integrity manifested by blurring of the intracellular structures and loss of the sarcolemma. We therefore feel that the tissue should be placed in the appropriate fixative at room temperature as soon as it is retrieved. It is beyond the scope of this discussion to review the variety of specific fixation techniques. Most diagnostic questions can be addressed, however, if adequate amounts of tissue are preserved in formalin and glutaraldehyde, and one to two specimens are fresh-frozen for immunologic studies. The recommended sample collections for specific diseases are elaborated at the end of this chapter. Finally, it goes without saying that the technique is only as good as the pathologist interpreting the specimen. For many pathologists, the evaluation of cardiac biopsy material rather than autopsy material will be a new experience. Most will require several cases before feeling comfortable with their interpretations.

Optimal Technique Performance

Right Ventricular Biopsy: Internal Jugular Vein Approach

The usual approach for right ventricular biopsy is thru the right internal jugular vein, although the femoral vein has also been used.[3,4,9] The procedure is performed using fluoroscopy. The patient is instructed to take only liquids by mouth for the previous 6 hours. Usually no presedation is required, however small amounts of a short-acting benzodiazapine can be used. For the right internal jugular approach, the patient is positioned on the fluoroscopy table in the supine position and the patient's head is turned completely to the left, bringing both the lateral and medial bellies of the sternocleidomastoid muscle anterior (Fig. 5). We raise the legs approximately 40 cm with soft cushions. The neck is then prepared from the chin to approximately 3 cm below the clavicle and draped using sterile technique, exposing the entire triangle bordered by the two bellies of the sternocleidomastoid and the clavicle. Local anesthesia is accomplished with 1% lidocaine without epinephrine with both superficial and deep soft tissue anesthetized down to but not en-

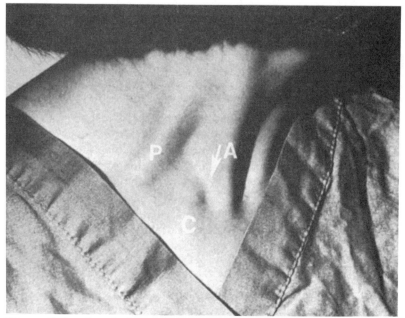

Figure 5. *Landmarks for needle entry into the right internal jugular vein are demonstrated. Note the triangle created by the anterior (A) and posterior (P) heads of the sternocleidomastoid muscle and the clavicle (C). The needle entry point (small arrow) is just lateral to the anterior head, approximately 3 cm above the clavicle.*

tering the carotid sheath. Injection of lidocaine into the carotid sheath may tamponade the internal jugular vein, making it difficult to cannulate. The entry site is along the lateral border of the medial belly of the sternocleidomastoid, approximately 2 cm above the clavicle. The skin is incised approximately 3 mm along the skin lines with a No.11 scalpel blade, and the subcutaneous tissue is spread with a mosquito clamp. The needle is directed toward the right nipple at an angle of approximately 30° off the skin. A 20- or 21-gauge, 1.5-inch needle may be used to locate the internal jugular vein, which is then punctured by an 18-gauge, thin-walled needle through which a 0.035-inch guidewire is passed. The guidewire is advanced into the internal jugular vein to the high right atrium, and its position confirmed by fluoroscopy. A 9 French sheath with sidearm, hemostasis valve, and dilator are advanced over the guidewire, and the guidewire and dilator are removed. The sheath must have a valve at its proximal portion to prevent both bleeding through the sheath and embolization of air. The bioptome utilized at this institution is the Caves-Schulz 9F instrument. Prior to insertion, the bioptome is carefully examined to ensure that its jaws approximate tightly and the 90° bend on the shaft is lined up with the bioptome handle. This enables the operator to know precisely where the bioptome tip is in the vertical (anteroposterior) plane during fluoroscopy.

The side portion of the catheter sheath is flushed with heparinized saline prior to and between every bioptome insertion. The patient is asked to suspend respiration, and the bioptome is inserted (Fig. 6). The tip is then directed laterally along the superior vena cava and right atrium. One-half to two-thirds of the length down the right atrial chamber, the bioptome tip is rotated anteriorly across the tricuspid valve and then medially into the right ventricle. As the bioptome is advanced into the right ventricle, the tip is gradually rotated posteriorly so that when the tip approaches the right ventricular apex, it is fully posterior. The tip of the bioptome is then gently abutted against the endocardium (Fig. 7), which is appreciated both fluoroscopically and by feeling the cardiac impulse. The tip is then retracted 1 cm, the jaws are opened (Fig. 8), the bioptome advanced again to the endocardial surface, and the jaws closed. A brisk but gentle tug removes the endocardial sample. The bioptome is removed during apnea and the endomyocardial sample is teased gently from the open jaws (Fig. 9).

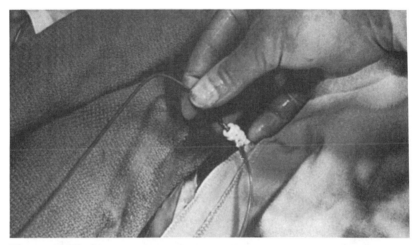

Figure 6. *The bioptome is inserted into the sheath as the patient suspends respiration.*

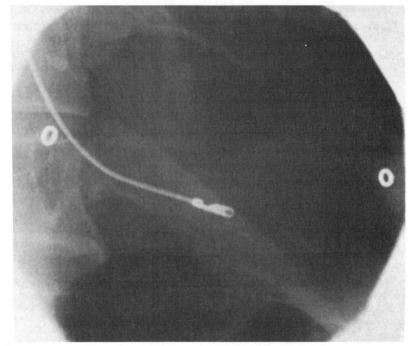

Figure 7. *The bioptome, with jaws closed, is seen under the fluoroscope.*

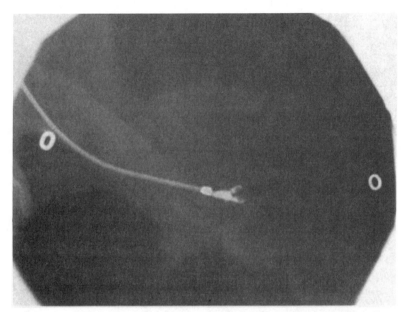

Figure 8. *The jaws of the bioptome are open in preparation for sampling.*

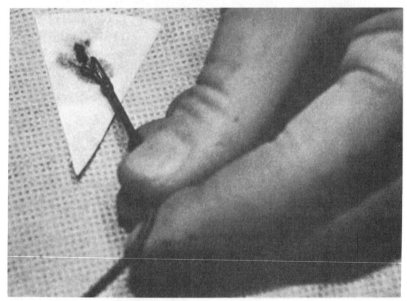

Figure 9. *An endomyocardial sample is gently teased from the open jaws of the bioptome onto a small piece of filter paper.*

Right Ventricular Biopsy: Femoral Vein Approach

Although described initially by Konno and colleagues[3] and later by Richardson,[4] the femoral vein approach to endomyocardial biopsy is less widely used than venous access from the upper extremities or jugular approaches. More recently, Anderson and Marshall presented a technique for right heart biopsy from the femoral vein, using a shaped long sheath catheter system.[9] They reported using the technique in 35 patients with only one minor complication. The technique used in this institution is a modification of the long sheath method. The right groin is prepared and draped, using sterile technique. Local anesthesia is accomplished with 1% lidocaine. The entry site for the femoral vein is below the inguinal ligament, just medial to the femoral artery. The skin is opened approximately 3 mm with a No. 11 scalpel blade, and the subcutaneous tissue spread with a blunt clamp. The femoral vein is entered using a thin-wall, 18-gauge needle through which a 0.035-inch, 125-cm long Teflon-coated guidewire is inserted and advanced, guided by fluoroscopy, into the right atrium.

The bioptome used for this technique is the Cordis 7 French left ventricular biopsy forceps (Cordis Corp., Miami, FL). It is modified by putting a 30° bend 2 cm from the tip. The sheath used is a 7 French Mullins sheath (USCI Division, C.R. Bard Inc., Billerica, MA), which is also modified by removing a portion of the end of the sheath to convert the 180° curve to 90°. Figure 10 demonstrates the modified bioptome and sheath system. A 7 French Lehman catheter is inserted into the sheath and the sheath and catheter inserted over the guidewire and advanced into the right atrium. The catheter is manipulated across the tricuspid valve and into the right ventricle, with the tip of the sheath at the tricuspid valve annulus. The Lehman catheter is removed and the sheath flushed carefully. The bioptome is then inserted through the sheath. As the sheath is not across the tricuspid valve, the bioptome is carefully manipulated into the right ventricle by rotating the sheath anteriorly to permit the bioptome to pass across the tricuspid valve. Once the bioptome is advanced near the right ventricular apex, the sheath is rotated clockwise, directing the tip posteriorly to ensure that the bioptome is directed toward the interventricular septum. The advantage of not having the sheath positioned more distally is that the bioptome itself can be manipulated to slightly different positions so that biopsies can be obtained from multiple sites.

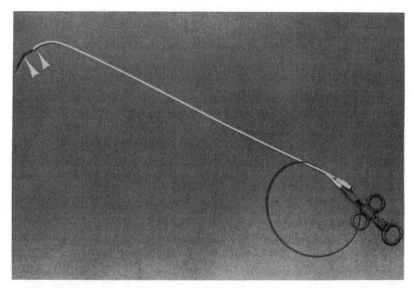

Figure 10. *The bioptome and sheath system used for right ventricular endomyocardial biopsy from the femoral vein. Note the shortened sheath and the bend in the bioptome approximately 2 cm from the tip for anteroposterior positioning (arrows).*

We have used this technique successfully on 32 patients with one instance of cardiac perforation on the second patient. The disadvantages of this technique are (1) it is more time consuming and (2) biopsies obtained using this bioptome are substantially smaller (1 mm) and therefore require more samples. For these reasons, we use this approach only if the internal jugular vein is not usable.

Left Ventricular Biopsy

Biopsy of the left ventricle has several theoretical advantages over right ventricular biopsy. First, the majority of myocardial diseases appear to affect the left ventricle functionally to a greater extent than the right, biopsy of the most severely affected chamber makes intuitive sense. In fact, certain disease states such as hypertrophic cardiomyopathy and endomyocardial fibroelastosis may show pathologic abnormalities only in the left ventricle.[27,28] Second, because of the more uniform thickness of the left ventricle, cardiac perforation should be less common. The disadvantages include the necessity for intra-arterial access with its potential complications as well as the concern of systemic arterial embolization.

In fact the need for left ventricular biopsy in our institution has been quite limited. Congenital myopathic disease that appears to primarily affect the left heart, the documentation of left ventricular endomyocardial fibroelastosis, and left ventricular masses have been the primary indications.

The technique is quite similar to routine arterial catheterization. The right or left femoral artery is cannulated with a 18-gauge Seldinger needle and a 0.035-inch 125-cm Teflon-coated guidewire is inserted and directed to the diaphragm under fluoroscopy. After the arteriotomy is dilated, a 7 French pigtail and sheath combination (Cordis Co., Miami, FL) is inserted over the guidewire and advanced to the abdominal aorta. The wire is removed and the patient anticoagulated with intravenous heparin (10 units/lb body weight) and the catheter is flushed. The catheter-sheath is then advanced across the aortic valve and into the left ventricle. The pigtail catheter is removed, leaving the sheath in the body of the left ventricle. A Cordis 104-cm, 7 French biopsy forceps is then advanced through the sheath into the left ventricle for sampling. The sheath is flushed carefully after each pass of the biopsy forceps to prevent thrombus formation.

Recommended Sample Collection for Specific Diseases

A. *Recent-onset dilated cardiomyopathy, rule out myocarditis:* Four to five specimens in 10% formalin for light microscopy (H&E, Masson's trichrome) should be obtained, due to the focal nature of the inflammation; one specimen fresh frozen for immunofluorescence; one specimen in glutaraldehyde to hold for potential electron microscopy may be useful in differentiating cell types (i.e., lymphocytes from endothelial cells).

B. *Restrictive/hypertrophic cardiomyopathy, rule out infiltrative disease:* Three to four specimens in 10% formalin for light microscopy (H&E, Masson's trichrome). In addition to standard stains, iron, PAS, and congo red (or equivalent) stains should be requested; one specimen in glutaraldehyde for electron microscopy is frequently helpful for confirming amyloid.

C. *Rule out anthracycline (daunorubicin, doxorubicin) toxicity:* One specimen in 10% formalin (H&E, Masson's trichrome); four to five specimens in glutaraldehyde for electron microscopy as severity of cardiac involvement is an electron microscopic diagnosis.

D. *Rule out cardiac allograft rejection:* Three specimens in 10% formalin for light microscopy (H&E, Masson's trichrome). As these patients require multiple biopsies, there is a problem obtaining specimens free of prior biopsy sites. Three adequate specimens are a compromise between the need to eliminate sampling error and the need to preserve right ventricular endocardium.

Conclusions

Endomyocardial biopsy has become a useful clinical tool in the evaluation and diagnosis of myocardial disease, chemotherapy toxicity, and the diagnosis of cardiac allograft rejection. Overall, it is a procedure with a low incidence of complications in experienced hands. A major potential complication is inadequate sampling, handling, and the interpretation of specimens.

References

1. Sutton DC, Sutton GC, Kent G: Needle biopsy of the human ventricular myocardium. Bull Northwest Univ Med Sch 30:213, 1956.
2. Bercu B, Heinz J, Choudhry AS, et al: Myocardial biopsy: a new technique utilizing the ventricular septum. Am J Cardiol 14:675, 1964.
3. Sakakibara S, Konno S: Endomyocardial biopsy. Jpn Heart J 3: 537, 1962.
4. Richardson PJ: King's endomyocardial bioptome. Lancet 1:660, 1974.
5. Caves PK, Schulz WP, Dong E Jr, et al: New instrument for transvenous cardiac biopsy. Am J Cardiol 33:264, 1974.
6. Ali N: Transvenous endomyocardial biopsy using the gastrointestinal biopsy (Olympus GFB) catheter. Am Heart J 87:297, 1974.
7. Lurie PR, Fujita M, Neustein HB: Transvascular endomyocardial bi-

opsy in infants and small children: description of a new tech-nique. Am J Cardiol 42:453, 1978.

8. Mason JW: Techniques for right and left ventricular endomyocardial biopsy. Am J Cardiol 41:887, 1978.

9. Anderson JL, Marshall HW: The femoral venous approach to endo-myocardial biopsy: comparison with internal jugular and transarterial approaches. Am J Cardiol 53:833, 1984.

10. Brooksby IAB, Swanton RH, Jenkins BS, et al: Long-sheath technique for introduction of catheter tip manometer or endomyocardial bioptome into left or right heart. Br Heart J 36:908, 1974.

11. Edwards WD: Endomyocardial biopsy and cardiomyopathy. Cardiovasc Rev Rep 4:820, 1983.

12. Nippoldt TB, Edwards WD, Holmes DR, et al: Right ventricular en-domyocardial biopsy. Clinicopathologic correlates in 100 consecutive patients. Mayo Clin Proc 57:407, 1982.

13. Mason JW, Billingham ME, Ricci DR: Treatment of acute inflammatory myocarditis assisted by endomyocardial biopsy. Am J Cardiol 45:1037, 1980.

14. Edwards WD, Holmes DR, Reeder GS: Diagnosis of active lymphocytic myocarditis by endomyocardial biopsy. Quantitative criteria for light microscopy. Mayo Clin Proc 57:419, 1982.

15. Lorell B, Aldrman EL, Mason JW: Cardiac sarcoidosis. Diagnosis with endomyocardial biopsy and treatment with corticosteroids. Am J Cardiol 42:143, 1978.

16. McFalls EO, Hosenpud JD, McAnulty JH, et al: Granulomatous myo-carditis. Diagnosis by endomyocardial biopsy and response to cortico-steroids in two patients. Chest 89:509, 1986.

17. Schroeder JS, Billingham ME, Rider AK: Cardiac amyloidosis. Diag-nosis by transvenous endomyocardial biopsy. Am J Med 59:269, 1975.

18. Short EM, Winkle RA, Billingham ME: Myocardial involvement in idiopathic hemochromatosis. Morphologic and clinical improvement fol-lowing venesection. Am J Med 70:1275, 1981.

19. Edwards WD, Hurdey HP, Partin JR: Cardiac involvement by Gauch-er's disease documented by right ventricular endomyocardial biopsy. Am J Cardiol 52:654, 1983.

20. Sugrue DD, Holmes DR Jr, Gersh BJ, et al: Cardiac histologic findings in patients with life-threatening ventricular arrythmias of unknown origin. J Am Coll Cardiol 4:952, 1984.

21. Strain JE, Grose RM, Factor SM, et al: Results of endomyocardial biopsy in patients with spontaneous ventricular tachycardia but without ap-parent structural heart disease. Circulation 68:1171, 1983.

22. Hosenpud JD, McAnulty JH, Niles NR: Unexpected myocardial disease in patients with life threatening arrhythmias. Br Heart J 56:51, 1986.

23. McKillop JH, Bristow MR, Goris ML, et al: Sensitivity and specificity of radionuclide ejection fractions in doxorubicin cardiotoxicity. Am Heart J 106:1048, 1983.

24. Fowles RE, Mason JW: Endomyocardial biopsy. Ann Intern Med 97:885, 1982.

25. Richardson PJ: Endomyocardial biopsy technique. In HD Bolte (ed):

Myocardial Biopsy, Diagnostic Significance. New York, Springer Verlag, 1982, p 3.
26. Castellanos A, Ramirez AV, Mayorga-Cortes A, et al: Left fascicular blocks during right heart catheterization using the Swan-Ganz catheter. Circulation 64:1271, 1981.
27. Neustein HB, Lurie PR, Fujita M: Endocardial fibroelastosis found on transvascular endomyocardial biopsy in children. Arch Pathol Lab Med 103:214, 1979.
28. Olsen EGJ: Myocardial biopsies. In J Hamer (ed): Recent Advances in Cardiology. Edinburgh, Churchill Livingstone, 1977, p349.

Chapter 7

Complications of Diagnostic Cardiac Catheterization in Infants and Children

Michael J. Silka

Introduction

"No patient should be denied the opportunity for precise diagnosis and possible cure or improvement because he is 'too small' or because functional severity of his lesion appears so great that death might occur during or after catheterization. For such a patient the greatest hazard lies in continuing failure to make an exact diagnosis upon which effective treatment may be based."[1]

The ability to precisely define anatomy and physiology or provide physiologic palliation or correction remains the goal of cardiac catheterization in the patient with congenital heart disease. Major improvements in invasive technology along with the development of noninvasive diagnostic techniques have evolved since the comments of Doctor Sones three decades ago. However, in spite of these new techniques and technologies, patient complications and problems related to cardiac catheterization persist. This chapter addresses the process of cardiac catheterization in the infant or child with heart disease, and discusses recognized or potential complications of each aspect. Specifically emphasized are the identification of patients at increased risk for complications and physiologic considerations that render the newborn infant particularly vulnerable.

From *Complications of Cardiac Catheterization and Angiography: Prevention and Management* edited by Jack Kron, M.D. and Mark J. Morton, M.D. © 1989, Futura Publishing Inc., Mount Kisco, NY.

Analysis of Catheterization-Related Complications

An understanding of the risks of cardiac catheterization in the young patient is necessary for the physician to determine when catheterization is warranted, and for the parents to give informed consent. Quantitation of the risk associated with the procedure is difficult, however, as many variables affect risk. Factors such as the severity of the congenital heart defect, physician experience, catheterization technique, and surgical options at a given institution profoundly influence the outcome in a given patient. Accordingly, the results of studies of catheterization complications vary (Table 1).

The high level of catheterization-related mortality in the newborn will vary according to the manner in which mortality is defined. If death within 24 hours hours of the study, from any cause, is the standard utilized, mortality rates of 6% to 14% are recognized. However, if only deaths within the catheterization laboratory are counted, the risk would appear to be less than 1% in recent studies. Similar difficulties apply in the analysis of other complications associated with cardiac catheterization, particularly in critically ill patients. It is difficult to list a complication that has not previously been reported during cardiac catheterization. A perspective must be maintained when evaluating the major and minor complications of catheterization and to determine whether their occurrence is due to the hemodynamic-angiographic study or represents an anticipated incident in the course of a critically ill patient. The major and frequent minor complications will be addressed as they could be expected to occur during the course of cardiac catheterization. Complications associated with interventional procedures will be discussed in the following chapter.

Precatheterization Assessment of the Potential for Complications

The Committee on Cardiac Catheterization and Angiocardiography of the American Heart Association reported in 1953 that catheterization was used "to complete the identification of specific congenital or acquired lesions, to establish their functional significance, to trace their physiologic course, and finally to evaluate the

Table 1
American Heart Association–Cooperative Study (1968)[2]

Age Group	Cardiac Catheterization No.	Death Within 24 Hours of Study* No. Percent		Death Due to Study No. Percent	
0–30 days	325	20	6.2	17	5.2
31–60 days	155	9	5.8	7	4.5
2–12 months	681	8	1.2	4	1.1
1–14 years	2,889	3	0.1	3	0.1

University of California–San Francisco (1974)[3]

Age Group					
0–30 days	218	33	14.7	2	0.9
31–60 days	26	0	0	0	
2–12 months	195	1	0.5	0	
1–14 years	683	1	0.2	1	0.2

Hospital for Sick Children–Toronto (1978)[1]

Age Group					
0–30 days	1470	98	6.6	NA	
31–90 days	1073	9	0.8	NA	
3–12 months	1869	6	0.3	NA	
1–15 years	7843	4	0.05	NA	

New England Regional Infant Cardiac Program (1985)[4]

Age Group					
0–30 days	155	10	6.4	1	0.6
31–60 days	52	1	1.8	0	–
2–12 months	105	1	0.95	0	–

* Death within 24 hours of study from all causes has been included with specific age groups.

results of surgical procedures."[5] These general indications would appear to continue to be applicable today, although much of the anatomic or functional data may be obtained with noninvasive methods. The decision to perform cardiac catheterization in any specific patient must be based on a consideration of the potential benefit versus risk of the procedure. The risks associated with catheterization are increased in recognized specific subsets of patients. More serious, however, is the failure to establish the correct or complete diagnosis, which may result in major surgical morbidity or mortality or failure to perform a necessary procedure.

Precatheterization Identification of the High Risk Infant and Child

The increased risk of complications associated with cardiac catheterization in the newborn infant is definite[1-4] and should be clearly communicated to parents when obtaining consent for cardiac catheterization. In 1974, Stanger and co-workers defined the following risk stratification for the neonate undergoing catheterization, based on assessment of the potential for deterioration during the procedure.[3]

1. *Low risk:* nondistressed nonacidotic neonate with (a) PaO_2 > 25 mmHg and (b) controlled congestive heart failure,
2. *Medium risk:* (a) Hypoxemic neonate with PaO_2 < 25 mmHg and (2) neonates with severe congestive heart failure, poorly controlled with digitalis and diuretics.
3. *High risk:* (a) ventilatory assistance, (b) profound hypoxemia with acidosis, and (c) poor perfusion resulting in shock or severe acidosis (pH < 7.1).

These criteria continue to be applicable to the precatheterization assessment of the newborn with congenital heart disease. Three additional factors deserve comment in the assessment of risk of catheterization in the neonate:

1. The impact of echocardiographic and Doppler techniques has perhaps been greatest in the newborn with congenital heart disease.[6-8] Accurate identification of anatomy and physiology

may be clearly established in the critically ill neonate utilizing these methods (e.g., critical aortic stenosis), allowing determination of the requirements for medical or surgical therapy. However, certain aspects of noninvasive diagnosis continue to require definition by catheterization before major decisions are made concerning therapy.[9,10]

2. The successful development of E-type prostaglandins (PGE) for use in the infant with critical congenital heart disease has been proven to improve oxygenation or cardiac output in ductus arteriosus-dependent lesions.[11]

The correction of profound hypoxemia or acidosis should be a priority prior to cardiac catheterization. However, the use of prostaglandin E_1 is itself associated with specific side effects,[12] specifically respiratory depression, which may be difficult to detect during cardiac catheterization. Although dramatic clinical improvement may occur with prostaglandin administration, cardiac catheterization should still be considered a high-risk procedure in these patients owing to the nature of the congenital defect and the potential for complications secondary to PGE_1.

3. With improved pre- and neonatal care, an increasing number of premature infants with congenital heart disease are being recognized. Limited experience regarding catheterization in these patients would suggest that their delicate physiology and anatomy would place them at high risk for deterioration during catheterization and that this procedure should be considered of significant risk.

Beyond the neonatal period, the anticipated risk of diagnostic cardiac catheterization declines significantly in the patient with congenital heart disease. Certain groups of patients continue to manifest an increased complication rate during catheterization, particularly after angiography, and they must be recognized prior to study.

The hazards of cardiac catheterization in children with pulmonary vascular obstructive disease are well established.[13,14] Statistically, this may represent the "highest" risk patient during catheterization. Similar caution is warranted in the patient with severe aortic stenosis. Accordingly, aortic valve surgery has increasingly been recommended on the basis of combined noninvasive studies without antecedent cardiac catheterization.[15,16] Increased risks of catheterization are present in patients with severe pulmonary oligemia: hypercyanotic spells, bradycardia, and death have been reported following study.[17,18] Lastly, patients with polyvalvar stenosis or coronary artery anomalies also present an increased risk of major complication during catheterization.[19]

Irrespective of the specific anatomic defect, left ventricular dysfunction (ejection fraction < 30%) and severe functional limitation (functional Class IV) are associated with a tenfold increased mortality rate during catheterization in adults.[20] Comparable data for children have not been established, but likely represent an equal risk. Lastly, patients with severe noncardiac disease, such as renal or pulmonary insufficiency, appear to have an increased incidence of major catheterization- related complications.

Contraindications to cardiac catheterization in children must be considered relative, rather than absolute. Previously, myocarditis and Ebstein's anomaly were considered unwarranted indications for cardiac catheterization. With the ability to diagnose and treat active inflammation based on endomyocardial biopsy in the patient with myocarditis[21] and the recognition of multiple accessory atrioventricular connections in the patient with Ebstein's anomaly,[22] catheterization has become invaluable in these patients. The indications for catheterization in the patient with active infective endocarditis remain controversial and require individualized consideration. The patient with known allergic reaction to contrast will be discussed in Chapter 9.

Precatheterization Considerations

The correction of treatable metabolic abnormalities prior to catheterization should be a priority. The value of treatment of severe ventricular dysfunction with inotropic agents, normalization of acid-base balance and electrolytes, and correction of anemia in the critically ill patient, cannot be underestimated. Once again, it must be emphasized that the severity of the patient's illness is the best correlate of the occurrence of a major complication during catheterization. Prior to catheterization, the objectives of the study should be clearly established. Physiologic measurements, in general, precede angiography in most cases; however, the most important question should be addressed first, such as the definition of pulmonary artery anatomy in the patient with pulmonary atresia. Systemic heparinization, if used, should be planned at the onset of left heart catheterization (50–100 IU/kg) so that this procedure is not overlooked. Also, in the patient with anticipated severe aortic or mitral stenosis the ability to perform transseptal catheterization should be available, if retrograde study is not feasible. Catheterization in the patient with congenital heart disease should be preceded by echocardiographic definition of as much of the anatomy and physiology as possible. However, data during catheterization should be interpreted objectively as the catheter course may be unexpected, perhaps entering a persistent left superior vena cava or anomalous pulmonary vein. Failure to do so may result in an error in diagnosis or a major complication during catheter manipulation.

The procedure of catheterization should be explained to the older child prior to sedation. Specifically, the transient sensory effects following angiography should be discussed. Mild sedation is advisable for all children over 1 month of age undergoing catheterization owing to the fear and discomfort associated with the procedure. Although a number of precatheterization sedation protocols have been established, I have found chloral hydrate, 50–75 mg/kg orally 30 minutes before catheterization, to be effective and associated with no significant complications. Sedation, as other aspects of catheterization, should be modified according to patient physiology. Morphine sulfate may be preferable in the patient with severe volume-overload congestive heart failure, whereas ketamine may be best for the patient with shunt-dependent pulmonary blood flow.

Potential Complications Inherent in Cardiac Catheterization

Patient monitoring and the maintenance of physiologic homeostasis during cardiac catheterization assume priority upon patient transfer to the laboratory. Heart rate and rhythm monitoring should be established prior to transfer and displayed continuously. Patient temperature should be determined and monitored by rectal probe and thermistor in the patient under 1 year of age. It is recommended that cardiac catheterization be terminated if the patient's temperature approaches 40°C or that a hypothermic patient be rewarmed before proceeding further with the catheterization.[23] These considerations are of paramount importance in the newborn in whom catheterization should be performed in a neutral thermal environment (31°–34°C). Undiagnosed hypothermia in the newborn may manifest as apnea, bradycardia, hypoglycemia, or acidosis. Assessment of the adequacy of ventilation, either spontaneous or mechanical, should be assessed clinically with subsequent determination of arterial blood gases once vascular access is established. Blood pressure should be monitored continuously from an arterial catheter, if possible, or at least every 30 minutes by sphygmomanometry.

Catheter Insertion

In general, catheterization is performed from the femoral vessels in children, except for the umbilical approach in the newborn and the upper extremity approaches in electrophysiologic studies and endomyocardial biopsy. Following sterile preparation, the area is infiltrated with 0.5% to 1% lidocaine. Although local anesthesia is required, excess infiltration may result in direct toxicity, manifest as seizures,[24] or circulating therapeutic levels of this antiarrhythmic drug during electrophysiologic study.[25] The total dose of lidocaine should not exceed 2.5 mg/kg. Serum levels of lidocaine should be determined if unexplained seizures occur during study or if the patient's electrophysiologic profile changes following administration of the drug. Serum levels of lidocaine peak 1 hour after dermal injection. The potential for either impaired atrioventricular conduction or increased ventricular response to atrial flutter or fibrillation following lidocaine must also be considered.[26,27]

Vasovagal reactions, although uncommon in infants, may occur in older children and may be catastrophic. Most commonly, they are elicited by pain in the tense, anxious patient and are manifest as bradycardia, hypotension, and nausea. The proposed mechanism involves sudden peripheral vasodilation of arterioles and venules unaccompanied by an increase in cardiac output.[28] If recognized early, the response to atropine (0.015 mg/kg) along with volume administration is prompt. Persistent hypotension, and bradycardia, however, may result in clinical deterioration in the patient with right to left shunt or severe valvar stenosis.

Local Vascular Complications

Catheterization of the arterial and venous systems may produce a variety of local complications, with a reported incidence between 3% to 40% in children.[29,30] The highest rates occur in infants weighing less than 10 kg.[31] As the etiologies, significance, and treatments of arterial and venous complications differ, they will be discussed separately. Surgical treatment of vascular injuries will be discussed in Chapter 11.

Venous catheterization can be performed using the percutaneous technique, saphenous vein cutdown, or umbilical vein cannulation in the newborn. Catheterization via a patent umbilical vein provides the easiest entry during the first week of life. This approach also conserves the femoral veins for future study, if necessary. However, bacteremia, the possibility of portal vein thrombosis, and trauma to the fragile ductus venosus are recognized complications of umbilical vein catheterization.[32] Catheter manipulation may be quite difficult when the umbilical vein is used, especially if access to the right ventricle is required. This problem was emphasized by Porter[33] in a study comparing the three techniques of venous access. Two cases of complete atrioventricular block were attributed to the manipulation required to pass the catheter across the tricuspid valve; along with one instance of left ventricular perforation during the attempt to position the catheter prior to angiography. Particular care must be exercised to be sure the catheter is not trapped behind the posterior papillary muscle prior to left ventriculography during umbilical vein catheterization (Fig. 1).

Saphenous vein cutdown to provide venous access in the child has gradually been replaced by the Seldinger technique[34] and subsequent modifications in the past decade.[35] Venotomy is preferred by some, however, and may be associated with a lower incidence of subsequent iliac vein-inferior vena cava thrombosis than with the percutaneous technique.[36] Major complications associated with venotomy include extensive scarring at the incision site, blood loss, infection, and loss of the vessel for future study. Ligation of the common femoral vein will result in subsequent venous obstruction and possible thrombus propagation and must be avoided.[37]

The percutaneous insertion of vascular sheaths has provided a major improvement in the performance of cardiac catheterization

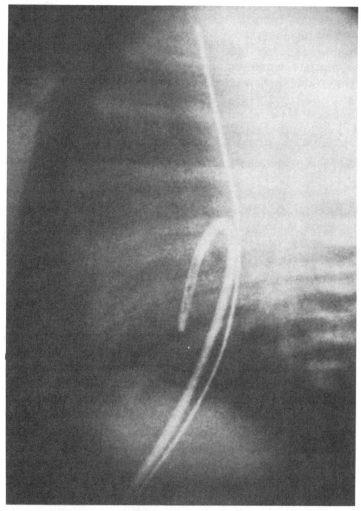

Figure 1. *Prograde catheterization of the left ventricle, umbilical vein approach (lateral projection). Catheter is positioned behind the posterior papillary muscle, rather than at the more anterior apex of the left ventricle.*

in small children. The use of venous sheaths reduces manipulation and local trauma at the entry site, preserving vein integrity. In addition, nontapered catheters can be readily exchanged to meet specific catheterization objectives.[38] Local bleeding, infection, and subsequent venous thrombosis remain potential complications. Angiographic documentation of femoral or iliac vein occlusion should be performed when suspected to confirm the diagnosis and prevent future attempts at cannulation of the vein (Fig. 2).

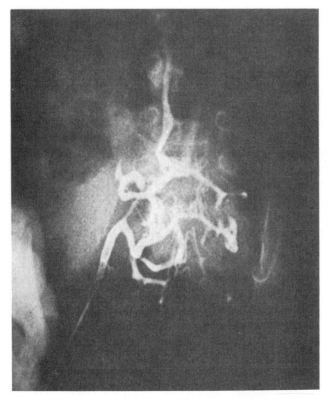

Figure 2. *Iliac vein occlusion following previous catheterization as a newborn. Collateral venous return to the lumbar plexus and left-sided inferior vena cava with situs inversus is evident in this patient. Demonstration of this anatomy precluded further attempts at guidewire passage from this vein.*

Arterial catheterization is commonly employed in studies of patients with congenital heart disease to monitor pressure and saturation, evaluate the hemodynamics of the systemic ventricle, and perform angiography. Percutaneous catheterization of the femoral artery is used in the majority of children, although umbilical artery cannulation is performed in the neonate, whereas brachial artery catheterization may be indicated in certain instances. Arterial thrombosis with subsequent vascular compromise is the primary concern in arterial catheterization, although blood loss, hematoma, and infection also present potential problems.

The incidence of vascular complications associated with arterial catheterization must be considered in view of the following variables:

1. method of arterial entry,
2. site of arterial entry,
3. catheter size and manipulation, and
4. use of heparin.

Comparative analysis of the percutaneous technique, puncture of an isolated artery, and arteriotomy by Stanger,[3] demonstrated the relative safety of the percutaneous method of entry. Brachial arteriotomy was associated with the highest incidence (16%) of vascular complications in patients with coarctation of the aorta leading to subsequent recommendations to avoid this approach, if possible. There were no arterial complications in the 89 infants with umbilical artery catheterization in Stanger's study. This relative safety of umbilical artery catheterization in the newborn has been long recognized.[39] Arterial puncture and the consequences of thrombosis following intimal trauma are avoided with this approach, although catheter manipulation must be gentle to avoid intimal perforation or dissection. The potential for infection from the umbilical stump and age limitations in the use of this technique present the major restraints. In general, umbilical artery patency is present in the newborn infant for up to 5 to 7 days of age.

The recent advent of transarterial balloon dilation procedures has been accompanied by a marked increase in the incidence of femoral artery thrombosis.[40] This has been attributed to the large size and irregular surface of these catheters and associated intimal trauma during manipulation. Infants less than 10kg have also

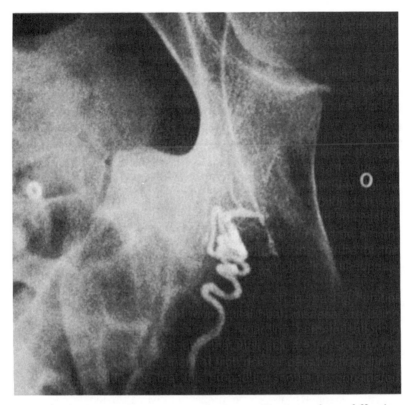

Figure 3. *External iliac artery occlusion at 20 years of age following arterial catheterization as an infant. Clinically, bounding femoral pulses were palpable, but guidewire advancement was not feasible. The tortuous collateral anatomy is evident.*

been identified as the other major group at risk for arterial compromise following catheterization. The postulated mechanisms of thrombosis in this group once again are intimal trauma and vascular stasis distal to the catheter/sheath, with thrombus propagation.[41] The use of systemic heparinization during arterial catheterization has been reported to reduce the incidence of subsequent thrombosis in children and thus may be warranted.[42] However, the recommended doses of heparin have varied between 30 and 100 IU/kg in children; other factors such as viscosity, hemodynamics, and duration of catheterization may affect the incidence of subsequent arterial compromise. Also, a large study of adult patients did not demonstrate that heparinization decreased the complication rate of cardiac catheterization.[43]

Late sequelae of arterial catheterization in children with congenital heart disease are well known. Return of distal pulses following arterial catheterization does not necessarily imply patency of the artery,[44] as illustrated in Figure 3. Reduced limb growth and claudication caused by arterial insufficiency remained poorly defined late complications.[45] It would appear that poor pedal pulses remain the best correlate of femoral arterial thrombosis following arterial catheterization.

Radiation Exposure During Cardiac Catheterization

The potential consequences of radiation exposure during cardiac catheterization are inherent to the procedure. Quantitative interpretation of this risk is difficult, however, as the radiation absorbed dose (rad) relationship to the roentgen (R) unit of exposure is based on multiple variables such as mass density, location of tissues, and total body area. Regardless, radiosensitivity is proportional to cell reproduction rate, rendering the child more susceptible to radiation than the adult.[46] Due to their smaller size, increased exposure from internal scatter also occurs in children.

The sensitivity of the head to ionizing radiation is clearly established in children,[47] although the radiation exposure to this area is generally quite low and related to scatter. Conversely, significant thyroid exposure to radiation during catheterization may be associated with thyroid tumors and hypothyroidism,[48] and may be difficult to eliminate during cardiac catheterization, especially if visualization of the aortic arch is required in a small infant. The development of collimation has reduced the "scatter" of the primary beam, although it remains difficult to define the field to include the aortic arch and still avoid the thyroid.

Perhaps the most frequently overlooked area of potential damage from ionizing radiation is the gastrointestinal tract. Waldman reported an average exposure of 150 mR during catheterization and subsequently recommended placement of a lead shield with the cephalad edge just below the level of the diaphragm to limit abdominal exposure.[49]

The heart, as the target organ of cardiac catheterization, and thorax are exposed to large doses of radiation during catheterization, 7–8 rad, according to the data of Waldman, which is approximately 15 times the recommended yearly exposure.[50] The cumulative effects of multiple cardiac catheterizations and subclinical damage that may become apparent only decades later still need to be clarified.

Given these considerations, the use of two-dimensional (2-D) echocardiography to define anatomy prior to catheterization should result directly in a reduction in catheter manipulation and radiation exposure. In conjunction with precatheterization echocardiographic evaluation, attention to limited field size during catheter manipulation and adequate shielding of the abdomen are recommended. In complex anatomy, an initial ventriculogram may define great artery relationships and defect locations, allowing a significant reduction in the time required for catheter manipulation. In specific situations such as pulmonary artery wedge angiography or left superior vena cava injection, filming speed is 30 frames/sec may allow the operator to reduce the dose of radiation without losing detail.

During axial angiography the heart is frequently superimposed on the liver, which is radiodense. Therefore, for adequate penetration during fluoroscopy and cineangiography, the dose of radiation to the patient must be increased. The greatly increased diagnostic accuracy afforded by this technique justifies the increased exposure. However, catheter manipulation should be performed in standard AP position, employing angled views only during angiography. Conscious efforts should be made to limit radiation exposure during catheterization; however, this must not be done at the expense of diagnostic accuracy or completeness.

Complications Associated with Techniques of Cardiac Catheterization

The standard approach to cardiac catheterization in the child consists of a prograde venous approach to the right heart, with subsequent left heart study via a patent foramen ovale or atrial septal defect when possible. With an intact interatrial septum, a retrograde arterial study or transseptal approach is required, depending on the specific defect(s) under consideration. The major potential complications during these types of catheter manipulation in children may be classified as perforation of the heart or great vessels, thromboembolism, dysrhythmias, or catheter-related complications.

Prograde Venous Catheterization of the Right and Left Heart

Before proceeding with right heart catheterization, preshading the woven Dacron catheter to a gentle 180°-bend with steam allows the operator to pass it directly from the right atrium into the ventricle. Subsequently, as the catheter softens in the ventricle some straightening will occur so that it can be passed to the pulmonary artery. If the catheter tip remains at the apex of the right ventricle, slow pullback with clockwise rotation under biplane fluoroscopic control will demonstrate migration toward the right ventricular outflow tract. In general, the course of the catheter from the inferior vena cava across the tricuspid valve and its subsequent passage to the pulmonary artery should be a relatively direct one rather than a series of acute angles. (Fig. 4). Deviation from this course may indicate catheter entrapment within the right ventricle or its passage to an anatomic variant, as discussed below. Biplane definition of the catheter's position, measurement of pressure and oxygen content, and a small, hand injection of contrast should define the catheter's position. If an unusual position is recognized, the catheter must not be advanced until its location has been defined.

A discussion of the variations of congenital heart defects and subsequent catheter courses is beyond the scope of this text.[51] However, catheterization must be performed with a systematic approach guided by echocardiographic findings and a knowledge of associated malformations. The common variants of a persistent left superior vena cava to the coronary sinus, patent ductus arteriosus, atrial septal defect, or infrahepatic interruption of the inferior vena cava with azygous continuation and their corresponding catheter courses must be recognized promptly (Figs. 5 and 6).

Continuous phasic pressure should be displayed at all times during catheter manipulation with the sole exception of the brief use of a soft guidewire to assist in catheter placement. A dampened

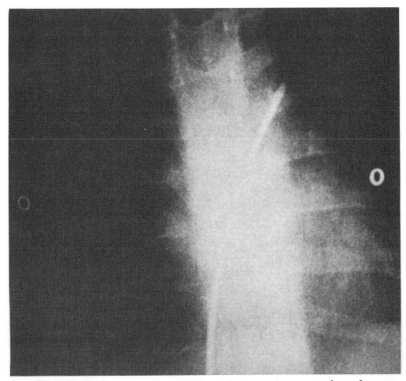

Figure 4. *The catheter course from the inferior vena cava to the pulmonary artery demonstrates the relatively direct course of passage through these structures.*

pressure should be taken to represent either catheter entrapment, partial occlusion by thrombus, or passage beyond a point of severe anatomic stenosis. Gentle aspiration and flushing of the catheter should allow differentiation of the above.

Balloon flotation catheters have gained wide acceptance in the catheterization of children.[52] In particular, catheterization of the pulmonary artery in the small infant and in the patient with transposition of the great arteries has been facilitated. Certain limitations regarding the use of balloon flotation catheters are recognized:

1. Balloon rupture, despite inflation with CO_2, may result in significant embolic sequelae.[4]

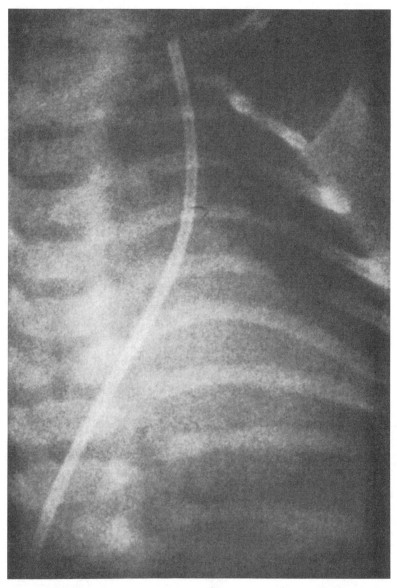

Figure 5. *The catheter has an initial course similar to that shown in Figure 4. However, atrial phasic pressure was maintained and a very posterior catheter course was evident on lateral fluoroscopy. Passage from the coronary sinus to a persistent left superior vena cava is demonstrated.*

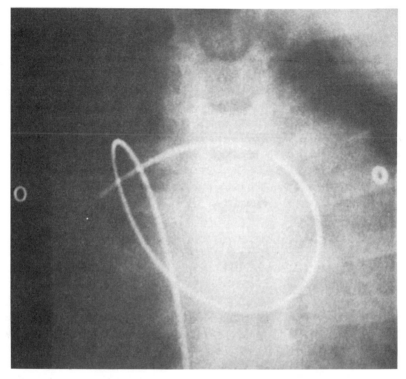

Figure 6. *Infrahepatic interruption of the inferior vena cava. Catheter passage from an azygous vein, subsequent junction with the superior vena cava, and eventual passage through a common atrium and ventricle to the right pulmonary artery are demonstrated in this patient.*

2. In certain types of anatomy, e.g., ventricular inversion, specific catheter manipulation is required for entry into the pulmonary circulation. This may not be possible with balloon flotation catheters as they are not shapeable and lack torque control.
3. Critical obstruction may be produced by the balloon in the pulmonary or aortic outflow tract, resulting in severe hypoxemia or hemodynamic compromise.

Despite these considerations, balloon catheters have contributed to the safety of cardiac catheterization in children, particularly in performing angiography in the small child. However, they should not be considered as substitutes for standard woven catheters, especially in fellowship training programs.[53]

Following complete right heart catheterization, the interatrial septum should be probed with the catheter to determine the patency of the foramen ovale or the presence of an atrial septal defect. This should be done only under biplane fluoroscopy, monitoring pressure constantly. Passage to the left atrium should be confirmed by oximetry. Subsequent passage to the left ventricle usually requires a soft guidewire formed to allow passage to the somewhat anterior and inferior apex of the left ventricle. Again, this manipulation should be done only with biplane fluoroscopy since posterior passage from the left atrium to the left lower pulmonary vein may not be recognized. An intact atrial septum necessitates either transseptal or retrograde approach to the left heart.

Transseptal Left Heart Catheterization in Pediatrics

The transseptal approach to left heart catheterization was introduced in 1959 by Cope[54] and Ross[55] but modified by Brockenbrough in 1960.[56] Application of this technique to smaller pediatric patients was limited until a successful modification was introduced by Mullins in 1978.[57] With the development of the Transseptal Introducer Set®, manufactured by United States Catheter Incorporated, Billerica, MA, the technical drawbacks of the original Brockenbrough catheter have been largely overcome and the transseptal introducer catheter has been applied increasingly in pediatric catheterization.

The largest experience to date using the Transseptal Introducer Set has been reported by Mullins,[58] who described results in 520 consecutive attempts using this technique. Of the patients studied, there were only 4 unsuccessful attempts at direct entry to the left atrium. The major reported complications, hemopericardium with tamponade, occurred in 2 patients; in both instances the tamponade was recognized and the patients stabilized in the catheterization laboratory prior to surgery. The pericardium was entered by needle only in 28 cases, an incidence of 6%. No complications were recognized in association with *isolated needle perforation* of the right or left atrium, and the catheterization was completed in all cases.

Transseptal catheterization in children has proved safe, given certain definite precautions. Perhaps most important is operator familiarity with this technique and ability to perform the procedure expeditiously. Mullins' report includes appropriately, a detailed technical description of this procedure. Briefly, the following aspects are emphasized:

1. The length relationship of the sheath, dilator, and transseptal needle must be measured in each case.
2. The sheath and dilator are positioned within the superior vena cava and the transseptal needle subsequently positioned within the dilator.
3. The system is withdrawn to a position midway down the atrial septum, corresponding to the region of the fossa ovalis; at this point the needle is advanced beyond the tip of the dilator and firmly advanced to the left atrium.
4. The transseptal needle must allow recording of a reliable left atrial pressure before the Introducer Set is advanced.
5. If there is any doubt about the position of the catheter, a brief hand injection of contrast is given to define its location.

Biplane fluoroscopy to allow three-dimensional (3-D) assessment of the position of the needle tip relative to the aorta, atrial septum, and left atrial free wall is essential, especially in patients with congenital heart malformations. A "learning curve," that is, fewer complications with greater experience with this technique has been reported to occur by several authors[59] and would be substantiated by personal experience.

The indications for transseptal left heart catheterization as opposed to retrograde study are in part determined by individual experience with the two techniques and the specific defect requiring catheterization. Our current indications for the transseptal approach are:

1. Evaluation of mitral and aortic valve stenosis.
2. Evaluation of mitral and aortic valve prostheses (Fig. 7).
3. Direct measurement of left atrial pressure in conditions associated with pulmonary hypertension.
4. Pulmonary vein wedge angiography in conditions such as pulmonary atresia (Fig. 8).
5. Performance of blade atrial septectomy.
6. Evaluation of multiple left-sided obstructive lesions.

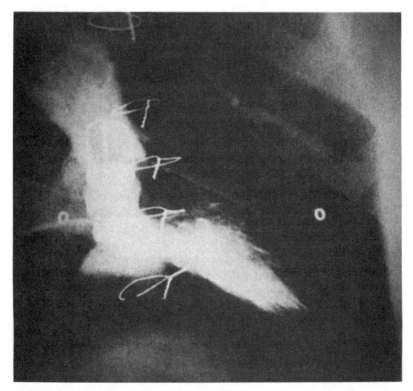

Figure 7. *Transseptal left ventriculography in a patient with a Starr-Edwards aortic valve prosthesis. The transseptal catheter is seen coursing thru the left atrium, across the mitral valve, and into the left ventricle.*

The transseptal technique may be used for angiographic delineation of aortic coarctation or to allow left ventricular electrophysiologic study, although the retrograde approach is still favored by some. Once again, physician proficiency with this technique should define the approach used.

Absolute and relative contraindications to the transseptal approach have been defined. Absolute contraindications include:

1. Left atrial thrombus or myxoma,
2. Inferior vena cava obstruction,
3. Interatrial baffle or patch.

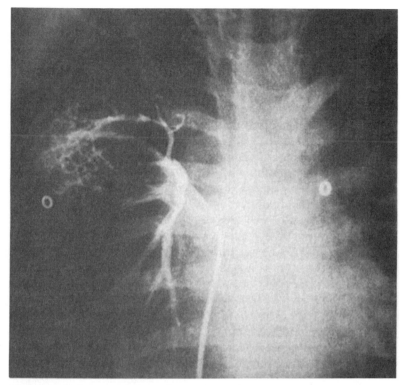

Figure 8. *Pulmonary vein wedge angiography in a patient with pulmonary atresia, ventricular septal defect, and an intact atrial septum. Access to the left atrium was transseptal, following brief injections to demonstrate a left superior vena cava, an enlarged overriding aorta, and a small left atrium. Retrograde angiography of the right pulmonary arterial system is demonstrated.*

A number of relative contraindications that do not preclude the transseptal approach but which require greater caution have also been defined:

1. A very large or small left atrium,
2. An enlarged aortic root,
3. Large coronary sinus (with persistent left SVC),

4. Cardiac malpositions,
5. Systemic anticoagulation or bleeding diathesis.

We advise that the precise anatomic relationships of an enlarged aorta and small left atrium be determined angiographically in anatomy such as pulmonary atresia with ventricular septal defect prior to transseptal puncture. Aortic root puncture can be avoided during transseptal catheterization by using biplane fluoroscopy to ensure the course of the needle is posterior to the aortic root.

Lastly, when the left femoral vein is used, it is often difficult to engage the atrial septum with the transseptal needle. Moderately bending the patient's thorax to the right may place the interatrial septum more perpendicular to the tip of the transseptal needle. As the transseptal needle will frequently traverse the atrial septum in a more anterior position than usual, passage directly to an upper pulmonary vein must be excluded.

Although the transseptal technique is somewhat more complex than retrograde left heart catheterization, it provides reliable access to the left atrium and ventricle and may avoid arterial complications attendant with the retrograde approach. The increased complexity of this approach and the potential for perforation of vascular or cardiac structures should not be underestimated. Therefore, transseptal catheterization should be performed **only** by those experienced with the technique. With experience and caution, transseptal catheterization has become an essential technique in pediatric catheterization.

Retrograde Arterial Catheterization of the Left Heart

Physiologic data and angiographic access to the left heart are frequently obtainable via a patent foramen ovale in the infant and young child. However, the atrial septum is often intact in the older child, particularly when pulmonary venous return is increased. Thus, in these patients, left heart information is obtained using the retrograde approach in most centers.[60] The first report of retrograde catheterization of the arterial circulation in study of the human heart was provided by Zimmerman, Scott, and Becker in 1950.[61] However, initial attempts were complicated by significant patient morbidity and mortality along with frequent inability to pass a catheter retrograde across the aortic valve. The initial problems with this technique resulted in delayed general acceptance until 1960.[62-63] The first large pediatric series in which this approach was used was provided by Vlad, Hohn, and Lambert in 1964.[64] In this series, 542 retrograde catheterizations were attempted and the left ventricle was successfully entered in 499 cases (92%), which included 115 patients with aortic stenosis. All studies were performed by brachial or superficial femoral arteriotomy. Failures to cross the aortic valve were significantly higher with the femoral approach than with brachial arteriotomy.

Application of the Seldinger technique to arterial catheterization and the subsequent development of the sheath-introducer system allowing catheter exchange, increased the use of this technique in femoral artery catheterization. With experience, it was also recognized that the brachial approach resulted in consistently higher local arterial complication rates,[65,66] particularly in the presence of coarctation of the aorta.[4] Currently, retrograde left heart catheterization in children is indicated when hemodynamic or angiographic data regarding the left ventricle or aorta are needed. It remains the method of choice for selective coronary angiography and, in general, provides easy access to the left ventricle without requiring extensive catheter manipulation. Despite the ease of the technique, certain limitations are recognized concerning its application in children. Difficulty crossing the aortic valve in congenital stenosis has given rise to a large number of methods due to the eccentric nature of the aortic orifice.[67-69] Most of these techniques require significant catheter manipulation and exchange with inherent risk of aortic perforation or thromboembolism. Second, although techniques for retrograde entry to the left atrium have been described,[70] uniform success has not been achieved, especially when mitral stenosis is present. Third, in the patient with coarctation of the aorta, intimal injury, perforation, or occlusion of a spinal injury during retrograde catheterization has been reported.[71,72] The severity of obstruction in coarctation may not be anticipated when major collaterals are present (Fig. 9). Lastly, catheterization in the patient with a prosthetic aortic valve deserves comment. Direct retrograde catheterization may be feasible in the patient with a homograft or xenograft prosthesis even though this approach is not recommended because valve perforation is a risk. Although the technique for retrograde crossing of a mechanical prosthesis has been de-

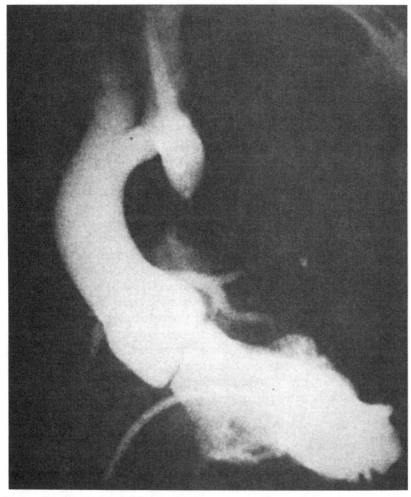

Figure 9. *Transseptal left ventriculogram in a 3-year-old referred for evaluation of coarctation of the aorta. Interruption of the aortic arch is evident; attempts at retrograde catheterization could have resulted in aortic perforation.*

scribed,[73,74] the risk of catheter entrapment as well as disturbed hemodynamic status caused by catheter disturbance of the prosthesis closure limit this technique. For these reasons, the transseptal sheath approach is an indispensable option in patients with left-sided obstructive lesions and aortic or mitral valve prostheses.

In the absence of left-sided obstruction, retrograde arterial catheterization and angiography using a pigtail catheter provides direct access to the left ventricle, allows good angiographic quality,[75] and has a low potential patient risk. The potential for a major complication associated with a specific technique as well as the ability to acquire the required information must be considered in planning each catheterization.

Perforation of the Heart or Great Vessels

Perforation of the heart or great vessels was both a common and serious complication, as reported by the Cooperative Study on Cardiac Catheterization.[2] It was recognized that perforation could occur both during catheter manipulation and contrast injection, with the latter causing more serious consequences. With the subsequent development of biplane fluoroscopy and softer woven Dacron catheters, Stanger reported only one recognized case of catheter perforation in 1,160 cases.[3] The subsequent development of balloon flotation catheters and precatheterization echocardiographic assessment of anatomy have contributed further to the decline in incidence of this complication. However, these improvements have not completely eliminated catheter perforation as a complication.

Perforation should be suspected if there is a sudden change from positive to negative pressure from the catheter, and verified by the failure to withdraw blood or by the aspiration of serous fluid. The injection of a small amount of contrast should follow to confirm the diagnosis. If the perforation occurred in an atrium or outflow tract, the catheter should be left in place so that the surgeon may repair the tear in a relatively bloodless field. Perforation of a ventricle by a catheter may be less serious since the muscular walls may effectively minimize blood loss. In any case, clinical evidence of tamponade is an immediate indication for pericardiocentesis and preparation for surgery. The aspiration of pericardial fluid with infusion into the femoral vein has been reported as a technique to maintain circulating volume while the patient is awaiting surgery.[76]

The development of guidewires to assist in catheter manipulation may have resulted in an increased incidence of unrecognized perforation of the heart or great vessels, although documentation for this is lacking. Very soft guidewires and minimal force in manipulation should limit the occurrence of occult perforation. Catheter molding by steam to attain the desired shape remains preferable to passing a guidewire out the end of a catheter. Particular care must be used if a guidewire is manipulated in the ductus arteriosus, given the friable nature of this structure.

Myocardial perforation secondary to the injection of contrast material as well as myocardial staining are related to catheter position in the heart at the time of pressure injection. Optimal catheter position during angiography will be discussed subsequently.

Any suspicion of a catheter defect, particularly bending at one of the sideholes, warrants catheter replacement prior to angiography. The risks of embolization of catheter fragments are greatest during power injection of contrast media.[77]

Cardiac Dysrhythmias and Conduction Disturbances

Major cardiac dysrhythmias, defined as those requiring cardioversion or cardiac pacing, are the most common major complications reported in association with cardiac catheterization. Nine of the 55 deaths reported in the Cooperative Study were directly attributed to severe bradycardia, heart block, or tachycardia in children, with Stanger subsequently reporting 17 major arrhythmias in 1,160 cases.

Bradycardia during catheterization may be an ominous sign of clinical deterioration and demands correction before the catheterization proceeds further. Continuous electrocardiographic monitoring during catheterization is mandatory and must be of sufficient quality to allow precise rhythm analysis. Critically ill infants are particularly vulnerable to bradycardia during catheterization, emphasized by the fact that seven infant deaths were due to bradycardia in the Cooperative Study. As the newborn has limited ability to increase stroke volume, cardiac output is heart rate dependent and bradycardia imposes severe hemodynamic consequences. These hemodynamics occur in the setting of vagal predominance, present in normal newborns,[78] which may be exaggerated if hypoxemia or hypothermia are allowed to occur during the course of catheterization.

The ability to institute cardiac pacing must be available to the physician who performs cardiac catheterization. Temporary pacing is required if bradycardia is not responsive to atropine or isoproterenol. Concurrent with treatment, the cause for bradycardia must be established. Arterial blood gas analyses and the differentiation of heart block from sinus bradycardia should be performed immediately (Fig. 10).

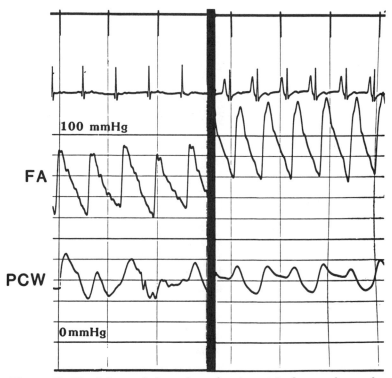

Figure 10. *The left panel shows loss of atrioventricular synchrony due to sinus slowing and junctional escape rhythm in a 2-year-old with a restrictive cardiomyopathy. Arterial pressure falls 20 mmHg with the loss of atrial kick compared to the right panel in which sinus rhythm is present. FA = Femoral Artery Pressure; PCW = Pulmonary Capillary Wedge pressure.*

Third degree AV block may occur following catheter manipulation in the area of the bundle of His. After the catheter is removed, block is usally transient, lasting from 1–10 minutes. However, clinical perfusion will depend on the anatomic substrate and institution of temporary pacing may be necessary. Congenital heart malformations associated with an increased frequency of heart block during catheterization are ventricular inversion, atrioventricular septal defects, and defects resulting in profound cyanosis.[79,80] The rare pediatric patient with complete left bundle branch block also is at risk because conduction to the ventricles is solely by the right bundle branch, which may be readily traumatized during right heart catheterization.

Sinus bradycardia or transient AV block may be anticipated following angiography may be anticipated because of the direct depressant effects of contrast material and secondary vagomimetic effects. Patients particularly at risk are those with severe right or left heart obstructive lesions or pulmonary hypertension.

Tachydysrhythmias

Isolated atrial and ventricular premature beats are common during catheter manipulation within the heart and are reported to occur in up to 95% of cases.[1] The incidence of these premature beats has been reduced with the introduction of balloon flotation catheters and biplane fluoroscopy and are not of major concern in the young patient.

Excluding electrophysiologic cases, the reported incidence of supraventricular tachycardia (SVT) during catheterization approximates 4% in most series.[2–4] The frequency of SVT is highest in the newborn[3] owing to AV node reentry or reciprocating tachycardias.[81] Most episodes are nonsustained or terminated with catheter induced extrastimuli or vagal maneuvers. Although well tolerated in most cases, SVT may result in severe compromise in patients with poor ventricular function or subpulmonic outflow obstruction.[82] Immediate termination of the tachycardia by overdrive pacing or synchronized DC cardioversion is indicated in patients with hemodynamic compromise.

Atrial flutter is commonly induced during catheterization, primarily in patients who have had prior cardiac surgery. Severe hemodynamic compromise may occur in the presence of 1:1 AV

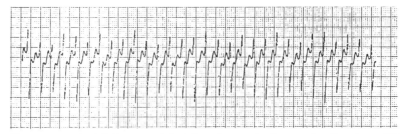

Figure 11. *Atrial flutter with 1:1 atrioventricular conduction in a 15-year-old patient following the Mustard procedure. Immediate synchronized cardioversion was performed.*

conduction in children (Fig. 11) and requires immediate cardioversion. If AV block is present, we prefer overdrive pacing, as described by Waldo,[83] to terminate atrial flutter. Any atrial dysrhythmia induced during catheterization should be terminated prior to further hemodynamic measurements or angiographic procedures. Very high degreees of AV block associated with atrial flutter following angiography have also been observed.

Repetitive ventricular ectopic beats most frequently occur during ventriculography or catheter manipulation in the area of the right ventricular outflow tract. The spontaneous occurrence of ventricular ectopy during catheterization may signal that the patient's metabolic status is deteriorating and requires evaluation. Care must also be exercised in patients with severe aortic or pulmonary obstruction since subendocardial ischemia may predispose to slow conduction and establish the substrate to maintain ventricular tachycardia or degenerate to ventricular fibrillation.

Ventricular fibrillation has been reported to occur in children during cardiac catheterization in the following settings: atrial fibrillation in the patient with pre-excitation[3]; following ventriculography or selective coronary angiography[84,85]; and as the result of an electrical current passing across a "two-ground" system.[86] All electrical outlets in a catheterization laboratory should be connected to a common ground to avoid the development of a potential difference. DC countershock remains the standard treatment for ventricular fibrillation during cardiac catheterization.

Critical Obstruction During Cardiac Catheterization

Critical obstruction of a stenotic orifice may result during catheter passage across a severely restrictive semilunar valve or vascular channel. The recognized potential to precipitate a severe hypoxic-acidotic spell in the patient with tetralogy of Fallot or critical pulmonary stenosis has resulted in the general recommendation that no attempt whatever be made to enter the pulmonary artery in these patients. Severe bradycardia and hypotension have been described during retrograde catheter passage across the aortic valve in severe aortic stenosis.[2] Accordingly, the transseptal approach to the left ventricle is the preferred approach in these patients.[58]

Obstruction of blood flow to coronary ostia or across a restrictive ductus arteriosus may also occur during catheter manipulation. Constant electrocardiographic and pressure monitoring during catheter manipulation should alert the physician to this possibility. Perhaps less easily recognized during retrograde catheterization is critical obstruction of the aorta in the patient with coarctation and the potential of ischemic injury to the abdominal viscera.[87]

If critical obstruction is recognized, prompt withdrawal of the catheter usually improves the situation. Stanger reported the unusual complication of the inability to withdraw the catheter from the left coronary artery in a 4-year-old child.[3] At surgery, the catheter was found to have fractured forming an acute angle, resulting in entrapment.

Peripheral Embolism

Emboli to cerebral, coronary, and vascular systemic beds constitute a well known, albeit infrequent complication of cardiac catheterization.[88,89] Fibrin-platelet emboli constitue the most common source, although catheter fragment and air emboli are also recognized, particularly in the patient with right-to-left intracardiac shunt. The development of clinically manifest emboli has not been eliminated completely by systemic heparinization, although the CASS study reported an incidence of less than 1 per 1,000 adult patients.[90] The proposed mechanism for most embolic events is the formation of thrombus along the inner surface of the catheter, possibly in association with a guidewire, with subsequent dislodgement during catheter exchange or angiography.[91] Systemic heparinization, careful wiping of guidewires, and limiting the use of indwelling wires to a total of 2 minutes should reduce but not eliminate the risk of emboli. When an arterial or venous sheath with a sideport is used, meticulous aspiration and flusing must be repeated every few minutes to prevent the formation of thrombus between the catheter and sheath.

Balloon rupture with latex fragment embolization may occur during atrial septostomy or with the use of flow-directed catheters. Catheter fracture and knotting are rare complications that should be avoided during catheter manipulation. The potential for catheter fracture and subsequent embolization during angiography is discussed in the next section.

Complications of Angiography in the Child

Inital reports of angiography in the child with congenital heart disease were provided provided by Castellanos and co-workers, working in Cuba in the 1930s.[92] Utilizing techniques of injecting contrast into either the antecubital vein or carotid artery, accurate descriptions of the common forms of congenital heart disease were presented. The subsequent development of ventriculography and aortography, along with an understanding of the principles of the use of radiographic and cineangiographic equipment represented the major developments of the next decades in the angiography of congenital heart disease.[93] New developments have added to both the diagnostic accuracy and the safety of angiography in the child, and have changed the approach to the delineation of intracardiac and great vessel anatomy. Axial angiography, described by Bargeron and colleagues, has evolved to become the standard for defining cardiac anatomy.[94,95] The development of two-dimensional echocardiography has enabled the physician to plan the angiographic procedure to define suspected lesions accurately and limit the total amount of contrast required. Lastly, the development of nonionic contrast media and new angiographic techniques such as balloon-occlusion aortography have reduced the hemodynamic burden of contrast media while preserving anatomic definition. A discussion of the potential complications associated with cardiac angiography in the infant or child is best approached by considering the physical properties of contrast media, the volume of contrast, and techniques of angiography.

Physical and Chemical Properties of Contrast Media

All radiographic contrast agents are iodinated compounds, yielding adequate radiographic density with an iodine concentration of between 320 and 400 mg/mL.[96] The major differences among the various contrast media are attributable to ionization in solution and sodium content, which result in hyperosmolar effects, and to the presence of stabilizing agents such as EDTA or sodium citrate. The conventional radiographic agents, such as Renografin-76 or Hypaque-76 are ionic monomers that dissociate in solution. Given their tri-iodinated benzene ring composition, and associated sodium content of 190 to 390 mEq/L, subsequent net osmolarity five times that of blood follows their injection. Attempts to reduce the consequences of hyperosmolarity have resulted in the development of dimeric (Hexabrix) or nonionic contrast media such as Metrizamide and Omnipaque. The pharmacologic effects of the various types of radiolucent media are reviewed in Chapter 9.

Given the concerns of hyperosmolarity and calcium chelation, new nonionic agents have gained increased acceptance in pediatric angiography. These media possess an osmolarity two to three times that of blood, and do not contain sodium. Preliminary studies in neonates[97,98] demonstrate reduced hemodynamic consequences and acceptable angiographic quality. These agents are considerably more viscous (13–16 cp at 37°C) than their ionic counterparts, (8 cp at 37°C) which must be considered when establishing delivery pressure and rates. The use of nonionic contrast media would appear to be an important consideration in the sick neonate.

Contrast Volumes and Injection Rates

The objective of angiography is to image cardiac or vascular structures with sufficient radiodensity to provide accurate anatomic definition and function. Radiodensity depends largely on iodine content and the volume and rate of delivery. Thus, a balance is required to obtain adequate angiographic assessment and avoid the complications related to excess pressure at the delivery site or to the volume administered. Congenital heart disease perhaps presents more complexities in determining adequate rates and volumes of contrast delivered than any other aspect of angiography. Intracardiac shunts, hypoplastic chambers or arteries, and rapid heart rates require each patient be handled individually. General guidelines include:

1. The total volume of contrast should not exceed 4 cc/kg in a case.
2. An attempt should be made to deliver the contrast in one heart beat.
3. The shortest but largest-diameter catheter requires the least pressure to deliver the contrast.

Regardless of the defect being considered, the injection of contrast should be preceded by:

1. A test injection during fluoroscopy to confirm that the catheter tip is positioned properly—i.e., away from valves, coronary ostia, and entrapment—and that the patient is positioned properly.
2. Adequate precautions to remove all air or potential thrombus from the catheter or injector.

In general, the following contrast volumes are recommended:

Cineangiogram	Volume cc/Kg
Ventriculography	1.5
Ventriculography with shunt or regurgitation	2.0
Ventriculography with outflow obstruction or dysfunction	1.0

Ventriculography in the presence of an intracardiac shunt may be inadequate to define the pulmonary artery or aortic arch, even with large volumes of contrast. Consequently, the balloon-occlusion angiographic technique has been increasingly applied for this purpose.[99,100] By preventing distal, "washout" an increased concentration of media is provided at a reduced volume. This technique is particularly applicable to newborn infants with aortic obstruction or ductal-dependent blood flow (Fig. 12). The increased use of bal-

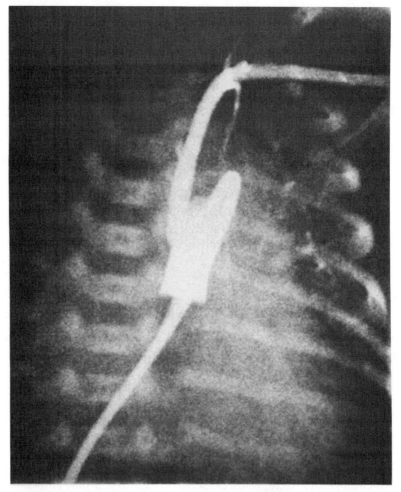

Figure 12. *Balloon-occlusion aortography, with the catheter passed through a patent ductus arteriosus. In this 1,800-g neonate, type B interrupted aortic arch is demonstrated; the balloon catheter occludes the descending aorta. Note the absence of contrast proximal to the left subclavian artery.*

loon-occlusion angiography should reduce neonatal angiographic complications and improve the quality of angiograms.

As discussed previously, perforation of a cardiac chamber or great vessel, or the related intramyocardial stain represent serious complications of angiography in children. The injection of contrast media was implicated in 10 of 24 cases of perforation of the heart or great vessels in children in the Cooperative Study, at a time when stiff Nylon-core catheters were used. Perforation was most frequent in the right ventricular outflow tract, or in patients with severe pulmonic stenosis or abnormal origin of the pulmonary artery. Stanger reported no instances of cardiac perforation during contrast injection, although several instances of intramyocardial injection of media (stain) were recognized as associated with ST- and T-wave changes. Cohn reported a similar incidence of myocardial stain, but no complete perforation secondary to contrast injection.

The reduced incidence of intramyocardial staining and perforation has been attributed to the balloon angiographic catheters, which prevent catheter entrapment in the small chamber.[101,102] Perhaps equally important, is the use of biplane fluoroscopy to position the catheter accurately within the ventricle, a small test injection to ensure rapid clearance of contrast, and the absence of induced ectopy.

The selection of catheter caliber and length are based on the size of the patient as well as the rate and volume of contrast agent to be delivered. With an automatic pressure injector, a maximal pressure of 600 to 700 psi should be used to limit the possibility of catheter rupture or inadvertent myocardial injection of contrast. The flow rates and corresponding equivalent pressures for given catheters, as recommended by their manufacturers, are given in Table 2. Due to the many variables involved (viscosity, temperature, lumen, consistency of pressure delivery), Table 2 provides only a general indication of pressures and flows and is not absolute. The data represent contrast media with viscosities of 8–16 centipoise (cp). Keane has reported preliminary results with a 3.2 French pigtail catheter in infants and small children.[60] These catheters were specifically tested for rupture, and found to rupture consistently at a pressure of 1,000 psi, at the junction of the shaft and hub. Angiographic quality was acceptable, except in cases in which low flow rates were chosen to allow measurement of ventricular volumes.

Table 2
Catheter Flow Rates and Equivalent Pressures

Catheter Manufacturer	Diameter (French)	Length (cm)	Flow Rate at Maximum Pressure (mL/sec)	Maximum Injection Pressure (PSI)
NIH	5	50	20	1,160
(USCI)	6	50	35	1,075
	7	100	35	920
Berman	5	80	6	600
(Critikon)	6	90	14	650
	7	90	20	700
Pigtail	5	65	11	500
(Cordis)	6	65	19	1,000
	6	80	16	1,000

Coronary Arteriography in the Child

The primary indication for selective coronary angiography in the pediatric age group may be defined as a nondiagnostic ascending aortogram in the patient with a suspected coronary anomaly, either congenital or acquired. The techniques of coronary arteriography and associated complications in children are similar to those in adults.[103,104] While the danger of complications in children may be lower due to the relative absence of atherosclerotic disease and because fewer projections are necessary, hazards associated with specific congenital anomalies are recognized. The risk in patients with aortic stenosis or a bicuspid valve is noteworthy, due to the short length of the left main coronary artery,[105] with passage of the catheter to a major branch. Selective injection into a single or dominant coronary artery, as in the Bland-Garland-White syndrome (anomalous left coronary artery) also may result in serious hemodynamic complications.

Precautions to avoid complications during coronary arteriography in infants and children include continuous electrocardiographic monitoring, accurate display of catheter-tip pressure, limited catheter time within the coronary ostium, and maintenance of a closed flushing system with free backflow to avoid emboli. Serial angiography should not be performed until ECG changes from the preceeding injection have normalized. In the presence of a superdominant left coronary system, the right coronary artery may be too small to safely catheterize. Coronary arteriography is associated with complications, but reports of fatal complications in children with coronary artery anomalies following cardiac catheterization and ascending aortography exist as well.[106,107] There are situations in which aortography will not clearly define coronary anatomy, and selective coronary angiography is required.

Electrophysiologic Catheterization in Pediatric Patients

In contrast to the vast literature available regarding the complications of hemodynamic and angiographic cardiac catheterization, few studies exist which address the complications of invasive cardiac electrophysiology, particularly in children. The electrophysiologic techniques and protocols used in infants and children have been largely derived from adult patients. However, unique catheters and equipment dedicated to use in small children must be available to ensure patient safety during the procedure.

A discussion of the potential complications of an electrophysiologic study must begin with the recognition that one of the main purposes of the study is to reproduce the patient's clinical dysrhythmia. Rapid hemodynamic deterioration may occur if the induced rhythm is not promptly terminated or restored to baseline. For this reason, patients with drug toxicity, metabolic abnormalities, or severe valvular heart disease, in whom the induction of a dysrhythmia may result in irreversible collapse, require careful evaluation before electrophysiologic study.[108]

Electrophysiologic catheters with a solid core are quite stiff compared to standard hemodynamic catheters and do not allow pressure monitoring. They should only be manipulated under biplane fluoroscopy, especially when it is necessary to enter the coronary sinus or the catheter is positioned in the right ventricular outflow tract. Recognized cardiac perforation was reported in 0.5% of patients undergoing electrophysiologic study in a recent multicenter study, with the warning that right ventricular perforation often may be asymptomatic.[109]

All electrical devices must be grounded and individual leakage currents must be less than 10m. An emergency cart that includes a monitor-defibrillator and pre-established emergency pacing cycles must be available before the study is initiated. Also, an established protocol for each study is required in order for the case to progress as expeditiously as possible. The presence of two physicians appears optimal.

With the above precautions, venous thrombosis is the most common complication reported in adult electrophysiologic studies.[110] As in other catheterizations, the probable mechanisms involve intimal trauma and temporary venous occlusion due to multiple catheter placement. The risk of embolus with right-to-left intracardiac shunt requires the patient to be fully heparinized. The incidence of complications in these studies appears to be acceptably low when performed with careful catheter techniques, and by individuals experienced in electrophysiology.

The Physician and Catheterization-related Complications

The various complications that may occur in the infant or child during cardiac catheterization are best evaluated in the context of the medical status of the patient, the skill and experience of the physician, and the current state of technology. In this chapter, the major and frequent minor complications recognized during catheterization have been discussed individually, in the context of the patient. However, as a highly technical procedure, the physician's role in the genesis or prevention of complications deserves comment.

The safety and efficacy of a laboratory require a caseload of adequate size to maintain the skill and efficiency of the staff. It has been recommended that in laboratories studying neonates and children a minimum of 150 examinations per year be performed.[111] Particularly to be discouraged is the occasional study of an infant or child in a laboratory remote from a pediatric cardiopulmonary surgical service. In spite of these sanguine recommendations, however, the quantitation of consistently safe numbers of studies per year, either per laboratory or per physician, has not proved feasible.

The impact of two-dimensional echocardiography on current practice, and training for future pediatric catheterization is complex. Precatheterization definition of anatomy has allowed angiography to be performed with greater precision and perhaps accuracy, as unsuspected associated lesions may be identified before catheterization. The two disciplines, catheterization and echocardiography, working in concert, have combined to improve presurgical definition of congenital heart defects.[112] Echocardiography has become the primary diagnostic modality before surgery in a number of defects, resulting in a reduced number of diagnostic catheterizations. The potential impact of a reduced number of studies per trainee on the future incidence of catheterization-related complications remains to be defined.

The ideal of catheterization should be a study free of complications and completely diagnostic. An error in diagnosis cannot be exonerated any more than a complication clearly related to the procedure of catheterization. The diagnostic catheterization of simple congenital defects will likely be replaced in the future by newer echocardiographic and digital subtraction techniques. Catheterization will be reserved for complex anatomic issues, electrophysiologic studies, or interventional procedures, as discusssed in the next chapter. In spite of changing techniques and applications, patient safety and diagnostic accuracy remain concerns of all physicians performing these studies. The importance of continued physician monitoring and communications regarding catheterization-related complications remain essential to all caring for children.

References

1. Kieth JD, Rowe RD, Vlad P: Heart Disease in Infancy and Childhood. New York, Macmillan, 1975, p 82.
2. Braunwald E, Swan HJC: Cooperative study on cardiac catheterization. Circulation 37 (Suppl III): , 1968.
3. Stanger P, Heymann MA, Tarnoff H, et al: Complications of cardiac catheterization of neonates, infants, and children. Circulation 50:595, 1974.
4. Cohn HE, Freed MD, Hellerbrand WF, et al: Complications and mortality associated with cardiac catheterization in infants under one year: a prospective study. Pediatr Cardiol 6:123, 1985.
5. Cournand A, Bing RJ, Dexter L, et al: Report of the committee on cardiac catheterization and angiocardiography of the American Heart Association. Circulation 7:769, 1953.
6. Rice MJ, Seward JB, Hagler DJ, et al: Impact of 2-dimensional echocardiography on the management of distressed newborns in whom cardiac disease is suspected. Am J Cardiol 51:288, 1983.

7. Smallhorn JF, Huhta JC, Adams PS, et al: Cross-sectional echocardiographic assessment of coarctation in the sick neonate and infant. Br Heart J 50:349, 1983.
8. Ueda K, Nojima K, Saito A, et al: Modified Blalock-Taussig shunt operation without cardiac catheterization: two-dimensional echocardiographic preoperative assessment in cyanotic infants. Am J Cardiol 54:1296, 1984.
9. Wolf WJ: Diagnostic features and pitfalls in the two-dimensional echocardiographic evaluation of a child with cor triatriatum. Pediatr Cardiol 6:211, 1986.
10. Marx GR, Allen HD: Accuracy and pitfalls of doppler evaluation of the pressure gradient in aortic coarctation. J Am Coll Cardiol 7:1379, 1986.
11. Freed MD, Heyman MA, Lewis AB, et al: Prostaglandin E_1 in infants with ductus arteriosus-dependent congenital heart disease. Circulation 64:899, 1981.
12. Lewis AB, Freed MD, Heyman MA, et al: Side effects of therapy with prostaglandin E_1 infants with critical congenital heart disease. Circulation 64:893, 1981.
13. Keane JF, Fyler DC, Nadas AS: Hazards of cardiac catheterization in children with primary pulmonary vascular obstruction. Am Heart J 96:556, 1978.
14. Young D, Mark H: Fate of the patient with Eisenmenger syndrome. Am J Cardiol 28:655, 1971.
15. Huhta JC, Latson LA, Gutgesell HP, et al: Echocardiography in the diagnosis and management of symptomatic aortic valve stenosis in infants. Circulation 70:438, 1984.
16. Hagler DJ, Tajik AJ, Seward JB, et al: Noninvasive assessment of pulmonary valve stenosis, aortic valve stenosis and coarctation of the aorta in critically ill neonates. Am J Cardiol 57:369, 1986.
17. Fellows KE, Smith J, Keane JF: Preoperative angiocardiography in infants with Tetrad of Fallot. Am J Cardiol 47:1279, 1981.
18. Lamberti JJ, Carlisle J, Waldman JD, et al: Systemic-pulmonary shunts in infants and children: early and late results. J Thorac Cardiovasc Surg 88:76, 1984.
19. Hawker RE, Bowdler JD, Celeamkyer JM, et al: Angiographic assessment of anomalous origin of the left coronary from the pulmonary artery in infancy and childhood. Pediatr Radiol 5:69, 1976.
20. Grossman W: Cardiac Catheterization and Angiography. Philadelphia, Lea and Febiger, 1986, p 31.
21. Mason JW, Billingham ME, Ricci DR: Treatment of acute inflammatory myocarditis assisted by endomyocardial biopsy. Am J Cardiol 45:1037, 1980.
22. Smith WM, Gallagher JJ, Kerr CC, et al: The electrophysiologic basis and management of symptomatic recurrent tachycardia in patients with Ebstein's anomaly of the tricuspid valve. Am J Cardiol 49:1223, 1982.

23. Giroud J, Pickoff AS, Garcia OL, et al: A method of maintaining thermal homeostasis during cardiac catheterization in the newborn. Cathet Cardiovasc Diagn 9:313, 1983.
24. Davison R, Parker M, Atkinson AJ Jr: Excessive serum lidocaine levels during maintenance infusions: mechanisms and prevention. Am Heart J 104:203, 1982.
25. Nattei S, Rinkenberger RL, Lehrman LL, et al: Therapeutic blood lidocaine concentrations after local anesthesia for cardiac electrophysiologic studies. N Engl J Med 301:418, 1979.
26. Gupta PK, Lichstein E, Chadda KD: Lidocaine induced heart block in patients with bundle branch block. Am J Cardiol 33:487, 1974.
27. Danahy DT, Aranow WS: Lidocaine induced heart rate changes in atrial fibrillation and flutter. Am Heart J 95:474, 1978.
28. Weissler AM, Warren JV: Vasodepressor syncope. Am Heart J 57:786, 1959.
29. Kirkpatrick SE, Takahashi M. Petry EL, et al: Percutaneous heart catheterization in infants and children. Circulation 42:1049, 1970.
30. Freed MD, Rosenthal AR, Fyler D: Attempts to reduce arterial thrombosis after cardiac catheterization: use of percutaneous technique and aspirin. Am Heart J 87:283, 1974.
31. Wessel DL, Keane JF, Fellows KE, et al: Fibrinolytic therapy for femoral arterial thrombosis after cardiac catheterization in infants and children. Am J Cardiol 56:347, 1986.
32. Porter CJ, Gillette PC, Mullins CE, et al: Cardiac catheterization in the neonate: a comparison of three techniques. J Pediatr 93:97, 1978.
33. Linde LM, Higashino SM, Berman G, et al: Umbilical vessel cardiac catheterization and angiography. Circulation 34:984, 1965.
34. Seldinger SI: Catheter replacement of the needle in percutaneous arteriography. Acta Radiol 39:368, 1953.
35. Sunderland CO, Nichols GAM, Henken DP, et al: Percutaneous cardiac catheterization and atrial balloon septostomy in pediatrics. Pediatr Cardiol 1:257, 1980.
36. Keane JF, Lang P, Newberger J, et al: Iliac vein-inferior vein thrombosis after cardiac catheterization in infancy. Pediatr Cardiol 1:257, 1980.
37. Nielsen G, Lorentzen JE: Venous blood flow in the leg after ligation of the femoral vein during cardiac catheterization in young children. Pediatr Cardiol 6:179, 1986.
38. Neches WH, Mullins CE, Williams RL, et al: Percutaneous sheath cardiac catheterization. Am J Cardiol 30:378, 1972.
39. Linde LM, Higashino SM, Berman G, et al: Umbilical vessel cardiac catheterization and angiocardiography. Circulation 34:984, 1966.
40. Wessel DL, Keane JF, Fellows KE, et al: Fibrinolytic therapy for femoral arterial thrombosis after cardiac catheterization in infants and children. Am J Cardiol 58:347, 1986.
41. Mortensson W, Hallbook T, Lundstrom NR: Percutaneous catheterization of the femoral vessels in children. Pediatr Radiol 4:1, 1975.

42. Freed MD, Keane JF, Rosenthal A: The use of heparin to prevent arterial thrombosis after percutaneous cardiac catheterization in children. Circulation 50:565, 1974.

43. Kennedy JW and the Registry Committee of the Society for Cardiac Angiography. Complications associated with cardiac catheterization and angiography. Cathet Cardiovasc Diagn 8:5, 1982.

44. Hurwitz RA, Franken EA, Girod DA, et al: Angiographic determination of arterial patency after percutaneous catheterization in infants and children. Circulation 56:102, 1977.

45. Adar R, Rubinstein N, Blieden L: Immediate complications and late sequelae of arterial catheterization in children with congenital heart disease. Pediatr Cardiol 4:25, 1983.

46. Adams FH, Norman A, Bass D, et al: Chromosome damage in infants and children after cardiac catheterization and angiography. Pediatrics 62:312, 1978.

47. Silverman C, Hoffman DA: Thyroid tumor risk from radiation during childhood. Prev Med 4:100, 1975.

48. Martin EC, Olson AP, Steeg CN, et al: Radiation exposure to the pediatric patient during cardiac catheterization and angiography. Circulation 64:153, 1981.

49. Waldman JD, Rummerfield PS, Gilpin EA, et al: Radiation exposure to the child during cardiac catheterization. Circulation 64:158, 1981.

50. Title 17, California Administrative Code, Chapter 5, Subchapter 4: No.30265-a.

51. Taketa RM, Sahn DJ, Simon AL, et al: Catheter positions in congenital cardiac malformations. Circulation 51:749, 1975.

52. Stanger P, Heyman MA, Hoffman JIE, et al: Use of the Swan-Ganz catheter in cardiac catheterization of infants and children. Am Heart J 83:749, 1972.

53. Rubenfire M: Injection of contrast media within the interatrial septum. (Letter) Cathet Cardiovasc Diagn 11:442, 1985.

54. Cope C: Technique for transseptal catheterization of the left atrium. J Thorac Surg 37:482, 1959.

55. Ross J Jr, Braunwald E, Morrow AG: Transseptal left atrial puncture: new technique for measurement of left atrial pressure in man. Am J Cardiol 3:653, 1959.

56. Brockenbrough EC, Braunwald E: A new technique for left ventricular angiography and transseptal left heart catheterization. Am J Cardiol 6:1062, 1960.

57. Duff DF, Mullins CE: Transseptal left heart catheterization in infants and children. Cathet Cardiovasc Diagn 4:213, 1978.

58. Mullins CE: Transseptal left heart catheterization: experience with a new technique in 520 pediatric and adult patients. Pediatr Cardiol 4:239, 1983.

59. O'Keefe JH, Vlietstra RE, Hanley PC, et al: Revival of the transseptal approach for catheterization of the left atrium and ventricle. Mayo Clin Proc 60:790, 1985.

60. Keane JF, Fellows KE, Lang P, et al: Pediatric arterial catheterization using a 3.2 French catheter. Cathet Cardiovasc Diagn 8:201, 1982.
61. Zimmerman HA, Scott RW, Becker NO: Catheterization of the left heart in man. Circulation 5:357, 1950.
62. Dotter CT, Gensini GG: Percutaneous retrograde catheterization of the left ventricle and systemic arteries in man. Radiology 75:171, 1960.
63. Voci G, Hammer NAJ: Retrograde arterial catheterization of the left ventricle. Am J Cardiol 5:493, 1960.
64. Vlad P, Hohn A, Lambert EC: Retrograde arterial catheterization of the left heart. Circulation 29:787, 1964.
65. Chahine RA, Herman MV, Gorlin R: Complications of coronary arteriography: comparison of the brachial to the femoral approach. Ann Intern Med 76:862, 1972.
66. Brener BJ, Couch NP: Peripheral arterial complications of left heart catheterization and their management. Am J Surg 125:521, 1973.
67. Baur HR, Mruz GL, Erickson DL, et al: New technique for retrograde left heart catheterization in aortic stenosis. Cathet Cardiovasc Diagn 8:299, 1982.
68. Laskey WK, Untereker WJ, Kusiak V, et al: A safe and rapid technique for retrograde catheterization of the left ventricle in aortic stenosis. Cathet Cardiovasc Diagn 8:429, 1982.
69. Lau KC, Leung MP, Lo RNS: Retrograde transfemoral catheterization of the left ventricle in children with aortic valve stenosis. Pediatr Cardiol 7:79, 1986.
70. Grossman W: Cardiac Catheterization and Angiography, 2nd Ed. Philadelphia, Lea and Febiger, 1980, p 48.
71. Gersony WM: Coarctation of the Aorta. In FH Adams, GC Emmanoulides (eds): Heart Disease in Infants, Children and Adolescents, 3rd Ed. Baltimore, Williams and Wilkins, 1983, p 195.
72. Talner NS, Berman MA: Postnatal development of obstruction in coarctation of the aorta: role of the ductus arteriosus. Pediatrics 56:562, 1975.
73. Karsh DL, Michaelson SP, Langou RA, et al: Retrograde left ventricular catheterization in patients with an aortic valve prosthesis. Am J Cardiol 41:893, 1978.
74. MacDonald RG, Feldman RL, Pepine CJ: Retrograde catheterization of the left ventricle through tilting disk valves using a modified catheter system. Am J Cardiol 54:1372, 1984.
75. Laskey WK: Retrograde left ventricular catheterization in aortic valve stenosis. Cathet Cardiovasc Diagn 12:75, 1986.
76. Moore JW, Bricker JT, Mullins CE, et al: Infusion of blood from the pericardial sac into femoral vein: a technique for survival until operative closure of a cardiac perforation during balloon septostomy. Am J Cardiol 56:494, 1985.
77. Schmierer JA, Isner JM, Konstam MA, et al: Catheter fragmentation: a source of catheter embolus. Cathet Cardiovasc Diagn 9:595, 1983.
78. Friedman WF, Lesch M, Sonnenblick EH: Neonatal Heart Disease.

79. Gillette PC, Busch V, Mullins CE, et al: Electrophysiologic studies in patients with ventricular inversion and "corrected transposition." Circulation 60:939, 1979.
80. Thiene G, Wenink ACG, Frescura C, et al: The surgical anatomy and pathology of the conduction tissues in atrioventricular defects. J Thorac Cardiovasc Surg 82:928, 1981.
81. Gillette PC: The mechanisms of supraventricular tachycardia in children. Circulation 54:133, 1976.
82. King SB, Franch RH: Production of increased right to left shunting by rapid heart rates in patients with tetralogy of Fallot. Circulation 44:265, 1971.
83. Waldo AL: Entrainment and interruption of atrial flutter with atrial pacing: studies in man following open heart surgery. Circulation 56:737, 1977.
84. Simon AL, Shabetai R, Lang JH: The mechanisms of production of ventricular fibrillation in coronary angiography. Am J Roentgenol 114:810, 1972.
85. Wolf GL: The fibrillatory properties of contrast agents. Invest Radiol 15:S208, 1980.
86. Mody SM, Richings M: Ventricular fibrillation resulting from electrocution during cardiac catheterization. Lancet 2:698, 1962.
87. Kern IB, Bowring AC, Cohen DH, et al: Spontaneous perforation of the colon following cardiac catheterization in the newborn. Med M Aust 2:1022, 1971.
88. Dimmick JE, Bove KE, McAdams AJ, et al: Fiber embolization—a hazard of cardiac catheterization and surgery. N Engl J Med 292:685, 1975.
89. Cha SD, Gooch AJ: Rupture of a catheter during left ventriculography. Cathet Cardiovasc Diagn 8:31, 1982.
90. Davis K, Kennedy JW, Kemp HG Jr, et al: Complications of coronary arteriography from the collaborative study of coronary artery surgery (CASS). Circulation 59:1105, 1979.
91. Nachnani GH, Lessin LS, Motomiya T, et al: Scanning electron microscopy of thrombogenisis on vascular catheter surfaces. N Engl J Med 286:139, 1972.
92. Castellanos A, Pereiras R: Countercurrent aortography. Rev Cubana Cardiol 2:187, 1939.
93. Christensen EE, Curry TS, Dowdy JE: An Introduction to the Physics of Diagnostic Radiology, 2nd Ed. Philadelphia, Lea and Febiger, 1978.
94. Bargeron LM, Elliot LP, Soto B, et al: Axial angiography in congenital heart disease. Circulation 56:1075, 1977.
95. Eliot LP, Bargeron LM, Bream PR, et al: Axial angiography in congenital heart disease. Section II: Specific lesions. Circulation 56:1084, 1977.
96. Hanley PC, Holmes DR, Julsrud PR, et al: Use of conventional and newer radiographic contrast agents in cardiac angiography. Prog Cardiovasc Dis 28:435, 1986.

98. Partridge JB, Scott O, Fiddler GI, et al: Angiography with Metrizimide in the neonate and infant. Clin Radiol 31:629, 1980.
99. Denham B: Aortography in infantile coarctation. (Letter) Br Med J 1:1282, 1978.
100. Keane JF, McFaul R, Fellows K, et al: Balloon occlusion angiography in infancy: methods, uses and limitations. Am J Cardiol 56:495, 1985.
101. Schwartz DC, West TD: Cardiac catheterization in infants and children. Heart Lung 3:404, 1974.
102. Kelly DT, Krovetz LJ, Rowe RD: Double lumen flotation catheter for use on complex cardiac anomalies. Circulation 44:910, 1971.
103. Formanek A, Nath PH, Zollikofer C, et al: Selective coronary arteriography in children. Circulation 61:84, 1980.
104. Bialostozky D, Luengo M, Magos C, et al: Coronary insufficiency in children. Am J Cardiol 36:509, 1975.
105. Johnson AD, Detwiller JH, Higgins CB: Left coronary artery anomaly in patients with bicuspid aortic valves. Br Heart J 40:489, 1978.
106. Noren GR, Raghib G, Moller JH, et al: Anomalous origin of the left coronary artery from the pulmonary trunk with special reference to the occurrence of mitral insufficiency. Circulation 30:171, 1964.
107. Sabiston DC Jr, Orme SK: Congenital origin of the left coronary artery from the pulmonary artery. J Cardiovasc Surg 9:543, 1968.
108. DiMarco JP: Intracardiac electrophysiology. In W Grossman (ed): Cardiac Catheterization and Angiography, 3rd Ed. Philadelphia, Lea and Febiger, 1986, p 339.
109. Horowitz LN: Safety of electrophysiologic studies. Circulation 73 (Suppl II):28, 1986.
110. DiMarco JP, Garan H, Ruskin JN: Complications in patients undergoing electrophysiologic procedures. Ann Intern Med 97:490, 1982.
111. Optimal resources for examination of the chest and cardiovascular system. Report of the Inter-Society Commission for Heart Disease Resources. Circulation 53:A-1, 1976.
112. Bierman FZ: Two-dimensional echocardiography and its influence on cardiac catheterization. Cardiovasc Interven Radiol 7:140, 1984.

Chapter 8

Complications of Interventional Catheterization Procedures in Congenital Heart Disease

Michael J. Silka

Introduction

Rubeo-Alvarez and Limon-Lason first described a single attempt at catheter relief of pulmonic stenosis in 1950.[1] However, in 1966 the creation of an atrial septal defect in a newborn with D-transposition of the great arteries by Rashkind and Miller is widely accepted as the basis of the use of cardiac catheterization for the treatment of congenital heart disease.[2] The current decade has witnessed a proliferation in the number of therapeutic catheter options available to the cardiologist; some have become widely accepted, such as balloon pulmonary valvuloplasty, while others, such as transcatheter patch closure of an atrial septal defect, remain restricted to a few centers on an investigational basis.

This chapter reviews the common reported difficulties and complications of interventional catheterization procedures and recent improvements in technology and technique.

From *Complications of Cardiac Catheterization and Angiography: Prevention and Management* edited by Jack Kron, M.D. and Mark J. Morton, M.D. © 1989, Futura Publishing Inc., Mount Kisco, NY.

The following procedures will be considered:

1. Balloon atrial septostomy.
2. Blade atrial septectomy.
3. Balloon pulmonary valvuloplasty.
4. Balloon dilatation of peripheral pulmonic stenosis.
5. Balloon angioplasty of coarctation of the aorta.
6. Endomyocardial biopsy.
7. Transvenous pacemaker insertion.

A complete listing and review of therapeutic interventional procedures would include balloon dilatation of mitral and aortic stenosis, transcatheter closure of atrial septal defects and the patent ductus arteriosus, and catheter ablation of the Bundle of His and foci of ectopic impulse formation. As these procedures are investigational at this time and limited data have been reported, they will not be discussed. Likewise, catheter retrieval of intravascular foreign objects will be considered in detail in Chapter 13.

Balloon Atrial Septostomy

Since the introduction of balloon atrial septostomy by Rashkind and Miller in 1966, the outlook for the infant with D-transposition of the great arteries has improved remarkably.[3] With improvements in both technique and understanding of the circulatory dynamics in congenital heart disease, the use of balloon atrial septostomy has been extended to patients with tricuspid atresia, total anomalous pulmonary venous connection, pulmonary atresia with intact ventricular septum, and complex defects with left atrioventricular valve atresia.[4] Although balloon atrial septostomy is performed with confidence and safety by pediatric cardiologists, related mortality and morbidity persist.[5,6]

The initial reviews of balloon atrial septostomy during the first 5 years following its introduction reported a procedure-related mortality rate of 10% to 17%.[7,8] Recognized complications included perforation of cardiac chambers or pulmonary veins, rupture or thrombosis of the inferior vena cava, and damage to the tricuspid or mitral valve apparatus. A significant incidence of catheter related problems, including balloon rupture and embolization, inability to deflate the balloon, and migration of the balloon along the catheter axis, were also reported.[9-12] Subsequent improvements in catheter design, and the ability to utilize percutaneous venous entry represented significant improvements which, combined with biplane fluoroscopy and echocardiography, have reduced the morbidity and mortality of this procedure.[13] Another factor that should be considered, however, is the early recognition and referral of the infant with D-transposition of the great arteries. In the initial 5 years of balloon atrial septostomy, only 50% of the patients with suspected D-transposition of the great arteries were referred in the first week of life; currently nearly 70% of infants are referred and undergo septostomy in the first *day* of life.[4] Prolonged hypoxemia and acidosis undoubtedly contributed to the early high mortality and morbidity reported in association with this procedure.

Current Diagnostic Approaches

The impact of two-dimensional echocardiography on the diagnosis of D-transposition of the great arteries has been profound, frequently eliminating the need for diagnostic catheterization[14,15] before therapeutic septostomy. A septostomy guided by echocardiography in conjunction with fluoroscopy has improved the efficacy and safety of the procedure, allows precise placement of the balloon catheter, avoids damage to the atrioventricular valves, and reduces radiation exposure. Echocardiography has been particularly helpful in guiding placement of the septostomy catheter in patients with relative hypoplasia of the left atrium, such as the mitral atresia complex. Echocardiography also allows the physician to immediately assess the anatomic adequacy of septostomy during the catheterization (Fig. 1). The recommended technique consists of placement of the balloon septostomy catheter in the left atrium under biplane fluoroscopy, confirmation of its position, subsequent inflation, and pullback under echocardiographic guidance and subsequent repositioning of the catheter in the left atrium under fluoroscopy.

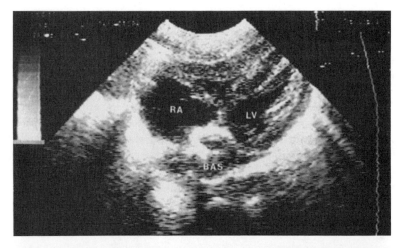

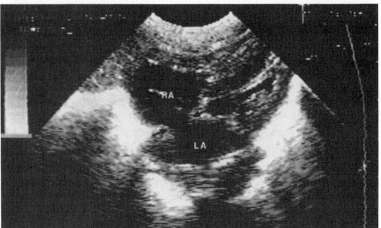

Figure 1. *Balloon atrial septostomy guided by two-dimensional echocardiography in a 1.7-kg infant with d-TGA. (Top) The balloon volume (1.5 mL) and position can be judged relative to the left atrium. (Bottom) Evaluation of defect size is possible immediately following atrial septostomy. LA = left atrium, RA = right atrium, LV = left ventricle, BAS = balloon septostomy catheter in left atrium.*

Vascular Access

In part, the early high complication rate associated with balloon atrial septostomy was attributable to the difficulties of vascular access and subsequent manipulation of the septostomy catheter. With the development of percutaneous vascular sheaths, local complications have been reduced,[16] although some authors continue to advocate the cutdown technique with subsequent vascular repair.[17]

Controversy exists regarding use of the umbilical vein as an access route for balloon atrial septostomy. The feasibility of this technique is established[18] in the term newborn infant with a patent ductus venosus. However, limited maneuverability of the septostomy catheter and inability to pass the catheter through the ductus venosus are common problems. One approach is to place a standard umbilical artery catheter in the umbilical vein and proceed to enter the femoral vein, utilizing the percutaneous technique. If this is not attained readily, the umbilical vein catheter is replaced with the septostomy catheter and the catheter advanced gently under biplane fluoroscopy.

Thrombosis of the inferior vena cava, iliac veins, or femoral veins is the most common recognized complication following balloon atrial septostomy.[19] The exact etiology is not clear, but has been attributed to the placement of a relatively large catheter in a small vein, resulting in intimal damage and vascular stasis with subsequent thrombosis.

Malpositions of the Septostomy Catheter

The position of the balloon atrial septostomy catheter in the left atrium must be established before septostomy is performed. Physicians who perform this procedure must be aware of the potential of juxtaposition of the atrial appendages in patients with D-transposition of the great arteries, especially patients with dextrocardia.[20] When conventional criteria are used, the balloon atrial septostomy catheter may appear to be in the left atrium; however, oximetry and angiography will confirm the levoposition of the right atrial appendage (Fig. 2). Echocardiography may predict the presence of this anatomic variant, which *must* be confirmed in the catheterization laboratory.[21] The other common malposition of the

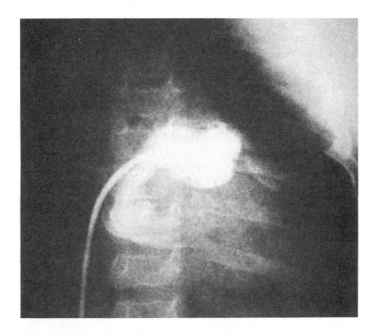

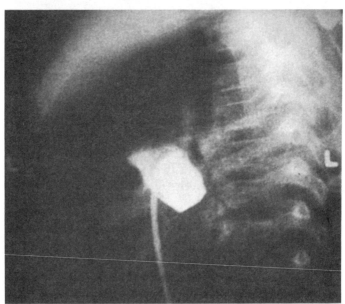

Figure 2.

septostomy catheter is its placement in the left upper pulmonary vein; slow filling of the balloon catheter will displace the balloon into the body of the left atrium. Echocardiography will identify this malposition of the balloon catheter reliably.

Precautions During Septostomy

The position of the catheter in the left atrium confirmed, the balloon is inflated with dilute angiographic material to at least a 15-mm diameter,[22] and withdrawn rapidly to the right atrium. It is extremely important to avoid introducing air bubbles when filling the balloon atrial septostomy catheter since these may embolize if the balloon ruptures. Another technical point worth mentioning is the preservation of the septostomy catheter stylette. If the balloon cannot be deflated, the first maneuver to attempt is to introduce the stylette into the catheter lumen supplying the balloon and remove any particulate matter obstructing the lumen. If it is impossible to deflate the balloon, perforating it with a transseptal needle is recommended.[23] To avoid this complication, use only clean syringes, saline, and contrast to fill the balloon.

Overdistention of the left atrium with rupture and death[24] is the most commonly reported serious complication of contemporary studies. Although the adequacy of septostomy is probably related to balloon volume at the time of balloon pullback, intracardiac trauma may result from excessive balloon volume. Particularly in the premature infant with D-transposition, the volume of the balloon must be viewed with respect to left atrial volume. By filling the balloon under echocardiographic control, the process can be visualized. Figure 3 shows the nonlinear relationship between balloon diameter and inflation volume.

Figure 2. *AP and lateral cineangiograms demonstrating left juxtaposition of the right atrial appendage in a patient with d-TGA. The leftward and somewhat posterior position of the catheter is similar to that of a catheter passed through the foramen ovale; however, presence within the right atrial appendage is confirmed by oximetry and angiography.*

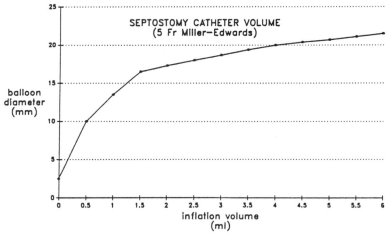

Figure 3. *The relationship between the volume of inflation and balloon diameter for the 5 F Edwards septostomy catheter is shown. The diameter increases proportional to the cube root of the volume, consistent with spherical geometry. For this reason, small increases in volume at low balloon diameters produce greater changes in diameter than similar increases in volume at greater diameter.*

Other Considerations

Dysrhythmias following balloon atrial septostomy include sinus bradycardia, advanced atrioventricular block, and supraventricular tachycardia.[25] Although the dysrhythmias usually are transient, the physician must be prepared to treat them as they occur, particularly to provide rate support in the event of bradycardia.

A final complication, difficult to define, is the inadequate balloon septostomy. As discussed, a certain balloon volume is required to produce rupture of the septum primum flap of the fossa ovalis. This must be performed as a single motion, withdrawing the catheter rapidly from the left atrium to the right atrial border of the inferior vena cava. Gradual and gentle withdrawal of the balloon across the foramen ovale results only in temporary distention of the fossa ovalis, which results in an inadequate septostomy. Also, regardless of the technique used, thick interatrial septum may make it impossible to achieve an adequate septostomy in the older infant, making blade septostomy the preferred initial approach.

Blade Atrial Septostomy

Although the efficacy of balloon atrial septostomy in the newborn is well established, a thick interatrial septum may preclude this procedure in older infants and children.[26,27] Moreover, repeat balloon septostomy is unlikely to be successful[26] and surgical creation of an atrial defect (Blalock-Hanlon procedure) carries a significant operative risk.[28,29] Given these considerations, Park and co-workers initially developed the blade atrial septostomy catheter.[30] Although technically more complex than balloon atrial septostomy, blade atrial septostomy provides the physician with greater control in the creation or enlargement of an interatrial defect with predictable success when it is performed with meticulous attention to detail.

The initial report on the clinical use of the blade septostomy catheter in 1978[31] indicated that an interatrial defect had been created successfully in seven patients, without significant complications. Following modifications in catheter design, a five institution collaborative study in which 52 patients underwent blade septostomy was reported in 1982.[32] This report described the technique of blade atrial septostomy in detail. One patient died, the right ventricle was perforated in another, and three developed neurologic complications. During the procedure, four patients required transfusion, which was attributed to a mismatch in size between catheter and percutaneous sheath.

Recently, Mullins and co-workers reported their results with blade and balloon atrial septostomy in 88 patients.[33] The blade catheter was placed in the left atrium by the transseptal technique in 41 of the 88 patients. Two deaths were reported, both in critically ill infants, and 36 patients showed significant clinical improvement. Thus, from the initial series reported, it would appear that the mortality and morbidity from blade atrial septostomy is comparable to that reported for balloon atrial septostomy.

The limited reported cases of mortality appear to be related to two specific anatomic features: (1) the unusual position of the interatrial defect resulted in blade placement adjacent to the free wall of the left atrium, and (2) a very small left atrium, the size of which was inadequate to allow safe extension of the blade catheter. The position of the interatrial defect *must* be clear to the physician before the blade catheter is extended. In our experience, it is mandatory that the anatomy of the left atrium and the position of the atrial defect be confirmed by angiography before proceeding with blade septostomy. Echocardiography may also be of assistance, especially in cases of cardiac malposition.[34] Figure 4 illustrates the posterior-superior atrial defect (sinus venosus) similar to that described in the single death in the Collaborative Study.[32] Determination of this catheter position indicates the need for transseptal placement of the blade catheter through the area of the fossa ovalis. When performing the transseptal puncture in association with blade and balloon septostomy, an atrial marker can be produced during the septostomy procedure by staining the atrial septum with contrast through the Brockenbrough needle. This permits the operator to determine the exact position of the blade catheter relative to the atrial septum during the procedure (Fig. 5).

Certain prerequisites are required prior to blade atrial septostomy. With these prerequisites the complication rate of this technique may be minimized:

1. a precise knowledge of the atrial anatomy,
2. the ability to perform transseptal catheterization,
3. an exact understanding of the mechanics of the Park blade catheter,
4. gentle manipulation and extension of the blade catheter once it is positioned in the left atrium,
5. applying gentle but steady force as the catheter is withdrawn to the right atrium, monitoring this step constantly by fluoroscopy,
6. partial extension of the blade catheter during the initial pullback, performed through an intact site in the atrial septum. This last precaution is advised because of the delicate nature of the blade apparatus.

One complication we have encountered during this procedure is the temporary inability to close the blade following pullthrough to the right atrium. This appears to have resulted from the rotation of components of the blade catheter about its axis during pullback. Once all components are realigned, the blade will close. Also, some blood loss, caused by the previously mentioned mismatch beween catheter and sheath, appears to be inevitable with this technique. Consequently, available replacement blood is mandatory.

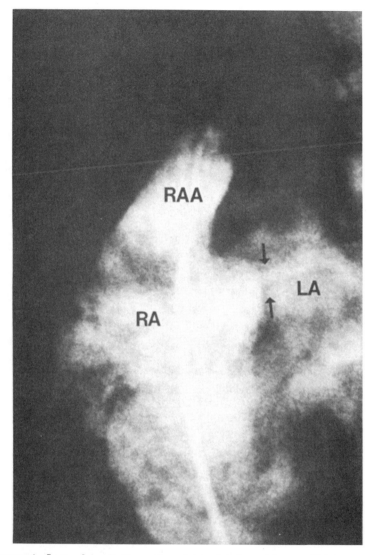

Figure 4. *Lateral projection of a right atrial angiogram (RAA) demonstrating a sinus venosus atrial septal defect (arrows) in a patient with tricuspid atresia. The angiographic catheter passes from the IVC to the right atrial (RA) appendage. A catheter passed through this defect would rest near the roof of the left atrium (LA) and pulmonary veins prohibiting safe extension of the blade catheter. Transseptal catheter passage across the fossa ovalis was performed in this case, with subsequent blade septostomy. RA = right atrium, LA = left atrium, RAA = right atrial appendage.*

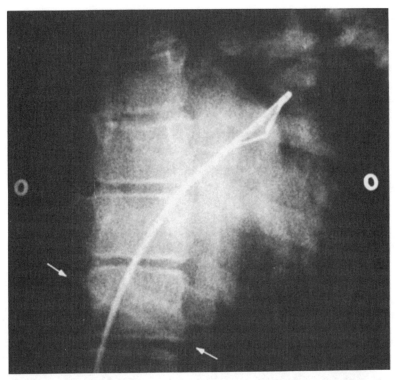

Figure 5. *Initial extension of the blade septostomy catheter within the body of an enlarged left atrium. An interatrial septal contrast stain (arrows) was injected during transseptal puncture, allowing fluoroscopic monitoring of the position of the blade catheter relative to the interatrial septum.*

Anatomy that precludes a femoral approach to catheterization (e.g., bilaterally thrombosed iliac veins, or absent infrahepatic segment of the inferior vena cava) prohibits use of this technique. Lastly, adequate patient anesthesia to eliminate excess motion during blade septostomy is mandatory. Blade septostomy is always followed by balloon atrial septostomy to ensure the creation of a maximal atrial defect.

Balloon Dilatation Procedures

Following the clinical reintroduction of the balloon angioplasty catheter treatment for congenital heart disease 5 years ago,[35] its subsequent acceptance and saftey have been both remarkable and ubiquitous. At certain centers, based on referral patterns, such procedures appear to constitute a significant percentage of all cardiac catheterizations performed.[36] Most of these procedures are still too new to identify all potential complications as well as contraindications, and significant differences in procedural technique exist.[37] Nevertheless, certain factors portending failure or complication with the commonly practiced applications appear to be emerging. Given the striking differences in success and complication rates, the various procedures will be considered separately. Limited data and experience at this time preclude discussion of all potential complications of balloon valvuloplasty of mitral or aortic stenosis.

Balloon Valvuloplasty for Pulmonary Valve Stenosis

Balloon pulmonary valvuloplasty has been established as the treatment of choice for isolated pulmonary valve stenosis beyond the neonatal period.[38] Although the exact number of patients who have undergone this procedure is unknown, there has been no reported fatality or major medical complication in an estimated 700 cases. The efficacy of the procedure also has been improved as balloons 20% to 40% larger than the pulmonary annulus have been used, compared to the initial use of balloons smaller than the pulmonary annulus.[39,40] In spite of the widespread use of this procedure, the potential for complication(s) must be kept in mind.

Infundibular Obstruction

Severe infundibular obstruction following balloon pulmonary valvuloplasty was reported by Ben-Shachar et al. in a 14-month-old child with suprasystemic right ventricular pressure preceeding valvuloplasty.[41] These authors postulate that the balloon pulmonary valvuloplasty resulted in unmasking severe infundibular stenosis, as has been observed following isolated surgical valvotomy.[42] Similar cases of increased right ventricular outflow tract gradients, which have undergone spontaneous regression following both balloon pulmonary valvuloplasty and surgical valvotomy, have been reported by other authors.[43,44] Right ventricular pressure must be determined after each balloon pulmonary valvuloplasty so that pharmacologic or surgical intervention may be employed, if indicated.[45] The potential to aggravate right ventricular outflow obstruction must be recognized and appreciated in severe pulmonary stenosis associated with a significant infundibular gradient.

Right Ventricular Outflow Tract Trauma

Balloon angioplasty catheters larger than the pulmonary valve annulus are acceptable. Experimental studies and surgical observations have provided some insight into possible complications caused by overdistension of the right ventricular outflow tract. Ring and co-workers reported the pathologic observations in newborn lambs subjected to overdilation of the pulmonary annulus.[46] Limited cardiac trauma was recognized, primarily in the right ventricle subjacent to the proximal end of the balloon. The major pathologic risk appeared to be right ventricular free-wall hemorrhage. Theoretically, such trauma has the potential to result in fibrosis and to establish an arrhythmogenic focus. The use of longer balloons was projected to result in greater trauma to this site. Surgical inspection at elective repair of associated intracardiac defects following balloon pulmonary valvuloplasty in 8 patients was reported by Wall.[47] No report of infundibular trauma or hemorrhage was indicated, although cusp avulsion, as opposed to commissural splitting, was reported in patients with infundibular stenosis. As the availability of the shorter (2–3 cm) angioplasty catheter increases, the risk of trauma to the right ventricular outflow tract may be reduced (Fig. 6). The passage of a catheter across the outflow tract following balloon pulmonary valvuloplasty should only be performed using the previously positioned guidewire (in the left pulmonary artery) due to the risk of outflow tract perforation.

Hemodynamic Consequences

During the sequence of balloon pulmonary valvuloplasty, there is an anticipated rise in right ventricular pressure and a fall in systemic arterial pressure as the pulmonary annulus is occluded. The noteworthy exception is the patient with an atrial septal defect (or patent foramen ovale). Balloon pulmonary valvuloplasty in these patients results in right-to-left shunting (orthodeoxyia) with subsequent reflex hyperventilation and sinus tachycardia, and relative

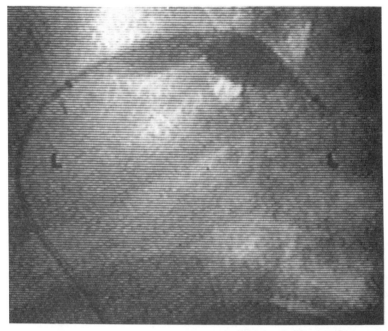

Figure 6. *Lateral fluoroscopic examination during balloon pulmonary valvuloplasty in a 6-month-old with discrete valvar pulmonic stenosis. Centering the "waist" before full inflation and relief of discrete stenosis is demonstrated. Catheter course was from the right atrium to the right ventricle, and across the pulmonary valve to the main and proximal left pulmonary artery. (The "L"s are external reference markers on the image intensifiers.)*

preservation of systemic arterial pressure. Right-to-left shunting in such patients has been documented by echocardiography[48] and presents the potential risk of paradoxical embolus during the procedure. The use of heparin in these patients is indicated, along with extreme caution to avoid air embolus. A complete right heart catheterization and probing of the atrial septum should be performed prior to balloon pulmonary valvuloplasty.

Concern regarding the hemodynamic compromise in patients undergoing balloon pulmonary valvuloplasty has led to attempts to utilize two balloons side by side, to try to split the stenotic valve along the commissural axis, while producing subtotal annular occlusion.[49] Although this technique may have greater application in balloon valvuloplasty of the aortic valve, it also provides an alternative when the diameter of a single angioplasty catheter is inadequate to perform valvuloplasty.

Dysrhythmias

Transient sinus bradycardia is an anticipated consequence during balloon pulmonary valvuloplasty. Acute distention of the right atrium and decreased perfusion of the sinus node have been suggested as mechanisms. Bradycardia may last for 30 seconds after the angioplasty catheter has been deflated. Spontaneous return to baseline heart rate or sinus tachycardia is the rule. Sustained ventricular tachycardia or ventricular fibrillation have not been reported following balloon pulmonary valvuloplasty, although frequent ventricular ectopy post procedure has been noted.[50] Prolongation of the electrocardiographic QTc interval following balloon angioplasty is recognized and continuous electrocardiographic monitoring is recommended following balloon pulmonary valvuloplasty.[51]

Vascular Injury

The introduction of the Medi-Tech (Watertown, MA) angioplasty catheter into the vein of a small child may present many of the vascular risks initially encountered during balloon atrial septostomy. Although the technique of balloon pulmonary valvuloplasty is well described, attention to the details of complete balloon deflation during its introduction and removal may reduce vascular trauma and the risk of femoral vein injury. Gradual dilation of the femoral vein with a dilator and heparin administration have been advocated. To date, no reports of significant vascular injury have been published. Because a vascular sheath is not used during this procedure, some bleeding should be anticipated during catheter exchange. Femoral arterial pressure should be monitored using the contralateral artery to avoid the risk of iatrogenic arteriovenous fistula.[52] Ipsilateral femoral artery and venous catheterization may also damage the arterial wall by compression between the two catheters during extensive manipulation of the large pulmonary valvuloplasty catheter.

Balloon Angioplasty of Stenotic or Hypoplastic Pulmonary Arteries

In distinction to balloon pulmonary valvuloplasty, balloon angioplasty of hypoplastic or stenotic pulmonary arteries remains a difficult procedure technically, with a recognized significant complication rate. Encouraged by the results of angioplasty in experimental branch stenosis in newborn lambs, clinical trials in this area were begun in 1981.[53,54] In the largest series to date, Ring and co-workers reported results in 52 attempted dilations.[55] Success was reported in 50% of patients undergoing this procedure, with one mortality related to the procedure. Subsequent data indicate that a mortality rate of 1% to 2% was associated with this procedure.[36] However, this risk must be viewed with consideration of the fact that operative management of lesions beyond the mediastinum are largely unsuccessful.

Given the definite risk, patient selection for balloon angioplasty must be precise. The procedure appears more successful in patients younger than 4 years of age, and in whom the stenotic site is not secondary to a previous vascular anastomosis. The current indications for this procedure are cyanosis, right heart failure, or systemic right ventricular pressure secondary to pulmonary arterial stenosis. Specific patients likely to benefit from this procedure are those who have undergone a Fontan procedure, or in whom there is a marked disparity of pulmonary blood flow between the lungs.

In the series reported by Ring, the one mortality was related to rupture of the balloon following inflation, with subsequent rupture of the pulmonary artery. A second case of pulmonary artery rupture was recognized intraoperatively and repaired without complication. Rocchini and co-workers subsequently reported perforation of a pulmonary artery during balloon angioplasty.[56] They also reported a second patient who developed severe hemoptysis and hypoxemia and subsequently expired following operative dilation of a stenotic pulmonary artery.

With experience, angiographic definition and catheter techniques have improved and recommendations have evolved which may improve patient selection and reduce complications. Prior to catheterization, a lung perfusion scan is performed to assess the inequalities of flow produced by the stenotic lesions. Precise angiographic definition of selective pulmonary arteries is performed, with an attempt to define the most severe stenosis, which is the first artery in which dilation is attempted. As passage of the angioplasty catheter may result in total obstruction of right ventricular output, passage over a nonlooped guidewire to the branch pulmonary artery is performed without first inflating the balloon. Once the diameter of the stenotic site is defined and measured, a balloon diameter three to four times the size of the narrowest site is utilized and the balloon centered at the narrowest segment along the axis of the balloon. The balloon is then inflated at low pressure to define the "waist"; subsequent inflation pressures should be 5 to 7 atmospheres for 30 seconds or until hemodynamic compromise occurs (Fig. 7).

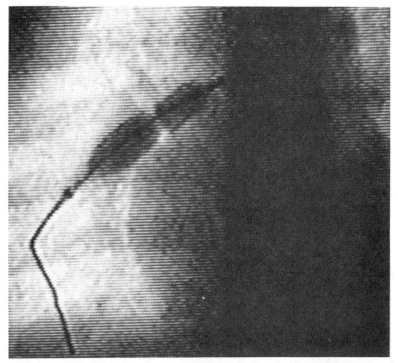

Figure 7. *AP fluoroscopic examination during balloon dilatation of peripheral pulmonic arterial stenosis. Following catheter passage from the right atrium, right ventricle, main and right pulmonary arteries, the catheter was centered across a distal arterial stenosis, and inflated to a volume adequate to produce a diameter four times the estimated diameter of the site of stenosis.*

Morphologic changes in the pulmonary arteries following balloon angioplasty have revealed intimal and medial tears, with subsequent formation of scar tissue.[57] Given the preservation of vascular integrity solely by the adventitia, catheter passage beyond the point of acute angioplasty should only be performed over a prepositioned guidewire. The risk of vascular perforation cannot be minimized. As a related complication, hemoptysis has been observed during pulmonary artery angioplasty and may reflect either rupture of collateral bronchial vessels or vasa vasorum.

Acute thrombosis of a pulmonary artery complicating angioplasty has been treated successfully with streptokinase.[58] The authors postulate that this unique complication was related to the sluggish, nonpulsatile flow in this patient following a Fontan procedure.

Femoral or iliac vein thrombosis has been recognized following pulmonary artery dilatation. Due to the significant catheter manipulation required during these cases and the relatively long duration of the procedure, systemic heparinization is recommended in any patient with right-to-left intracardiac shunting to reduce the risk of thromboembolic events. Individual judgement must be exercised in patients without this substrate, given the risk of significant bleeding associated with this procedure.

It must be recognized that certain forms of pulmonary arterial stenosis are not amenable to balloon dilatation. Nonetheless, given the lack of therapeutic alternatives, balloon angioplasty of stenotic or hypoplastic pulmonary arteries remains the only option for this difficult patient group.

Balloon Angioplasty of Coarctation of the Aorta

Although surgical repair of coarctation of the aorta has been performed since 1945, a significant incidence of recurrence, morbidity, and mortality is recognized, particularly if repair is performed in infancy.[59-61] Guided by postmortem and experimental studies indicating that certain forms of aortic coarctation may be amenable to balloon dilation,[62,63] attempts to relieve these congenital stenoses by angioplasty have evolved. Subsequently, differing success and complication rates have become apparent for angioplasty of native and recurrent coarctation with the morphology of the coarctation (discrete versus long segment) evolving as a significant factor as well.

The lack of long-term follow-up and the conflicting results currently available make it somewhat difficult to evaluate the results and complications of this procedure. The initial attempts at coarctation angioplasty in young infants were largely unsuccessful and were associated with two procedure-related deaths due to aortic tear or perforation.[64,65] Subsequent reports of angioplasty of recurrent coarctation were more encouraging, although one patient died from an unexplained episode of ventricular fibrillation 6 hours postprocedure.[66] Recognized procedural complications and sequelae, along with long-term concerns, have resulted in a somewhat restricted application of balloon angioplasty in the patient with coarctation of the aorta.

Coarctation angioplasty requires arterial catheterization with relatively large-diameter catheters. The risk of arterial damage or thrombosis is implicit in this procedure, as recently emphasized by Wessel, who reported a 39% incidence of femoral artery thrombosis in patients undergoing transarterial balloon dilation procedures.[67] It is postulated that initial arterial trauma is central to subsequent thrombus formation,[68] although the large size and irregular surface of the deflated catheters may be responsible for vascular trauma. Systemic heparinization following placement of hemodynamic catheters is indicated,[69] and careful pulse monitoring post angioplasty is mandatory as medical or surgical treatment of an ischemic limb may be necessary. Likewise, the risk of an arterial thromboembolic event increases as the duration of the procedure lengthens.

Since the goal of angioplasty is to produce an intimal and partial medial tear,[70] it is mandatory that the diameter of the coarctation and proximal aorta be defined precisely (Fig. 8). An angioplasty catheter balloon with a diameter 1–2 mm less than that of the proximal aorta appears to be the best size by current experience. Experimental assessment of aortic wall tears in infants indicates that an oversized balloon may rupture the aorta before bursting and that a balloon equal in size to the aorta may result in aortic dissection in the event the balloon ruptures.[71]

Given the risk of balloon rupture, inflation limited to 3 to 4 atmospheres is recommended, unless the stenotic area is eliminated at a lower inflation pressure. Once again, it is mandatory to center the balloon precisely.

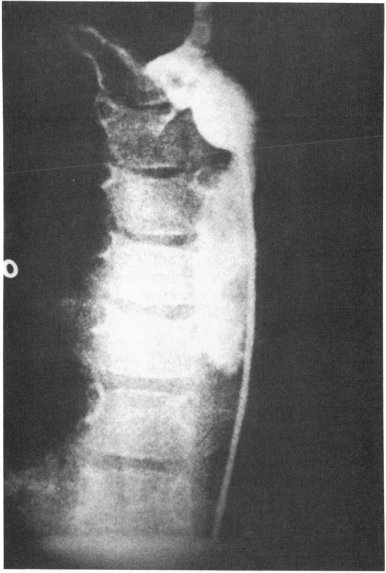

Figure 8. *Precise determination of the diameter of the proximal aorta prior to balloon dilatation is of paramount importance. Balloon diameter should be restricted to 2 mm less than the proximal aortic diameter, with inflation pressure limited to 3 to 4 atmospheres. This AP aortogram was referenced to an external grid not depicted in this illustration.*

Following the angioplasty procedure, any catheter manipulation in the aorta must be performed over an exchange wire.[72] Once intimal and medial tearing have occurred, guidewires and catheters may perforate this site with minimal resistance.

Considerable concern is present regarding late anuerysm formation following dilation of aortic coarctation in patients with previously unoperated coarctation.[73,74] The incidence and long-term significance remain to be determined, but indicate the need for re-evaluation of this procedure, particularly in the unoperated patient. The eccentric narrowing of a native coarctation may represent a less favorable substrate for dilation due to the transmission of balloon pressure to friable contralateral ductal tissue. Conversely, the scar tissue surrounding a previously operated coarctation site may be a safety factor during angioplasty, limiting any potential bleeding should aortic disruption occur.

Potentially, paradoxic hypertension and mesenteric arteritis may follow coarctation angioplasty, as has been reported following surgery.[75] The mechanisms of the postcoarctectomy syndrome are not completely delineated, and may relate to the duration of aortic cross-clamp time, as opposed to a response to increased pulse pressure.

The current status of balloon angioplasty of aortic coarctation must be viewed with respect to surgical alternatives, and an appreciation of the unknown long-term follow-up. As the risks of surgical repair of infantile coarctation are low (2% to 3%) and the long-term efficacy and complications of balloon angioplasty are unknown, operative repair would appear preferable in this patient group.[76] Conversely, the higher surgical risks associated with recurrent coarctation along with recent angioplasty results would suggest balloon dilation as the preferred therapeutic option in these patients.[77]

Endomyocardial Biopsy in Infants and Children

Endomyocardial biopsy has become the standard modality for the diagnosis of rejection following orthotopic heart transplantation. However, only limited experience and data are available in the literature regarding pediatric recipients. Endomyocaridal biopsy is described in detail in Chapter 6. The discussion in this chapter is limited to the unique aspects and results in pediatric patients.

Transvascular endomyocardial biopsy in infants and children was first reported by Lurie and co-workers in 1978.[78] Utilizing preformed catheters shaped to conform to intravascular anatomy, successful biopsies were obtained from the right ventricle consistently. However, minor complications or inability to attain retrograde access to the left ventricle occurred in three of ten patients. Ventricular ectopy, blood loss, or inability to obtain an adequate specimen were reported. Subsequently, Rios and co-workers reported results utilizing a femoral approach to introduce a long sheath to either the right or left ventricle, with subsequent introduction of the bioptome.[79] Utilizing a 6-French diameter bioptome, no complications were recognized in the first 20 patients, with a 95% success rate. All left ventricular samples were obtained by transseptal access to the left ventricle.[80] Other series have reported histologically adequate specimens in over 90% of biopsies.[81,82] Wiles has reported 11 serial biopsies in a single patient following heart transplantation at 8 months of age.[83] Management of acute rejection episodes in this patient was directed by biopsy results, because noninvasive testing and clinical assessment were not diagnostic.

The reported complications associated with endomyocardial biopsy in children have included ventricular perforation with subsequent tamponade, pneumothorax, biopsy of the tricuspid chordae, and transient arrhythmias.[81–83] Air embolism and transient nerve palsies have been reported in adults but not in children. The types and rates of biopsy-related complications in children and adults must be viewed considering the different vascular approaches (femoral versus jugular).

Undoubtedly there will be growing application of this technique in the near future as orthotopic heart transplantation increases in children. The indications for endomyocardial biopsy in infants and children with dilated cardiomyopathy are not clearly established, as results in these patients indicate ultrastructural abnormalities rather than an acute inflammatory process.[82]

Other current indications for endomyocardial biopsy include anathracycline cardiotoxicity and myocardial storage disease. Very limited data currently exist regarding the use of biopsy in these settings in pediatric patients.

Transvenous Cardiac Pacemakers

Temporary Cardiac Pacing

The ability to provide chronotropic support is a basic skill required of all pediatric cardiologists performing catheterization in infants and children. This skill is mandatory because the ability of the newborn's heart to increase stroke volume is limited and cardiac output therefore is dependent on heart rate. Although infrequent, specific complications are recognizably associated with the use of temporary pacing leads placed in a young patient.

In a series of 18 patients reported by Harris, two (11%) developed right ventricular perforation within 48 hours of placement.[84] This is contrasted with the 2% to 4% incidence of perforation reported in much larger adult series.[85,86] In both cases of perforation, the catheters were withdrawn without significant complication and no significant hemodynamic compromise occurred. It is postulated that the small 4 French pacing catheter may be predisposed to ventricular perforation. The evaluation of ventricular perforation by two-dimensional echocardiography has been reported[87] and should be considered in unexplained loss of capture of the myocardium or when a right bundle branch block paced morphology evolves, implying pacing from a left ventricular site.

Venous thrombosis following prolonged cannulation may occur in temporary transvenous pacing, along with a predisposition to ascending infection, especially if the femoral vein is utilized. Sudden loss of capture due to a change in patient position may result in profound bradycardia or asystole, as there may be overdrive suppression of the functioning escape pacemaker sites (Fig. 9). Given the above considerations, temporary transvenous pacing must be viewed as a limited-duration procedure, with definite guidelines established to indicate placement of a permanent pacing unit.

Specific emergencies may require transthoracic wire placement for cardiac pacing,[88] although this is uncommon. Pharmacologic restoration of an acceptable heart rate should always be attempted before transthoracic pacing, given the associated risks of coronary artery laceration and hemopericardium. It appears that external cardiac pacing will supplant transthoracic pacing during this decade, given the recent improvements in this technology (Chapter 5).

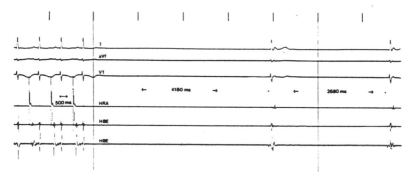

Figure 9. *Prolonged asystole occurred after atrial pacing was terminated during the evaluation of AV node conduction. Junctional escape rhythm with a His bundle electrogram preceding each QRS is evident. 1, aVF, V1 = surface electrocardiographic leads. HRA = high right atrium, HBE = His bundle electrogram. Time lines = 1 sec.*

Lastly significant electrolyte disturbance, particularly hypokalemia may preclude ventricular capture during attempts at emergency pacing, regardless of the method of lead placement.[89]

Permanent Transvenous Pacemakers

Among the interventional procedures performed by the pediatric cardiologist, the implantation of permanent transvenous pacemakers demands a somewhat different set of skills and training than the previously discussed procedures. The number of centers at which transvenous implants are performed in children is not documented but the numbers tend to be smaller than those for other interventions. Current experience confirms the safety and long-term efficacy of this approach to cardiac pacing in children,[90–92] with superior threshold and sensing lead characteristics compared to epicardial placement.[93] Initial concerns regarding lead fracture or dislodgement due to growth have not been confirmed, even with follow-up extending to 15 years.[94] In general, the indications for permanent cardiac pacing in children are similar to those for adults, although there are exceptions. Most transvenous pacemaker implants in children are for symptomatic bradydysrhythmias following surgery for congenital heart disease.

Before proceeding with endocardial lead placement, it is necessary to confirm vascular patency from the access site to the right atrium in the patient with prior surgery for congenital heart disease. If the patient has not undergone recent catheterization, a venogram, utilizing the antecubital vein of the ipsilateral side of the anticipated implant, may be performed to confirm vascular patency (Fig. 10). This is particularly important in patients who have undergone a

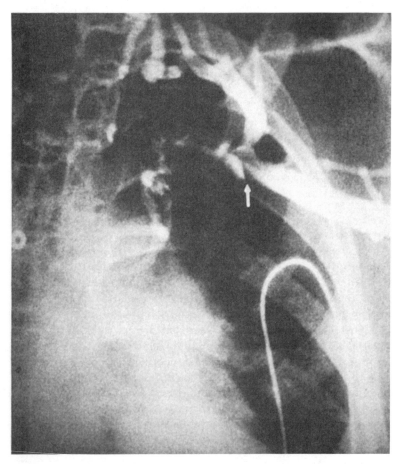

Figure 10. *Peripheral left antecubital venogram (AP projection) preceding transvenous pacemaker placement in a patient following the Mustard procedure. Left subclavian vein occlusion precluding the use of this site and collateral venous drainage are identified.*

prior Mustard procedure due to the frequency of systemic venous obstruction.[95]

The subclavian introducer technique has been the author's preferred approach to vascular access in children; however, cephalic vein cutdown is preferred by some.[96] Significant care must be exercised during the subclavian entry to avoid lung laceration or arterial puncture. The possibility of pneumothorax or hemothorax are inherent in the subclavian approach, and require evaluation both during and post procedure (Fig. 11). In small children the placement of a small Teflon wire or catheter in the subclavian vein, utilizing femoral or antecubital access, or limited angiography may guide subclavian vein entry under fluoroscopy (Fig. 12). This technique will permit subclavian entry almost invariably on the first attempt.

Cardiac dysrhythmias may occur during implantation, including both ventricular fibrillation and asystole.[97] Patients with significant bradycardia may exhibit temporary failure of intrinsic escape rhythm following termination of pacing to determine threshold for capture. Thus, measurement of the sensed atrial or ventricular electrogram should be performed before pacing is initiated.

Infection of the pacemaker pocket, endocardial lead, or both is estimated to occur in 1% to 13% of implants,[98–100] and represents the most serious complication of this procedure. Infection of the pacemaker pocket appears most commonly at the site of entry, with subsequent involvement of the pacing lead. Active infection mandates removal of the pacing system[101,102] either by thoracotomy or the transvascular approach.[103]

Thrombosis of the veins of the upper arm and shoulder may occur in up to 30% of patients with transvenous pacemakers; however, clinical evidence of peripheral edema is less than 5%.[104] Right atrial thrombi, and pulmonary embolism complicating permanent cardiac pacing have been the subject of many case reports.[105–107] Pathologic study indicates that thrombus formation around the pacing lead occurs soon after implantation, with subsequent endothelialization.[108] The actual incidence of this problem in children remains undefined. The use of transvenous polyurethane pacing leads may result in a reduced incidence of venous thrombosis.

Prophylaxis against endocarditis appears reasonable in the presence of an intravascular catheter. Definitive data are not available regarding this issue; however in terms of intracardiac position

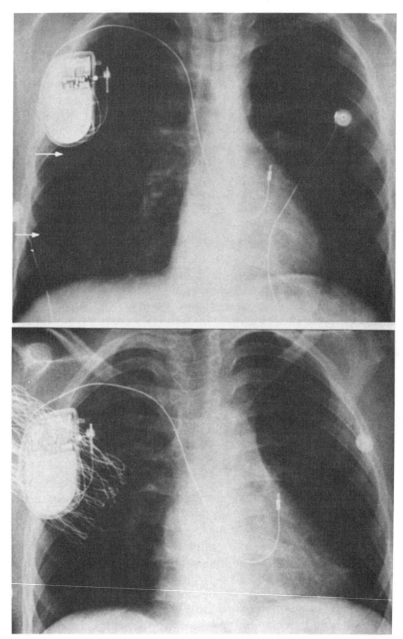

Figure 11.

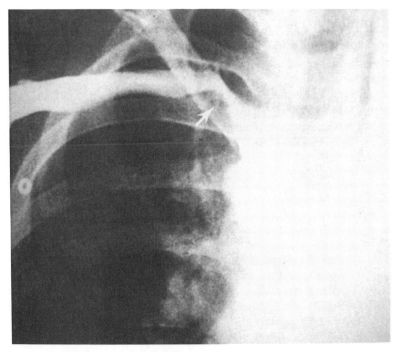

Figure 12. *Same patient as in Figure 10. In spite of the moderate stenosis of the right subclavian vein, subclavian puncture and pacemaker lead placement were performed without difficulty following angiographic vascular definition.*

Figure 11. *Twelve hours following transvenous AAI pacemaker placement, this patient became short of breath and demonstrated phrenic nerve pacing (top). The right pneumothorax and mediastinal shift present on this AP chest roentgenogram were not present immediately postimplant (bottom). Pacemaker lead placement is in the posterior left atrium following the Mustard procedure.*

and Venturi effects, the pacing electrode may result in hemodynamic alterations similar to common mild valvular abnormalities.[109]

Conclusions

The diagnostic and therapeutic approaches to the patient with congenital heart disease have evolved rapidly in the current decade. Precise noninvasive diagnosis with complimentary axial cineangiography is feasible, even in the premature infant. Primary intracardiac repair of congenital heart defects in infancy has become the operative standard in many defects. Currently, an increasing number of congenital heart defects have been treated with catheter directed interventions.

The improvement and development of new therapeutic catheter procedures for the treatment of congenital heart defects will continue to rely on research and technology dedicated to the cardiovascular system of the young patient, along with clinical follow-up of the current procedures. Some of the procedures discussed in this chapter may be abandoned in the future if late onset complications or unsatisfactory long-term results are found. New procedures, not described in this chapter, also will likely be developed and perfected in the near future.[110] The current status of interventional procedures for congenital heart disease cannot be considered to be perfected at this time. As any of the interventional procedures discussed in this chapter may incur patient morbidity or potential mortality, they must be used with discretion.[111] Increased experience and the reporting of early and late complications associated with these new procedures will benefit both the patient and the physician. An awareness of potential complications and continued technologic improvement are vital to progress in this area.

References

1. Rubeo-Alvarez V, Limon-Lason A: Treatment of pulmonary valvular stenosis and tricuspid stenosis with a modified cardiac catheter. Proceedings of the First National Conference on Cardiovascular Disease. Washington, DC, 1950.
2. Rashkind WJ, Miller WW: Creation of an atrial septal defect without thoracotomy: a palliative approach to complete transposition of the great arteries. J Am Med Assoc 196:991, 1966.

3. Rashkind WJ: Balloon atrioseptostomy revisited: the first fifteen years. Int J Cardiol 4:369, 1983.
4. Rashkind WJ: Interventional cardiac catheterization in congenital heart disease. In Cardiovascular Clinics: Invasive Cardiology. Philadelphia, FA Davis, 1983, p 303.
5. Moore JW, Bricker JT, Mullins CE, et al: Infusion of blood from pericardial sac into femoral vein: a technique for survival until operative closure of a cardiac perforation during balloon septostomy. Am J Cardiol 56:494, 1985.
6. Blanchard WB, Knauf DG, Victoria BE: Interatrial groove tear: an unusual complication of balloon atrial septostomy. Pediatr Cardiol 4:149, 1983.
7. Rashkind WJ: The complications of balloon atrioseptostomy. J Pediatr 44:649, 1970.
8. Scott O: A new complication of Rashkind balloon septostomy. Arch Dis Child 45:716, 1970.
9. Ellison RC, Plauth WH, Gazzaniga AB, et al: Inability to deflate catheter balloon: a complication of balloon atrial septostomy. J Pediatr 76:604, 1970.
10. Hawker RE, Celermajer JM, Cartmill TB, et al: Thrombosis of the inferior vena cava following balloon septostomy in transposition of the great arteries. Am Heart J 82:593, 1971.
11. Vogel JHK: Balloon embolization during atrial septostomy. Circulation 42:155, 1970.
12. Ehmke DA, Durnin RE, Lauer RM: Intra-abdominal hemorrhage complicating a balloon atrial septostomy for transposition of the great arteries. Pediatrics 45:289, 1970.
13. Powell TG, Dewey M, West CR, et al: Fate of infants with transposition of the great arteries in relation to balloon atrial septostomy. Br Heart J 51:371, 1984.
14. Bierman FZ, Williams RG: Prospective diagnosis of d-transposition of the great arteries in neonates by sub-xiphoid two-dimensional echocardiography. Circulation 60:1496, 1979.
15. Bass NM, Roche AHG, Brandt PWT, et al: Echocardiography in assessment of infants with complete d-transposition of great arteries. Br Heart J 40:1165, 1978.
16. Hurwitz RA, Girod DA: Percutaneous balloon atrial septostomy in infants with transposition of the great arteries. Am Heart J 91:618, 1976.
17. Jarmakani JM: Catheterization and angiography. In Adams FH, Emmanoulides GC (eds): Heart disease in Infants, Children and Adolescents, 3rd Ed. Baltimore, Williams and Wilkins, 1983, p 83.
18. Newfeld EA, Purcell C, Paul MH, et al: Transumbilical balloon atrial septostomy in 16 infants with transposition of the great arteries. Pediatrics 56:495, 1975.
19. Keane JF, Lang P, Newberger J, et al: Iliac vein-inferior caval thrombosis after cardiac catheterization in infancy. Pediatr Cardiol 1:257, 1980.

20. Tyrrell MJ, Moes CAF: Congenital levoposition of the right atrial appendage: its relevance to balloon atrial septostomy. Am J Dis Child 121:508, 1971.
21. Rice MJ, Tajik AJ, Hagler JB, et al: Echocardiographic recognition of left juxtaposition of the atrial appendages. J Am Coll Cardiol 1:1330, 1983.
22. Fisher EA, Paul MH: Transpostion of the great arteries: recognition and management. Cardiovasc Clin 2:211, 1970.
23. Hohn AR, Webb HM: Balloon deflation failure: a hazard of "medical" atrial septostomy. Am Heart J 83:389, 1972.
24. Sondheimer HM, Kavey RW, Blackman MS: Fatal overdistention of an atrioseptostomy catheter. Pediatr Cardiol 2:225, 1982.
25. Cohn HE, Freed MD, Hellerbrand WF, et al: Complications and mortality associated with cardiac catheterization in infants under one year: a prospective study. Pediatr Cardiol 6:123, 1985.
26. Baker F, Baker L, Zoltun R, et al: Effectiveness of the Rashkind procedure in transposition of the great arteries in infants. Circulation 43 (Suppl 1):I-1, 1971.
27. Meng CCL, Wells CR, Valdes-Pena M, et al: The anatomy of the foramen ovale in relation to the balloon atrial septostomy. (abstract) Pediatr Res 7:304, 1973.
28. Gutgesell HP, Garson AT, McNamara DG: Prognosis for the newborn with transposition of the great arteries. Am J Cardiol 44:96, 1979.
29. Litwin SB, Plauth WH, Jones JE, et al: Appraisal of surgical atrial septectomy for transposition of the great arteries. Circulation 43 and 44 (Suppl I):I-7, 1971.
30. Park SC, Zuberbuhler JR, Neches WH, et al: A new atrial septostomy technique. Cathet Cardiovasc Diagn 1:195, 1975.
31. Park SC, Neches WH, Zuberbuhler JR, et al: Clinical use of the blade atrial septostomy. Circulation 58:600, 1978.
32. Park SC: Blade atrial septostomy: collaborative study. Circulation 66:258, 1982.
33. Vick GW, Mullins CE, Nihill MR, et al: Blade and balloon atrial septostomy after transseptal atrial puncture. (abstract) J Am Coll Cardiol 7:117A, 1986.
34. Lin AE, DiSessa TG, Williams RG: Balloon and blade atrial septostomy facilitated by two-dimensional echocardiography. Am J Cardiol 57:273, 1986.
35. Kan JS, White RI Jr, Mitchell SE, et al: Percutaneous balloon valvuloplasty: a new method for treating congenital pulmonary valve stenosis. N Engl J Med 307:540, 1982.
36. Lock JE, Keane JF, Fellows KE: The use of catheter intervention procedures for congenital heart disease. J Am Coll Cardiol 7:1420, 1986.
37. Yeager SB: Occlusion time and inflation pressure in pulmonary valvuloplasty. Am J Cardiol 55:619, 1985.
38. Radtke W, Keane JF, Fellows KE, et al: Percutaneous balloon valvotomy of congenital pulmonary stenosis using oversized balloons. J Am Coll Cardiol 8:809, 1986.

39. Kan JS, White RI, Mitchell SE, et al: Percutaneous transluminal balloon valvuloplasty for pulmonary valve stenosis. Circulation 69:554, 1984.
40. Rocchini AP, Kveselis DA, Crowley D, et al: Percutaneous balloon valvuloplasty for treatment of congenital pulmonary valvular stenosis in children. J Am Coll Cardiol 3:1005, 1984.
41. Ben-Shachar G, Cohen M, Sivakoff MC, et al: Development of infundibular obstruction after percutaneous pulmonary balloon valvuloplasty. J Am Coll Cardiol 5:754, 1985.
42. Griffith BP, Hardesty RL, Siewers RD, et al: Pulmonary valvulotomy alone for pulmonary stenosis: results in children with and without muscular infundibular hypertrophy. J Thorac Cardiovasc Surg 83:577, 1982.
43. Currie PJ, Fyfe DA, Seward JB, et al: Acute subpulmonary stenosis following pulmonary valvuloplasty: serial noninvasive 2D/doppler echocardiographic assessment. Echocardiography 3:151, 1986.
44. Arendrup HC, Kruse-Anderson S, Alstrup P: Regression of infundibular hypertrophy after pulmonary valvulotomy without myocardial resection. Scand J Thorac Cardiovasc Surg 17:243, 1983.
45. Moulaert AJ, Buis-Liem TN, Glendo WC: The post valvulotomy propanolol test to determine reversibility in pulmonary stenosis. J Thorac Cardiovasc Surg 71:577,1982.
46. Ring JC, Kulik TJ, Burke B, et al: Overdilation of the pulmonary valve annulus with angioplasty balloons in the normal lamb. (abstract) Circulation 68 (Suppl):III-394, 1983.
47. Wall JT, Lababidi Z, Curtis JJ, et al: Assessment of percutaneous balloon pulmonary and aortic valvuloplasty. J Thorac Cardiovasc Surg 88:352, 1984.
48. Shuck JW, McCormack DJ, Cohen IS, et al: Percutaneous balloon valvuloplasty of the pulmonary valve: role of right to left shunting through a patent foramen ovale. J Am Coll Cardiol 4:132, 1984.
49. Butto F, Amplatz K, Bass JL: Geometry of the proximal pulmonary trunk during dilation with two balloons. Am J Cardiol 58:380, 1986.
50. Kveselis DA, Rocchini AP, Snider R, et al: Results of balloon valvuloplasty in the treatment of congenital valvar pulmonary stenosis in children. Am J Cardiol 56:527, 1985.
51. Martin GR, Stanger P: Transient prolongation of the QTc interval after balloon valvuloplasty and angioplasty in children. Am J Cardiol 58:1233, 1986.
52. Kron J, Sutherland D, Rosch J, et al: Arteriovenous fistula: a rare complication of arterial puncture of cardiac catheterization. Am J Cardiol 55:1445, 1985.
53. Lock JE, Niemi T, Einzig S, et al: Transvenous angioplasty of experimental branch pulmonary artery stenosis in newborn lambs. Circulation 64:886, 1981.
54. Lock JE, Castaneda-Zuniga WR, Fuhrman BP, et al: Balloon dilation angioplasty of hypoplastic and stenotic pulmonary arteries. Circulation 67:962, 1983.
55. Ring JC, Bass JL, Marvin W, et al: Management of congenital stenosis

of a branch pulmonary artery with balloon dilation angioplasty. J Thorac Cardiovasc Surg 90:35, 1985.

56. Rocchini AP, Kveselis D, Dick M, et al: Use of balloon angioplasty to treat peripheral pulmonary stenosis. Am J Cardiol 54:1069, 1984.

57. Edwards BS, Lucas RV, Lock JE, et al: Morphologic changes in the pulmonary arteries after percutaneous balloon angioplasty for pulmonary arterial stenosis. Circulation 71:195, 1985.

58. DiSessa TG, Yeatman LA, Williams RG, et al: Thrombosis complicating balloon angioplasty of left pulmonary artery after Fontan's procedure: successful treatment with intravenous streptokinase. Am J Cardiol 55:510, 1985.

59. Moss AJ, Adams FH, O'Loughlin BJ, et al: The growth of the normal aorta and of anastomotic sites in infants following surgical resection of coarctation of the aorta. Circulation 19:338, 1959.

60. Pelletier G, Davignon A, F-Ethier M, et al: Coarctation of the aorta in infancy: a postoperative follow-up. J Thorac Cardiovasc Surg 57:171, 1969.

61. Hesslien PS, MacNamara DG, Morriss MJH, et al: Comparison of resection versus patch aortoplasty for repair of coarctation of the aorta in infants and children. Circulation 64:164, 1981.

62. Sos T, Sniderman KW, Retter-Sos B: Percutaneous transluminal dilatation of coarctation of the aorta postmortem. Lancet 2:970, 1979.

63. Lock JE, Castenada-Zuniga WR, Bass L, et al: Balloon dilatation of excised aortic coarctation. Radiology 143:689, 1982.

64. Finley JP, Beaulieu RG, Nanton MA: Balloon catheter dilatation of coarctation of the aorta in young infants. Br Heart J 50:411, 1983.

65. Singer MI, Rowen M, Dorsey TJ: Transluminal aortic balloon angioplasty for coarctation of the aorta in the newborn. Am Heart J 103:131, 1982.

66. Kan JS, White RI, Mitchell SE, et al: Treatment of restenosis of coarctation by percutaneous transluminal angioplasty. Circulation 68:1087, 1983.

67. Wessel DL, Keane JF, Felloows KE, et al: Fibrinolytic therapy for femoral arterial thrombosis after cardiac catheterization in infants and children. Am J Cardiol 58:347, 1986.

68. Mortensonn W, Halbook T, Lundstrum NR: Percutaneous catheterization of the femoral vessels in children. Pediatr Radiol 4:1, 1975.

69. Freed MD, Keane JF, Rosenthal A: The use of heparin to prevent arterial thrombosis after percutaneous cardiac catheterization in children. Circulation 50:565, 1974.

70. Mitchell SE, Kan JS, White RI: Interventional techniques in congenital heart disease. Semin Roentgenol 20:290, 1985.

71. Waller BF, Girod DA, Dillon JC: Transverse aortic wall tears in infants after balloon angioplasty for aortic valve stenosis. J Am Coll Cardiol 4:1235, 1984.

72. Lababidi ZA, Daskalopoulis DA, Stoekle H: Transluminal balloon coarctation angioplasty: experience with 27 patients. Am J Cardiol 54:1288, 1984.

73. Marvin WJ, Mahoney LT: Balloon angioplasty of unoperated coarctation in young children. (abstract) J Am Coll Cardiol 5:405, 1985.

74. Marvin WJ, Mahoney LT, Rose EF: Pathologic sequelae of balloon dilation angioplasty for unoperated coarctation of the aorta in children. (abstract) J Am Coll Cardiol 7:117, 1986.
75. Sealy WC, Harris JS, Young WG: Paradoxical hypertension following resection of coarctation of the aorta. Surgery 42:135, 1957.
76. deLeval M: Coarctation of the aorta and interruption of the aortic arch. In Stark J, deLeval M (eds): Surgery for Congenital Heart Defects. Orlando, FL, Grune and Stratton, 1983, p 213.
77. Rocchini AP, Kveselis D: The use of balloon angioplasty in the pediatric patient. Pediatr Clin N Am 31:1293, 1984.
78. Lurie PR, Fujita M, Neustien HB: Transvascular endomyocardial biopsy in infants and small children: description of a new technique. Am J Cardiol 42:453, 1978.
79. Rios B, Nihill MR, Mullins CE: Left ventricular endomyocardial biopsy in children with the transseptal long sheath technique. Cathet Cardiovasc Diagn 10:417, 1984.
80. Mullins CE: Transseptal left heart catheterization: experience with a new technique in 520 pediatric and adult patients. Pediatr Cardiol 4:156, 1983.
81. Alboliras ET, Driscoll DJ, Mair DD, et al: Endomyocardial biopsy in infants and children. (Abstract) Am Heart J 110:710, 1985.
82. Lewis AB, Neustien HB, Takahashi M, et al: Findings on endomyocardial biopsy in infants and children with dilated cardiomyopathy. Am J Cardiol 55:143, 1985.
83. Wiles HB, Bricker JT, Cooley DA, et al: Repeated endomyocardial biopsy without complication in an infant after heart transplantation. J Thorac Cardiovasc Surg 91:637, 1986.
84. Harris JP, Nanda NC, Moxley R, et al: Myocardial perforation due to temporary transvenous pacing catheters in pediatric patients. Cathet Cardiovasc Diagn 10:329, 1984.
85. Hynes JK, Holmes DR, Harrison CE: Five year experience with temporary pacemaker therapy in the coronary care unit. Mayo Clin Proc 58:122, 1983.
86. Austin JL, Preis LK, Crampton RS, et al: Analysis of pacemaker malfunction and complications of temporary pacing in the coronary care unit. Am J Cardiol 49:301, 1982.
87. Gondi B, Nanda NC: Real-time, two-dimensional echocardiographic features of pacemaker perforation. Circulation 64:97, 1981.
88. Morriss JH, Gillette PC, Barrett FF: Atrioventricular block complicating meningitis: treatment with emergency cardiac pacing. Pediatrics 58:866, 1976.
89. O'Reilly MV, Murniaghan DP, Williams MB: Transvenous pacemaker failure induced by hyperkalemia. J Am Med Assoc 228:326, 1974.
90. Gillette PC, Shannon C, Blair H, et al: Transvenous pacing in pediatric patients. Am Heart J 105:843, 1983.
91. Hayes DL, Holmes DR, Maloney DJ, et al: Permanent endocardial pacing in pediatric patients. J Thorac Cardiovasc Surg 85:618, 1983.
92. Young D: Permanent pacemaker implantation in children: current status and future considerations. PACE 4:61, 1981.
93. Henglein D, Gillette PC, Shannon C, et al: Long-term follow-up of

pulse width thresholds of transvenous and myoepicardial leads. PACE 7:203, 1984.

94. Epstein ML, Knauf DG, Alexander JA: Long-term follow-up of transvenous cardiac pacing in children. Am J Cardiol 57:889, 1986.

95. Gillette PC, Wampler DG, Shannon C, et al: Use of cardiac pacing after the Mustard operation for transposition of the great arteries. J Am Coll Cardiol 7:138, 1986.

96. Littleford PO, Parsonnet V, Spector SD: Method for the rapid and atraumatic insertion of permanent endocardial pacemaker electrodes through the subclavian vein. Am J Cardiol 43:980, 1979.

97. Chung EK: Artificial Cardiac Pacing: Practical Approach, 2nd Ed. Baltimore, Williams and Wilkins, 1983, p 367.

98. Bluhm G, Julander I, Levander-Lindgren M, et al: Septicemia and endocarditis: uncommon but serious complications in association with permanent cardiac pacing. Scand J Thorac Cardiovasc Surg 16:65, 1982.

99. Imparato AM, Kim GE: Electrode complications in patients with permanent cardiac pacemakers: 10 years experience. Arch Surg 105:705, 1982.

100. Beder SD, Hanisch DG, Cohen MH, et al: Cardiac pacing in children: a 15 year experience. Am Heart J 109:152, 1985.

101. Bryan CS, Sutton JP, Saunders DE, et al: Endocarditis related to transvenous pacemakers: syndromes and surgical implications. J Thorac Cardiovasc Surg 75:758, 1978.

102. Rettig G, Doenecke P, Sen S: Complications with retained transvenous pacemaker leads. Am Heart J 98:587, 1979.

103. Byrd C: Transvascular removal of retained endocardial leads. (Abstract) PACE 8:109, 1986.

104. Stoney WS, Addlestone RB, Alford WC Jr, et al: The incidence of venous thrombosis following long term transvenous pacing. Ann Thorac Surg 22:166, 1976.

105. Krug H, Zerbe F: Major venous thrombosis: a complication of transvenous pacing electrodes. Br Heart J 44:158, 1980.

106. Nicolosi GL, Charmat PA, Zanuttini D: Large right atrial thrombosis: rare complication during permanent transvenous endocardial pacing. Br Heart J 43:199, 1980.

107. Kaulbach MG, Krukonis EE: Pacemaker electrode induced thrombosis in the superior vena cava with pulmonary embolization. Am J Cardiol 26:205, 1970.

108. Huang T, Baba N: Cardiac pathology of transvenous pacemakers. Am Heart J 83:469, 1972.

109. Phibbs B, Marriott HJL: Complications of permanent transvenous pacing. N Engl J Med 312:1428, 1985.

110. Fellows KE: Therapeutic catheter procedures in congenital heart disease: current status and future prospects. Cardiovasc Interven Radiol 7:170, 1984.

111. Lock JE: Now that we can dilate, should we? Am J Cardiol 54:1360, 1984.

Chapter 9

Pharmacologic and Anaphylactoid Reactions to Radiocontrast Media

Greg C. Larsen and Jeffery D. Hosenpud

Introduction

Reactions to the intravascular injection of radiocontrast media are among the most common complications encountered in routine cardiac angiography. Whereas major complications (e.g., death, myocardial infarction, serious arrhythmia, stroke, or vascular injury) from any cause have been estimated to occur in 1.8% to 3.4% of cases,[1] reactions requiring treatment and/or hospitalization attributed to radiocontrast media alone occurred in 1.5% of patients undergoing intra-arterial procedures in one large, prospective series.[2] The nature of these radiocontrast media-induced reactions is heterogeneous, however. One group of effects can be thought of as the body's generally predictable, dose-related responses to the agents acting as drugs. In addition, however, radiocontrast media occasionally produce anaphylactoid reactions, which are idiosyncratic, nondose-related pathophysiologic responses of the body to the agents acting as toxins. This review discusses the nature, recognition, and treatment of both types of reactions.

From *Complications of Cardiac Catheterization and Angiography: Prevention and Management* edited by Jack Kron, M.D. and Mark J. Morton, M.D. © 1989, Futura Publishing Inc., Mount Kisco, NY.

Physical Properties of Radiocontrast Agents

All of the radiocontrast media in current use are derivatives of tri-iodinated benzoic acids (Fig. 1). Iodine is used because it is an effective absorber of x-rays in the energy range generated by most clinical cardiovascular imaging systems; therefore, the concentration of iodine is an important determinant of each agent's opacifying ability. The agents predominantly used for cardiovascular imaging have iodine concentrations ranging from 320 to 400 mg/mL.

Cardiovascular radiocontrast media are categorized as ionic or nonionic, depending on whether or not they dissociate into charged particles in solution. Most ionic media are sodium and methylglu-

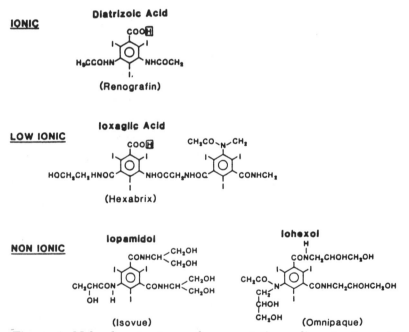

Figure 1. *Molecular structures of representative radiocontrast agents. The highlighted hydrogen atom of each ionic agent is replaced by a sodium or meglumine cation during synthesis. Each agent has three iodine atoms per molecule, except for ioxaglic acid, which has six. Brand names are shown in parentheses (see Table 1).*

Table 1
Chemical Properties of Selected Radiocontrast Agents

Agent	Iodine Content (mg/mL)	Sodium Content (mEq/L)	Osmolality (mOsm/kg)
Blood plasma	0	135–145	285
Standard ionic			
* Renografin-76 (sodium methylglu-camine diatrizoate)	370	190	1,940
† Hypaque M-75 (sodium methylglu-camine diatrizoate)	385	390	2,108
†† Conray-400 (sodium iothalamate)	400	1,050	2,300
†† Hexabrix (sodium methylgluca-mine ioxaglate)	320	150	600
Nonionic			
* Isovue-370 (iopamidol)	370	0	796
† Omnipaque-350 (iohexol)	350	0	844

* ER Squibb, Princeton, NJ; † Winthrop-Breon, New York, NY; †† Mallinckrodt Diagnostics, Inc., St. Louis, MO.

camine salts and have high osmolalities, from five to eight times the osmolality of blood. Nonionic media have lower osmolalities, approximately two to three and one-half times that of blood (Table 1). The higher osmolality of the ionic agents derives from the fact that dissociation of the salt produces approximately twice as many osmotically active particles in solution as the nonionic agents. One newer ionic agent, sodium methylglucamine ioxaglate (Hexabrix), is an exception. Because each of its molecules contains six iodine atoms, only about half the molecules are required to provide the iodine concentrations necessary for adequate radiographic imaging. Therefore, this agent, although ionic, has an osmolality only about twice that of blood. Because high osmolality appears to mediate several of the adverse pharmacologic effects of radiocontrast agents, the newer, low osmolality media may be safer for use in selected patients.

Pharmacologic Effects of Radiocontrast Media

Predictable dose-related effects of radiocontrast media occur when they are used for angiocardiography and these effects may be divided into seven general categories: (1) direct myocardial effects, (2) coronary and peripheral vascular effects, (3) intravascular volume effects, (4) arrhythmias and ECG changes, (5) renal effects, (6) hemostatic effects, and (7) miscellaneous effects. Renal effects are discussed in Chapter 10 of this text.

Direct Myocardial Effects

Selective injection of standard ionic radiocontrast media into the coronary arterial tree produces transient depression of myocardial function in laboratory animals and in man. These changes have been ascribed to the hypertonicity of these agents, to excessive amounts of their monovalent cations sodium and methylglucamine, and to local hypocalcemia induced by their calcium-chelating preservative, EDTA disodium, and buffer, sodium citrate.[2-11]

Hyperosmolality may not be as important a factor in radiocontrast-associated myocardial depression as was originally thought. For example, Popio et al. and Newell and colleagues have shown that intracoronary injection of nonionic hypertonic solutions, such as glucose or mannitol, in concentrations up to 1,800 mOsm/kg, produced a slight increase in myocardial contractile performance in dogs.[6,12] However, injection of a 900 mOsm/kg sodium chloride solution profoundly reduced myocardial function. Thus, the ionic nature of the hypertonic solution, and particularly its very high sodium ion concentration, appears to determine its negative ionotropic effect. By extension, intracoronary injection of sodium containing ionic contrast media shows similar depression, while injection of nonsodium-containing nonionic contrast agents produces no myocardial depressant effects.[3,5,13,14] The low osmolality ionic agent ioxaglate, which has a lower sodium content than standard media, produces myocardial depressant effects intermediate to those of standard ionic and nonionic agents.[13,14]

High sodium ion concentration is not the only reason for the cardiodepressant action of ionic radiocontrast agents, however. Transient hypocalcemia in coronary sinus blood has been demonstrated following intracoronary injection of various standard radiocontrast agents,[8,9] presumably caused by the sodium citrate used as a buffer and the chelating agent EDTA disodium used as a preservative in these media. This decrease in ionized calcium concentration peaks 6 to 8 seconds after injection, persists for 10 to 15 seconds, and parallels peak declines in systolic blood pressure and maximum dP/dt as well as peak rise in left ventricular end-diastolic pressure. When calcium is added to the contrast medium in concentrations adequate to restore postinjection coronary sinus blood calcium levels to normal (approximately 2 mEq/L), myocardial function improves but is not fully restored, suggesting that both sodium hypertonicity and myocardial hypocalcemia contribute to the cardiodepressant effects of standard ionic contrast agents. Of interest, higher concentrations of intracoronary calcium (6 to 40 mEq/L) demonstrate additional positive ionotropic activity and can restore myocardial function to normal or even supernormal levels.[6,9]

Significant coronary sinus hypocalcemia is not seen following intracoronary injection of the nonionic agents iohexol, metrizoate or iopamidol.[4,9,13] This is believed due in large part to the fact that these media use a different form of EDTA, calcium disodium EDTA, as a preservative and contain no sodium citrate buffer. Calcium disodium EDTA does not have the same chelating avidity for calcium ions that EDTA disodium does, thereby reducing its effect on coronary sinus calcium levels and thus, on myocardial contractility.

In summary, standard ionic contrast media such as Renografin-76 reduce myocardial contractile function, whereas the nonionic agents do not. This reduction reflects a transient imbalance in the ratio of myocardial extracellular sodium to calcium ions caused by the relatively high sodium content of standard ionic media coupled with a transient reduction in calcium levels produced by their preservatives. These extracellular disturbances presumably alter cardiac contractile performance by disturbing intracellular calcium and sodium kinetics at the myocyte cellular membrane and the sarcoplasmic reticulum.

Coronary and Peripheral Vascular Effects

The early studies of Kloster et al. in patients with and without coronary artery disease demonstrated decreases in coronary vascular resistance and increases in coronary blood flow of between 20% and 35% within 1 to 3 minutes of selective left coronary injection with standard ionic contrast media.[15] Coronary hemodynamics were altered for 5 to 7 minutes and the magnitude of these changes was not related to the extent of coronary stenosis present.

Recent studies in experimental animals have shown that changes in coronary blood flow following radiocontrast injection are actually biphasic. Both the standard ionic agent Renografin-76 [16] and the newer nonionic agent iohexol[17] cause a two- to threefold reduction in coronary blood flow 2 to 5 seconds after onset of left coronary artery injection. This early reduction is brief, and coronary flow rates of up to three and one-half times control values occur in dogs by 20 seconds after injection.[18] Because computer-aided videodensitometry can now be used in conjunction with coronary angiography to assess coronary blood flow, it is important to understand the effects of contrast on coronary hemodynamics so that pharmacologic effects of these agents can be separated from physiologic behavior of the coronary arterial tree.

Marked decreases in regional vascular resistance and increases in blood flow have also been demonstrated after selective injection of radiocontrast media into the canine femoral artery.[18,19] This response occurs using other hypertonic materials and persists after ganglionic denervation, suggesting that it is mediated through a direct effect of hypertonicity on the blood vessel wall. The mechanism of coronary dilation may be similar since hypertonic nonradiocontrast materials also produce a significant decrease in coronary vascular resistance.

In humans, significant peripheral vasodilation occurs within seconds of direct intracoronary radiocontrast injection. This effect appears to be mediated via cholinergic chemoreceptors and mechanoreceptors because it can be abolished with vagolytic doses of atropine.[20,21] This reflex response is most marked after selective right coronary artery contrast injection, begins 1 to 10 seconds after injection, peaks approximately 10 seconds later, and last up to 2 minutes. Left ventriculography with standard ionic radiocontrast media also produces marked vasodilation of the peripheral arterial tree, but this seems to be due to direct peripheral vascular effects of hyperosmolality.[22]

In summary, there is a biphasic change in coronary blood flow following intracoronary radiocontrast injection, consisting of an initial 5- to 10-second reduction in flow followed by a more prolonged increase. Peripheral vascular resistance is decreased following intracoronary radiocontrast injection, presumably mediated via coronary reflex mechanisms. Exposure of the peripheral vasculature to larger amounts of radiocontrast media, such as occurs following ventriculography, also causes peripheral vasodilation mediated by the direct vascular effects of hypertonicity.

Intravascular Volume Effects

The high osmolality of conventional contrast media causes significant fluid shifts when these agents are injected into the cardiac chambers or vascular tree. Aortography performed in human subjects, using 40 mL of 75% sodium methylglucamine diatrizoate (75% Hypaque-M, 2,108 mOsm/kg), has been associated with a mean rise in plasma volume at 2 minutes, of 8.2% or approximately 215 mL.[23] Left ventriculography performed using 40 to 60 mL of 76% sodium methylglucamine diatrizoate (Renografin-76, 1,940 mOsm/kg) increased mean plasma volume by 16.5% or 480 mL at 2 minutes after injection.[24] In both studies the changes resolved toward normal over 30 minutes.

Studies in dogs have demonstrated that increases in plasma osmolarity of up to 25% occur within seconds after left ventriculography, using sodium iothalamate (Angio-Conray, 2,400 mOsm/kg), inducing substantial shifts of interstitial and cell water into the vascular space during the first pass of this high osmolarity plasma through the peripheral capillary network.[25] Increased plasma volume in turn elevates venous flow to the right heart, leading to subsequent increases in end-diastolic ventricular volumes, pressures and stroke volumes, beginning 15 to 30 seconds after initial contrast injection. Importantly, cardiac volume changes do not appear to occur during the first six beats of ventricular opacification with contrast, ensuring that left ventricular volume and ejection fraction measurements obtained early during angiocardiography accurately represent baseline ventricular performance.[26,27]

Relatively less is known about acute intravascular volume changes attending aortography and left ventriculography performed with nonionic contrast agents. Because the osmolality of these agents is only one-half to one-third that of conventional agents, significantly smaller increases in plasma volume can be assumed. This assumption has not yet been substantiated, however.

Arrhythmias

Bradycardias

Intracoronary contrast injections produce substantial slowing of the sinus rate in humans, with onset of action in 2 to 3 seconds, peak effect at 8 to 15 seconds and resolution of effect by 40 to 60 seconds. [5,7,9,28,29] Injection of the right coronary artery generally produces a greater effect than that of the left, presumably because the right coronary artery supplies the sinus node artery in 55% and the atrioventricular (AV) nodal artery in 90% of patients. [28]

Although contrast media depresses Purkinje fiber, sinus and AV nodal tissues directly, the predominant contribution to sinus slowing after intracoronary injection is provided by a vagus nerve-mediated reflex response. [28] The same vagal response can produce transient second-degree AV nodal block, especially in patients who have been taking calcium channel blockers. [30] The primary trigger of this vagal reflex response appears to be the hypertonicity of the radiocontrast agent rather than its specific cation, calcium or iodine composition. [29]

Ventricular Arrhythmias

During coronary angiography, and to a lesser extent during ventriculography, standard ionic radiocontrast media lower the ventricular fibrillation threshold in animals and man; the effect lasts approximately 1 minute. [31] A suspected mechanism for this effect involves an acute lowering of the ionized calcium concentration in myocardial capillaries and interstitial fluid caused by chelating agents used as preservatives in the media. The fibrillatory threshold in the dog is lowered in a dose-dependent manner by increasing the total volume of contrast injected or by prolonging the injection time into the coronary artery. Addition of calcium ions to ionic contrast media helps return the fibrillatory threshold towards normal. [32,33] Recently animal experiments by Murdock et al. have shown that QT intervals and repolarization potentials are markedly prolonged and disorganized in the local myocardial region supplied by the coronary artery injected with ionic radiocontrast.[34] This regional effect on repolarization appears to provide the substrate necessary for microreentry, which can lead to ventricular fibrillation in the presence of a spontaneous extrasystole. Murdock and co-workers also noted a marked decline in fibrillatory activity when ionized calcium was added to the contrast media.

The sodium concentration of ionic contrast media has also been shown to have an important effect on the ventricular fibrillation threshold of experimental animals; either the absence of sodium ions or too high a sodium ion concentration lowers the fibrillatory threshold.[35-37] The reason for this is unclear but, for myocardial electrical stability, it may reflect the importance of maintaining a balance between extracellular sodium and calcium ion concentrations.[38] As a result, all ionic media in current use contain some sodium, the exact concentration depending on the nature of the iodine-containing anion and on the concentration of methylglucamine, the companion cation to sodium in all standard ionic contrast agents.

In humans the occurrence rate of ventricular fibrillation during coronary angiography has been reported to be between 1 and 12 episodes/1,000 patients. A recent large review from the Mayo Clinic reports 39 episodes of ventricular tachycardia or ventricular fibrillation among 7,915 patients undergoing diagnostic coronary angiography, for a rate of 5/1,000.[39] In the Mayo Cinic series the "typical" patient with ventricular arrhythmia had normal ventricular function (79%), developed arrhythmia during right coronary artery injection (62%), and had onset within 10 seconds after coronary injection was completed (95%). In half the patients arrhythmia was initiated by a single ventricular premature beat (VPB), which occurred during the T wave of the preceding beat, without associated bradycardia or marked QT prolongation. Interestingly, when the arrhythmia was associated with bradycardia and QT prolongation, all but one injected vessel had no obstructing coronary disease.

Substantial experimental evidence in animals has demonstrated less depression of the ventricular fibrillatory threshold with nonionic contrast media, as compared with standard ionic agents.[33] Large scale human studies are lacking, however, and smaller series suggesting a trend toward a decreased risk of ventricular fibrillation with these agents require further confirmation.[40]

ECG Changes

Surface electrocardiographic changes routinely occur during coronary injection of standard ionic contrast media.[41-45] Changes appear within 5 seconds of injection, peak at 8 to 12 seconds, and generally resolve within 1 to 3 minutes. As discussed above, intracoronary injection of ionic contrast media has pronounced effects on sinoatrial and AV nodal conduction, leading to sinus bradycardia and prolonged PR interval. These effects are predominantly mediated via vagal reflex mechanisms and can be ameliorated with atropine. Slight widening of the QRS complex is common and transient bundle branch block is occasionally seen. Repolarization abnormalities are also common. ST-segment elevation or depression may occur. The T-wave amplitude is often markedly increased, and deep T-wave inversions may be seen, especially after right coronary artery injection.[43] These changes can be described, using vector analysis, as a shift in the mean QRS vector toward, and the T-wave vector away from, the artery being injected, resulting in marked widening of the QRS-T vector angle.

The QT interval is prolonged over baseline in virtually all patients. It has been suggested that the risk of ventricular fibrillation may be proportional to the degree of QT prolongation, especially in those patients without obstructive coronary disease.[39]

Nonionic radiocontrast media have significantly less effects on the surface ECG during coronary angiography than do standard ionic contrast agents. Heart rate is generally not reduced. The QT interval may show slight lengthening but on average appears to increase by no more than 5% above baseline.[41,46] ST-segment and T-wave amplitude changes are similarly blunted. Nonionic contrast agents are, however, still associated with ventricular fibrillation during coronary angiography; thus the clinical importance of these ECG findings remains unclear.

Figure 2, modified from the study of Gertz et al.,[41] summarizes the ECG changes produced by representative ionic and nonionic contrast agents.

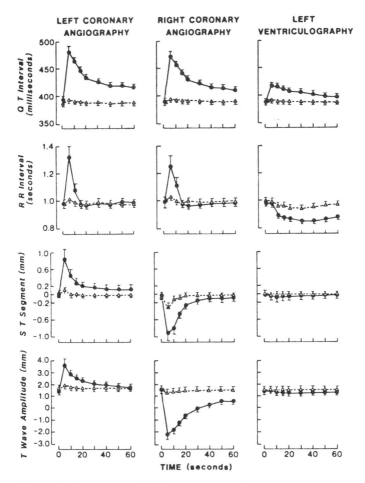

Figure 2. *Summary of ECG changes produced by ionic (closed circles) and nonionic (open triangles) contrast media during coronary angiography and left ventriculography. (Modified from Gertz EW, Wisneski JA, Chiu D, et al: Clinical superiority of a new nonionic contrast agent [iopamidol] for cardiac angiography. J Am Coll Cardiol 5:250, 1985.*[41] Reproduced with permission of the Journal of the American College of Cardiology.)

Integrated Hemodynamic Consequences of Radiocontrast Administration

The following summary reflects the reported experience of several studies in patients with coronary disease and preserved left ventricular ejection fractions. Different responses are likely in other patient groups.

Left Ventriculography

In the first 20 seconds after an injection of standard ionic media into the left ventricular cavity, left ventricular end-diastolic pressure rises 1 to 2 mmHg. There is no change in left ventricular end-diastolic volume, end-systolic volume, or ejection fraction during the first six cardiac cycles. The systolic arterial and peak systolic left ventricular pressures begin to decline slightly. Isovolumic indices of contractility and diastolic relaxation do not change.

In the next 20 seconds, mild, direct depression of left ventricular contractile function occurs as radiocontrast perfuses the myocardium from the coronary circulation. This effect is accompanied by marked peripheral vasodilation, leading to a 20% to 30% lowering of systolic blood pressure and a reflex increase in heart rate. The mechanism of peripheral vasodilation may be a combination of direct peripheral vascular effects of hyperosmolarity as well as reflex loss of peripheral vascular tone. At the same time peripheral vasodilation is beginning, an increased blood volume is returning to the right heart as a result of fluid shifts brought on by the passage of hyperosmolar contrast through the body's capillary network. This results in increases in left ventricular end-diastolic pressure and volume. Ejection is further enhanced by reduced peripheral vascular resistance and lowered arterial pressure. All of these factors combine to offset the direct negative inotropic effect of the contrast.

By 1 minute after injection, left ventricular end-diastolic pressure has begun to rise; it reaches its maximum at 2 to 5 minutes. In patients without obstructive coronary artery disease the increase is small, generally 4 to 6 mmHg.[47] The increase is greater in patients with obstructive coronary lesions, ranging from 8 to 18 mmHg.[48] The magnitude of increase appears to be proportional to the severity of the patient's coronary disease.

Several causes for the rise in left ventricular end-diastolic pressure have been advanced, including increased volume returning to the left ventricle, a decline in the rate of diastolic left ventricular relaxation, and increased passive diastolic stiffness (turgor) of the left ventricular myocardium due to increased coronary blood flow. In addition, if coronary disease is severe, ischemia induced during ventriculography may lead to increased diastolic myocardial stiffness.

In conjunction with the rise in left ventricular end-diastolic pressure, pulmonary capillary wedge pressure also increases. The time course of this increase parallels the change in left ventricular end-diastolic pressure. In two studies performed in patients with normal left ventricular ejection fractions the average rise in pulmonary capillary wedge pressure was 5 to 6 mmHg.[49,50]

Changes in cardiac output and peripheral vascular resistance are maximal between 1 and 2 minutes, and by 2 minutes myocardial contractility has usually returned to normal. Blood pressure generally returns to baseline within 2 to 5 minutes, while cardiac output, heart rate and left ventricular end-diastolic pressure may take 5 to 15 minutes to recover.

The hemodynamic consequences of left ventriculography using nonionic contrast media are considerably attenuated when compared to those of standard ionic media. Systolic blood pressure drops an average 10% during the first 30 seconds but returns to normal or may slightly exceed baseline values 60 seconds after injection. Heart rate increases approximately 5%. Left ventricular end-diastolic pressure appears to rise to a lesser extent than with ionic contrast injection, averaging about 3 mmHg at 1 minute, and it remains elevated for a shorter period of time, generally 4 to 5 minutes.

Coronary Angiography

Ten to 20 seconds following injection of standard ionic contrast media into the left coronary artery, heart rate drops 15% to 20%, while systolic and diastolic blood pressures drop an average of 10% to 15%. These parameters return to baseline within 30 to 45 seconds of a single contrast injection. Left ventricular end-diastolic pressure usually does not change. Isovolumic indices of left ventricular contractility and diastolic relaxation suggest that a mild (10%) decrease in myocardial systolic function occurs within 20 seconds of injection and that the rate of early diastolic relaxation is similarly, mildly impaired.[5]

After right coronary injection, heart rate initially decreases by an average of 20%, while systolic blood pressure declines by 5% to 8% and left ventricular end-diastolic pressure remains unchanged. Isovolumic indices of systolic left ventricular performance remain unchanged, although the rate of early diastolic relaxation slows slightly. These hemodynamic changes return to normal within 30 seconds of injection, on average.

When nonionic contrast media are used for coronary angiography no significant changes have been shown in heart rate, systolic or diastolic blood pressure, left ventricular end-diastolic pressure or isovolumic indices of left ventricular systolic function. A slight slowing of the rate of early diastolic relaxation has been seen with right coronary artery contrast injection.

Hemostatic Effects

Standard ionic radiocontrast media have a moderate anticoagulant effect in vitro. This is in part caused by the chelation of calcium ions necessary for the activation of the clotting cascade, and in part by inhibition of both platelet aggregation and fibrin polymerization.[51,52] The effect on platelets is felt to be produced by binding of ionic radiocontrast molecules to platelet membrane proteins. It is not known exactly how fibrin monomers are inhibited from polymerizing, but the prior step of fibrinogen to fibrin conversion is unaffected by radiocontrast agents.

Generally, the anticoagulant effects of standard radiocontrast media do not have a clinically significant impact on patient hemostasis. However, prolonged bleeding times have been demonstrated following ventriculography and coronary angiography, [53] and disseminated intravascular coagulopathy has been reported.[54]

By comparison with standard agents, nonionic radiocontrast media have little anticoagulant effect in vitro.[51,52] The clinical significance of this finding remains undefined. Robertson filled syringes with ionic and nonionic contrast agents and then contaminated each with fresh blood.[55] After standing undisturbed for 30 minutes, a small clot was noted in one syringe filled with nonionic contrast but in none of the ionic contrast-filled syringes. Thus, the anticoagulant effect of standard ionic radiocontrast media may be of clinical benefit in some situations by preventing blood clot formation at the blood-radiocontrast interface in angiographic catheters and syringes, thereby decreasing the risk of arterial embolism during angiography. On the other hand, we are aware of no reports linking nonionic contrast agents to an increased incidence of embolic phenomena. In addition, any in vitro benefit of conventional ionic agents due to their anticoagulant properties may be offset by the greater in vivo potential of these agents to damage vascular endothelium because of their higher osmolarity, thus stimulating local platelet aggregation and possible thrombus formation.[51]

Given the above considerations, the manufacturers of nonionic contrast agents have urged that during radiographic procedures catheters be flushed frequently and that prolonged contact of blood with contrast in catheters and syringes be avoided.

Miscellaneous Effects

The hyperosmolality of all radiocontrast agents has effects on red blood cells, extracting intracellular water from them and thereby altering their shape and reducing their deformability. The pathophysiologic significance of these observations is not completely known but may contribute to the early reduction in coronary blood flow seen after intracoronary radiocontrast injection as well as to the nephrotoxicity induced by radiocontrast media.[17,56,57] Sickle cell crisis has been precipitated, as have rare instances of hemolytic anemia.

Hyperthyroidism has been induced after intravenous pyelography in patients from an area of endemic goiter and to a previously euthyroid patient with an autonomous thyroid nodule, presumably reflecting excess thyroid hormone production and release caused by sudden exposure of the gland to the large quantity of iodine contained in radiocontrast media (the Jod-Basedow phenomenon).[58]

Symptoms Associated With Radiocontrast Injection

Controlled comparisons of standard ionic contrast agents (usually Renografin-76) with nonionic and low osmolality ionic agents have demonstrated differences in the frequency of some commonly experienced symptoms. Pooled data from several such studies are listed in Table 2.[41,59-63]

Virtually all patients note a sensation of heat or warmth after left ventriculography with standard ionic radiocontrast media. This feeling is normally most pronounced in the chest, head, and face but often generalizes. Two studies using different scoring methods each showed significantly fewer complaints of unpleasant warmth with low osmolality agents (ioxaglate and iopamidol). There appears to be a similar trend toward decreased headache in the low osmolality group. Nausea with vomiting was provoked with roughly equal frequency in both groups, however, as was moderate to severe chest pain.

Reports of symptoms after coronary arteriography do not appear to favor one group of agents over the other; unfortunately the wide variety of scoring methods used make quantitative comparisons difficult.

Studies that evaluated symptoms associated with peripheral arteriography show striking differences in favor of a low osmolality agent (iopamidol in both studies) (see Table 3). These findings may have relevance to angiography performed to evaluate internal mammary artery bypass grafts, a procedure which in our experience is

---

Table 2
Symptoms During Left Ventriculography

Symptom	Standard Ionic (1600–2500 mOsm/kg)	Low Osmolarity (600–800 mOsm/kg)
Nausea with vomiting	11/148 (7%)	10/153 (7%)
Chest pain	8/68 (12%)	10/72 (14%)
Headache	12/68 (18%)	2/72 (3%)
Unpleasant warmth (2 studies)	24/48 (50%) 40 pts: mean pain score = 7/10	13/52 (25%) 41 pts: mean pain score = 4/10

Table 3
Frequency of Moderate or Severe Pain with Peripheral Arteriography

Vessels Studied	Standard Media	Iopamidol
Aortofemoral (2 studies)	59 / 132 (45%)	11 / 136 (8%)
Lower extremity (1 study)	27 / 58 (47%)	2 / 61 (3%)

often painful to patients when a standard ionic contrast agent is employed. We are aware of no formal studies comparing the use of high and low osmolality contrast media for this purpose, but anticipate that low osmolality media would generally be better tolerated.

When Should Nonionic Contrast Media Be Used?

When nonionic contrast media are used for coronary angiography and left ventriculography they produce fewer hemodynamic and electrophysiologic changes than standard ionic contrast agents (Table 4). If their costs were the same there would be little reason to persist in using the older agents. Unfortunately, at the present time the newer contrast agents are approximately 15 to 25 times more expensive than equal volumes of standard media, and there

Table 4
Indications for The Use of Contract Media

Severely depressed left ventricular function

Suspected severe obstructive valvular heart disease

Complex angiographic procedures requiring large contrast volumes

Chronic renal failure

Evaluation of internal mammary artery grafts

History of previous anaphylactoid contrast reaction

Sickle cell disease

?Calcium channel blockers

seems no reason to believe that their prices will soon drop. In addition, most patients tolerate angiocardiographic procedures using standard ionic agents without difficulty. Thus, some selectivity seems appropriate in the use of the newer agents.

The major adverse effects of high osmolality ionic contrast agents such as Renografin-76 have been detailed above and include increased left ventricular end-diastolic pressure, depressed myocardial contractility, hypotension, a decline in the ventricular fibrillation threshold and patient discomfort. Certain groups of patients, such as those with severely impaired left ventricular function and/or severe obstructive valvular heart disease may be particularly vulnerable to these adverse effects and may be candidates for nonionic contrast agents. In addition, patients in whom complex angiographic evaluations are anticipated requiring the infusion of large amounts of contrast (angioplasty patients or patients with complex congenital heart lesions, for example) may also be candidates, as might patients with chronic renal failure who are in fragile fluid balance. As mentioned above, evaluation of internal mammary artery bypass grafts may be better tolerated by patients in whom nonionic contrast agents are used. Patients with sickle cell disease will have less red blood cell rheologic changes with nonionic media and therefore run less risk of suffering sickle cell crisis following angiography with these agents. Finally, there is some evidence to suggest that patients who have had previous anaphylactoid reactions to standard ionic contrast media may be at less risk of recurrent reaction if a nonionic agent is used (see below).

Patients taking large doses of calcium channel blockers who are otherwise hemodynamically stable pose a potentially difficult decision. Two recent studies have noted exaggerated responses to ionic contrast media in both dogs and humans who were pretreated with calcium channel blockers. Excessive hypotension or marked bradycardia were noted after injection of ionic contrast but not after nonionic contrast. In a study by Higgins et al., dogs pretreated with verapamil demonstrated significantly more AV nodal conduction delay during intracoronary injection of Renografin-76 than with iohexol given in equal doses.[30] Another study by Morris and colleagues showed augmented hypotensive responses following left ventriculography when Renografin-76 or Hypaque-76 but not iopamidol was used in 125 patients receiving diltiazem or nifedipine.[64]

Although the hypotension described by Morris and colleagues

in patients receiving calcium channel blockers was statistically significant, it is important to point out that none of the patients who underwent left ventriculography with standard ionic contrast developed a clinical complication from the procedure. Thus in patients with preserved ventricular function and no complicating valvular heart disease, who are taking calcium channel blockers, the risk of using standard ionic contrast agents for left ventriculography may be small.

Anaphylactoid Radiocontrast Reactions

The American College of Radiology has defined three types of "adverse reactions" to radiocontrast media as an aid to physician reporting, record keeping, patient treatment and follow-up.[65] Minor reactions are those that cause the patient "some but not excessive discomfort or apprehension" and for which treatment is usually not required. Examples include nausea, vomiting, headache, chills, lightheadedness, mild urticaria, and nonspecific itching. Intermediate reactions are defined as "transient episodes of hypotension or bronchospasm and any slowly responsive or refractory skin reaction such as rash, urticaria or edema." Major reactions have been defined as "those which threaten life," for which treatment is "urgent and mandatory" and the outcome of which is not immediately predictable. Examples include shock, loss of consciousness, convulsions, pulmonary edema, cardiac arrhythmias or arrest, as well as laryngeal edema and bronchospasm.

It should be clear from the preceding discussion of the pharmacologic effects of intravascular radiocontrast media on the cardiovascular system that some of the reactions defined by the American College of Radiology, for example headache, nausea, and hypotension, are predictable, if undesireable, pharmacologic effects of these agents. Pharmacologic effects should therefore be distinguished from anaphylactoid reactions, the unpredictable, nondose-related reactions to radiocontrast media, which occasionally occur during angiocardiography. It should generally be possible to make this discrimination on the basis of symptomatic, electrocardiographic, and hemodynamic information available to the physicians in the cardiovascular angiography laboratory.

Definition and Incidence

Anaphylactoid contrast reactions can be thought of as unpredictable, nondose-related pathophysiologic responses to radiocontrast media which mimic IgE-mediated hypersensitivity allergic reactions. They include urticaria, angioedema, rhinitis, conjunctivitis, bronchospasm, and acute vasodilatory cardiovascular collapse.

The incidence of anaphylactoid reactions during cardiovascular administration of radiocontrast media is difficult to estimate. Most data on adverse reactions derive from studies of intravenous urography.[2,66] During this procedure anaphylactoid reactions of all types occur at a rate of approximately 2%, "severe" reactions of all types at a rate of 0.1%, and fatal reactions at a rate of 1/10,000 to 1/50,000. It appears that the incidence of anaphylactoid reactions during cardiovascular angiography may be somewhat less.[2]

The incidence of contrast reactions is increased in patients who have had previous reactions. However, the type and severity of recurrent reactions is not predictable. In two large series the frequency of allergic-type reactions to radiocontrast media among patients giving a history of previous reactions was about 16%, [66,67] and second reactions tended to be the same or less severe than the first. Urticaria and facial erythema or mild facial swelling were the most common clinical manifestations.

Patients who have a history of hypersensitivity states or clinical allergic diseases also appear to exhibit an increased incidence of reactions to radiocontrast media. Hay fever, asthma, hives, as well as allergic reactions to seafood, antibiotics, fruit, eggs, chocolate, and iodine all have been associated with a 4% to 12% incidence of radiocontrast reactions.[2] Importantly, the nature of these radiocontrast reactions is usually mild. There appears to be no increase in the frequency of severe or fatal reactions among these patients.

Pathogenesis of Anaphylactoid Reactions

The pathogenesis of anaphylactoid radiocontrast media reactions is not fully established.[68] It has long been known that histamine release is sometimes a feature of these reactions, a fact that in the past generated enthusiasm for an IgE-mediated pathophysiologic explanation of these events. Unfortunately, other substances besides IgE-antigen complexes can activate histamine release from mast cells and basophils, and several lines of evidence favor involvement of nonallergic mechanisms in the production of anaphylactoid radiocontrast media reactions. First, patients never before exposed to radiocontrast media develop anaphylactoid reactions. Second, patients with previous anaphylactoid reactions to radiocontrast media may often develop no reaction upon rechallenge with the same agent. Third, skin testing does not produce the wheal and flare response typical of IgE-mediated allergy, and the results of skin testing are of no value in predicting the likelihood of future anaphylactoid reactions.[69] Fourth, intravascular injection of radiocontrast media can induce endothelial cell injury, kallikrein production, and nonimmunologically mediated histamine release from mast cells without complement activation. Blood histamine levels are often elevated after radiocontrast injection, yet there is a poor correlation between blood histamine levels and the development of symptoms or reaction in individual patients.[70–73] Finally, complement activation occurs frequently during intravascular radiocontrast media injection, and it is known that the complement anaphylatoxins C3a and C5a can produce release of histamine, kallekrein, and other allergic mediators in the absence of IgE-antigen complexes. There is, however, a poor correlation between levels of complement, degree of C3a and C5a activation, and development of a contrast reaction.[70–72,74]

From the foregoing, it appears that the development of an anaphylactoid reaction in a given patient is the result of a complex series of events, which includes the patient's inherent pathophysiologic sensitivity to radiocontrast media, the amount of mediator (or mediators) released into the circulation upon exposure, the patient's responsiveness to the mediator once it has been released, and the rate at which the patient's body is able to reestablish homeostasis after being challenged by radiocontrast media injection.

Prevention of Radiocontrast Media-Induced Anaphylactoid Reactions

As mentioned above, there is an increased incidence of mild reactions to radiocontrast media among patients who have a documented history of various hypersensitivity states. Because there has been no documented increased risk of severe reactions or death among these patients, routine pretreatment with antihistamines or corticosteroids has not generally been recommended.[65,68,75,76]

Pretreatment is advised for patients with a past history of an anaphylactoid reaction to radiocontrast media administration because these patients are at increased risk for recurrent reaction and because pretreatment regimens are available that appear to reduce the chances of recurrence. In the most comprehensive series published to date, Greenberger and colleagues pretreated 743 patients undergoing 857 radiocontrast media procedures, all of whom had well-documented, true anaphylactoid reactions to previously administered radiocontrast agents.[75,76] Three pretreatment regimens were used and are listed in Table 5. The results shown in Table 6 are abstracted from Greenberger's data for the 695 procedures requiring intravascular administration of radiocontrast media.

Statistical analysis demonstrated that regimen 2 was more effective than regimens 1 or 3 in preventing contrast reactions. Regimen 3 was no better than regimen 1 in preventing reactions, implying that cimetidine provided no additional protection to the basic steroid plus antihistamine regimen. Finally, the route of contrast administration (intravenous versus intra-arterial) did not alter the frequency of reactions. Of the 68 contrast reactions that occurred, there were 57 mild reactions (predominantly localized ur-

---

Table 5
Pretreatment Regimens for Patients with Prior Anaphylactoid Reactions To Radiocontrast media

Regimen 1: Prednisone 50 mg orally 13, 7, and 1 hour before start of procedure, plus diphenhydramine 50 mg orally or intramuscularly 1 hour before start of procedure

Regimen 2: Regimen 1 plus ephedrine 25 mg orally 1 hour before start of procedure (not given to patients with unstable angina or uncontrolled hypertension)

Regimen 3: Regimen 2 plus cimetidine 300 mg orally 1 hour before start of procedure

Modified from Greenberger, et.al.[75]

Table 6
Effect of Prophylactic Regimens on the Incidence of Recurrent
Anaphylactoid Reactions in 695 Intravascular Procedures

Regimen*	Number of Procedures	Number of Reactions
1	415	45 (10.8%)
2	180	9 (5.0%)
3	100	14 (14.0%)
Totals	695	68 (9.8%)

* Regimens defined in Table 5.
Modified from Greenberger, et.al.[75]

ticaria), 8 episodes of generalized urticaria, and 3 serious reactions involving hypotension.

A substantial number of both intravascular and extravascular radiographic procedures were performed on patients whose prior anaphylactoid radiocontrast reactions were classified as "serious," defined as involving laryngeal edema, severe wheezing, hypotension or syncope in the supine position. The recurrence rate of reactions in this subgroup is shown in Table 7. Following prophylactic pre-

Table 7
Responses to Radiocontrast Media in Patients with Prior Serious*
Anaphylactoid Reactions

Regimen**	Procedures in Patients with Prior Serious* Reactions	Total Recurrent Reactions	Recurrent Serious Reactions
1	110	10 (9%)	1 (0.9%)
2	33	1 (3%)	0
3	13	0	0
Totals	156	11 (7.1%)	1 (0.6%)

* "Serious" = associated with hypotension or syncope in the supine position, laryngeal edema, or severe wheezing; ** Regimens defined in Table 5.
Modified from Greenberger, et.al.[74,75]

treatment, only one of 156 procedures was associated with a recurrent serious reaction, and the number of total recurrent reactions was small (11 of 156 or 7%), similar to the total incidence of recurrent reactions among all patients undergoing intravascular procedures (68 of 695 or 9.8%). Thus, in pretreated patients the risk of serious second reactions appears to be no different than the risk of serious reaction among all patients with any previous anaphylactoid response.

The incidence of a second anaphylactoid reaction after the pretreatment regimens reported by Greenberger and colleagues is substantially lower than the generally accepted 16% incidence of second reactions among the untreated population. Although their study understandably contained no patients randomized to an untreated control group and thus cannot claim to provide definitive proof of pretreatment efficacy, such efficacy is suggested when compared against previously published reports.

The newer, nonionic radiocontrast media may be associated with fewer idiosyncratic reactions than the standard media for which the above treatment regimens were developed and used. Both iohexol and iopamidol have been shown to cause less histamine release, complement activation, endothelial injury, kallikrein production and platelet aggregation in animals than do standard ionic contrast media.[73] Since all these mechanisms have been implicated in the pathogenesis of anaphylactoid reactions, there is reason to think that nonionic contrast media may be safer in this regard than standard media. Three reports in relatively small series of patients suggest that this is so; however, the numbers are as yet too small to allow definite conclusions.[77-79]

Recommendations

In patients with a history of clinical hypersensitivity but no prior contrast reactions, pretreatment is not indicated to prevent serious radiocontrast reactions. In patients with a history of a previous anaphylactoid radiocontrast reaction, the incidence of recurrence is increased over that of the general population and pretreatment seems warranted because it appears to reduce the chances of recurrent reaction. For normotensive patients without unstable angina, resting claudication, or unstable hemodynamic state, regimen 2 listed above may be appropriate, since it appears to be the most effective in reducing recurrent reactions in high-risk patients. In any patient for whom ephedrine may be contraindicated, regimen 1 would be the appropriate choice. In addition, use of an a nonionic contrast agent should be considered for these patients.

References

1. Grossman W: Cardiac catheterization and angiography, 3rd Ed. Philadelphia, Lea and Febiger, 1986, p 30.
2. Shehadi WH: Adverse reactions to intravascularly administered contrast media. Am J Roentgenol 124:145, 1975.
3. Higgins CB, Sovak M, Schmidt WS, et al: Direct myocardial effects of intracoronary administration of new contrast materials with low osmolality. Invest Radiol 15:39, 1980.
4. Gerber KH, Higgins CB, Yuh Y-S, et al: Regional myocardial hemodynamic and metabolic effects of ionic and nonionic contrast media in normal and ischemic states. Circulation 65:1307, 1982.
5. Mancini GBJ, Atwood JE, Bhargava V, et al: Comparative effects of ionic and nonionic contrast materials on indexes of isovolumic contraction and relaxation in humans. Am J Cardiol 53:228, 1984.
6. Popio KA, Ross AM, Oravec JM, et al: Identification and description of separate mechanisms for two components of Renografin cardiotoxicity. Circulation 58:520, 1978.
7. Gertz EW, Wisneski JA, Neese R, et al: The effects of iopamidol on myocardial metabolism: a comparison with Renografin-76. Invest Radiol 19:S191, 1984.
8. Higgins CB, Schmidt W: Alterations in calcium levels of coronary sinus blood during coronary arteriography in the dog. Circulation 58:512, 1978.
9. Bourdillon PD, Bettmann MA, McCracken S, et al: Effects of a new nonionic and a conventional ionic contrast agent on coronary sinus ionized calcium and left ventricular hemodynamics in dogs. J Am Coll Cardiol 6: 845, 1985.
10. Higgins CB: Mechanism of cardiovascular effects of contrast media: evidence for transient myocardial calcium ion imbalance. J Am Coll Cardiol 6:854, 1985.
11. Zipfel J, Baller D, Blanke H, et al: Decrease in cardiotoxicity of contrast media in coronary angiography by addition of calcium ions: a combined experimental and clinical study. Clin Cardiol 3:178, 1980.
12. Newell JD, Higgins CB, Kelley MJ, et al: The influence of hyperosmolality on left ventricular contractile state: disparate effects of nonionic and ionic solutions. Invest Radiol 15:363, 1980.
13. Thomson KR, Evill CA, Fritzsche J, et al: Comparison of iopamidol, ioxaglate, and diatrizoate during coronary arteriography in dogs. Invest Radiol 15:234, 1980.

14. Tragardh B, Lynch PR: Cardiac function during left coronary arteriography in canines with ioxaglate, nonionic compounds, and diatrizoate. Invest Radiol 15:449, 1980.
15. Kloster FE, Friesen WG, Green GS, et al: Effects of coronary arteriography on myocardial blood flow. Circulation 46:438, 1972.
16. Hodgson JM, Mancini GBJ, Legrand V, et al: Characterization of changes in coronary blood flow during the first six seconds after intracoronary contrast injection. Invest Radiol 20:246, 1985.
17. Friedman HZ, DeBoe SF, McGillem MJ, et al: The immediate effects of iohexol on coronary blood flow and myocardial function in vivo. Circulation 74:1416, 1986.
18. Gerber KH, Higgins CB: Comparative effects of ionic and nonionic contrast materials on coronary and peripheral blood flow. Invest Radiol 17:292, 1982.
19. Marshall RJ, Shepherd JT: Effect of injections of hypertonic solutions on blood flow through the femoral artery of the dog. Am J Physiol 197:951, 1959.
20. Zelis R, Caudill CC, Baggett K, et al: Reflex vasodilation induced by coronary angiography in human subjects. Circulation 53:490, 1976.
21. White CW, Eckberg DL, Kioschos JM, et al: A study of coronary artery reflexes in man.(abstract) Circulation 48 (Suppl IV):IV-65, 1973.
22. Kloster FE, Bristow JD, Porter GA, et al: Comparative hemodynamic effects of equiosmolar injections of angiographic contrast materials. Invest Radiol 2:353, 1967.
23. Iseri LT, Kaplan MA, Evans MJ, et al: Effect of concentrated contrast media during angiography on plasma volume and plasma osmolality. Am Heart J 69:154, 1965.
24. Morissette M, Gagnon RM, Lamoureux J, et al: Effects of angiographic contast media on colloid oncotic pressure. Am Heart J 100:319, 1980.
25. Bristow JD, Porter GA, Kloster FE, et al: Hemodynamic changes attending angiocardiography. Radiology 88:939, 1967.
26. Vine DL, Hegg TD, Dodge HT, et al: Immediate effect of contrast medium injection on left ventricular volumes and ejection fraction: a study using metallic epicardial markers. Circulation 56:379, 1977.
27. Hammermeister KE, Warbasse JR: Immediate hemodynamic effects of cardiac angiography in man. Am J Cardiol 31:307, 1973.
28. Eckberg DL, White CW, Kioschos MJ, et al: Mechanisms mediating bradycardia during coronary arteriography. J Clin Invest 54:1455, 1974.
29. Higgins CB: Effects of contrast media on the conducting system of the heart. Radiology 124:599, 1977.
30. Higgins CB, Kuber M, Slutsky RA: Interaction between verapamil and contrast media in coronary arteriography: comparison of standard ionic and new nonionic media. Circulation 68:628, 1983.
31. Wolf GL, Kraft L, Kilzer K: Contrast agents lower ventricular fibrillation threshold. Radiology 129:215, 1978.
32. Thomson KR, Violante MR, Kenyon T, et al: Reduction in ventricular fibrillation using calcium-enriched Renografin-76. Invest Radiol 13:238, 1978.

33. Wolf GL, Mulry CS, Kilzer K, et al: New angiographic agents with less fibrillatory propensity. Invest Radiol 16:320, 1981.
34. Murdock DK, Euler DE, Becker DM, et al: Ventricular fibrillation during coronary angiography: an analysis of mechanisms. Am Heart J 109:265, 1985.
35. Snyder CF, Formanek A, Frech RS, et al: The role of sodium in promoting ventricular arrhythmia during selective coronary angiography. Am J Roentgenol 113:567, 1971.
36. Simon AL, Shabetai R, Lang JH, et al: The mechanism of production of ventricular fibrillation in coronary angiography. Am J Roentgenol 114:810, 1972.
37. Almen T: Effects of metrizamide and other contrast media on the isolated rabbit heart. Acta Radiol (Suppl) 335:216, 1973.
38. Fischer HW, Thomson KR: Contrast media in coronary arteriography: a review. Invest Radiol 13: 450, 1978.
39. Nishimura RA, Holmes DR, McFarland TM, et al: Ventricular arrhythmias during coronary angiography in patients with angina pectoris or chest pain syndromes. Am J Cardiol 53:1496, 1984.
40. Tragardh B, Lynch PR: ECG changes and arrhythmias induced by ionic and nonionic contrast media during coronary arteriography in dogs. Invest Radiol 13:233, 1978.
41. Gertz EW, Wisneski JA, Chiu D, et al: Clinical superiority of a new nonionic contrast agent (iopamidol) for cardiac angiography. J Am Coll Cardiol 5:250, 1985.
42. MacAlpin RN, Weidner WA, Kattus Jr AA, et al: Electrocardiographic changes during selective coronary cineangiography. Circulation 34:627, 1966.
43. Grendahl H, Eie H, Nordvik A, et al: Electrocardiographic changes during selective coronary angiography. Acta Med Scand 191:493, 1972.
44. Wolf GL, Hirshfeld Jr JW: Changes in QTc interval induced with Renografin-76 and Hypaque-76 during coronary arteriography. J Am Coll Cardiol 1:1489, 1983.
45. Kyriakidis M, Jackson G, Jewitt D: Contrast media during coronary arteriography: electrocardiographic changes in the presence of normal coronary arteries. Br J Radiol 51:799, 1978.
46. Ciuffo AA, Fuchs RM, Guzman PA, et al: Benefits of nonionic contrast in coronary arteriography: preliminary results of a randomized double-blind trial comparing iopamidol with Renografin-76. Invest Radiol 19:S197, 1984.
47. Hamby RI, Aintablian A, Wisoff BG, et al: Effects of contrast medium on left ventricular pressure and volume with emphasis on coronary artery disease. Am Heart J 93:9, 1977.
48. Slutsky R, Higgins C, Costello D, et al: Mechanism of increase in left ventricular end-diastolic pressure after contrast ventriculography in patients with coronary artery disease. Am Heart J 106:107, 1983.
49. Mancini GBJ, Ostrander DR, Slutsky RA, et al: Intravenous vs. left ventricular injection of ionic contrast material: hemodynamic implications for digital subtraction angiography. AJR 140:425, 1983.

50. Mancini GBJ, Bloomquist JN, Bhargava V, et al: Hemodynamic and electrocardiographic effects in man of a new nonionic contrast agent (iohexol): advantages over standard ionic agents. Am J Cardiol 51:1218, 1983.
51. Dawson P, Hewitt P, Mackie IJ, et al: Contrast, coagulation, and fibrinolysis. Invest Radiol 21:248, 1986.
52. Stormorken H, Skalpe IO, Testart MC: Effects of various contrast media on coagulation, fibrinolysis, and platelet function: an in vitro and in vivo study. Invest Radiol 21:348, 1986.
53. Verdirame JD, Davis JW, Phillips PE: The effect of radiographic contrast agents on bleeding time and platelet aggregation. Clin Cardiol 7:31, 1984.
54. Zeman RK: DIC following intravenous pyelography. Invest Radiol 12:203, 1977.
55. Robertson HJF: Blood clot formation in angiographic syringes containing nonionic contrast media. Radiology 163:621, 1987.
56. Hanley PC, Holmes DR, Julsrud PR, et al: Use of conventional and newer radiographic contrast agents in cardiac angiography. Prog Cardiovasc Dis 28:435, 1986.
57. Dawson P, Harrison MJG, Weisblatt E: Effect of contrast media on red cell filtrability and morphology. Br J Radiol 56:707, 1983.
58. Blum M, Weinberg U, Shenkman L, et al: Hyperthyroidism after iodinated contrast medium. N Engl J Med 291:24, 1974.
59. Hirshfeld, Jr JW, Laskey W, Martin JL, et al: Hemodynamic changes induced by angiography with ioxaglate: comparison with diatrizoate. J Am Coll Cardiol 2:954, 1983.
60. Bonati F: European experience with iopamidol. Invest Radiol 19:S175, 1984.
61. Newman TJ: Evaluation of iopamidol in peripheral arteriography and coronary arteriography with left ventriculography. Invest Radiol 19:S181, 1984.
62. Lyons J, Brooks N, Cattell M, et al: Comparison of Hexabrix 320 and Conray 420 for left ventriculography in patients with coronary artery disease. Br J Radiol 57:209, 1984.
63. Gwilt DJ, Nagle RE: Contrast media for left ventricular angiography: a comparison between Cardio-Conray and iopamidol. Br Heart J 51:427, 1984.
64. Morris DL, Wisneski JA, Gertz EA, et al: Potentiation by nifedipine and diltiazem of the hypotensive response after contrast angiography. J Am Coll Cardiol 6:785, 1985.
65. Prevention and Management of Adverse Reactions to Intravascular Contrast Media. Committee on Drugs, Commission on Public Health and Radiation Protection, The American College of Radiology, 1977.
66. Witten DM: Reactions to urographic contrast media. J Am Med Assoc 231:974, 1975.
67. Shehadi WH: Contrast media adverse reactions: occurrence, recurrence, and distribution patterns. Radiology 143:11, 1982.
68. Greenberger PA: Radiographic contrast media. In Patterson R (ed):

Allergic Diseases: Diagnosis and Management, 3rd Ed. Philadelphia, JB Lippincott, 1985, p 627.

69. Fischer HW, Doust VL: An evaluation of pretesting in the problem of serious and fatal reactions to excretory urography. Diagn Radiol 103:497, 1972.

70. Siegle RL, Lieberman P: Measurement of histamine, complement components and immune complexes during patient reactions to iodinated contrast material. Invest Radiol 11:98, 1976.

71. Cogen FC, Norman ME, Dunsky E, et al: Histamine release and complement changes following injection of contrast media in humans. J Allergy Clin Immunol 64:299, 1979.

72. Simon RA, Schatz M, Stevenson DD, et al: Radiographic contrast media infusions: measurement of histamine, complement, and fibrin split products and correlation with clinical parameters. J Allergy Clin Immunol 63: 281, 1979.

73. Dawson PR: Chemotoxicity of contrast media and clinical adverse effects: a review. Invest Radiol 20:S84, 1985.

74. Arroyave CM, Bhat KN, Crown R: Activation of the alternative pathway of the complement system by radiographic contrast media. J Immunol 117:1866, 1976.

75. Greenberger PA, Patterson R, Tapio CM: Prophylaxis against repeated radiocontrast media reactions in 857 cases. Arch Intern Med 145:2197, 1985.

76. Greenberger PA, Patterson R, Radin RC: Two pretreatment regimens for high-risk patients receiving radiographic contrast media. J Allergy Clin Immunol 74:540, 1984.

77. Dahlstrom K, Shaw DD, Claus W, et al: Summary of US and European intravascular experience with iohexol based on the clinical trial program. Invest Radiol 20:S117, 1985.

78. Holtas S: Iohexol in patients with previous adverse reactions to contrast media. Invest Radiol 19:563, 1984.

79. Rapaport S, Bookstein JJ, Higgins CB, et al: Experience with metrizamide in patients with previous severe anaphylactoid reactions to ionic contrast agents. Radiology 143:321, 1982.

Chapter 10

Contrast Nephropathy: Recognition and Management

Lawrence Elzinga and Thomas A. Golper

Introduction

Contrast nephropathy may be broadly defined as acute renal dysfunction following exposure to radiographic contrast media, provided that other potential causes for the renal functional impairment have been excluded. Although the overall incidence of contrast nephropathy in selected patient populations appears to be quite low, a group of patients at particular risk has been identified and account for the majority of cases of acute renal failure. Contrast agents rank third, behind low renal perfusion states and major surgery, as a cause for hospital-acquired acute renal failure, exceeding aminoglycoside antibiotics.[1] Current estimates indicate that contrast nephropathy is responsible for approximately 10% of all cases of acute renal failure.[1] Because of the increased use of radiographic contrast studies it is important to identify patients at risk for contrast nephropathy. Such identification will aid in the recognition and management of this complication and may decrease its incidence.

Incidence

Acute impairment of renal function is a recognized complication of any radiographic procedure in which iodinated contrast agents are used. However, the actual incidence is unknown, and

From *Complications of Cardiac Catheterization and Angiography: Prevention and Management* edited by Jack Kron, M.D. and Mark J. Morton, M.D. © 1989, Futura Publishing Inc., Mount Kisco, NY.

estimates reported by several groups of investigators vary widely due to differences in the types of radiographic procedures performed, patient selection, definition of renal failure, and the duration of surveillance (Table 1).

Most of the reported series on contrast nephropathy involve intravenous pyelography or noncardiac angiography. In a retrospective study of hospitalized patients undergoing intravenous pyelography, Van Zee and co-workers[2] reported acute renal failure in only 1 of 169 patients (0.6%) without pre-existing renal disease (serum creatinine < 1.5 mg/dL). However, in patients with nondiabetic renal disease (serum creatinine ≥ 1.5 mg/dL), the incidence was 5.6% and rose to 58% in diabetics with renal disease. Furthermore, there was a direct correlation between the preprocedure serum creatinine level and the incidence of renal dysfunction following contrast exposure. Swartz et al.,[3] in a retrospective review of 109 consecutive noncardiac angiographic procedures, identified 13 cases (12%) of acute renal failure (an elevated serum creatinine of 50% or 1 mg/dL, or a 20 mg/dL or 50% increase in BUN, within 48 hours). Renal failure was severe in approximately one-third of cases, some of which received dialysis support; but recovery of renal function occurred in 90%. In addition, they identified a number of associated conditions that appeared to be risk factors (see Risk Factors).

In response to this seemingly excessive incidence, Eisenberg and co-workers[4] conducted a prospective study of 100 consecutive patients undergoing cerebral, abdominal, or peripheral angiography and found no cases of acute renal failure despite the presence in 23 patients of 2 or more of the "risk factors" proposed by Swartz et al. Although their acute renal failure criteria were more restricted and they followed patients for only 1 day, they attributed their success to a hydration regimen that included saline infusion at an average rate of 800 mL/hr throughout the procedure. This same group subsequently reported that in their study of 537 consecutive patients who underwent angiography, none developed postangiographic renal failure.[5] This low incidence of postangiographic renal failure was confirmed by Kumar et al.[6] in a prospective study of 100 consecutive patients in which only one patient developed acute renal failure (> 0.5 mg/dL increment in serum creatinine). The patient was an elderly man with advanced chronic renal insufficiency (serum creatinine = 6.5 mg/dL). In another prospective

Table 1
Reported Incidence of Contrast Nephropathy (CN)

Author	Number of Patients	Procedure	Incidence (%)	Comments
Retrospective Studies				
Van Zee et al., 1972[2]	377	IVP	4.8 (N 0.6, RI 5.6, DRI 58.3)	Subclinical CN likely excluded
Diaz-Buxo et al., 1975[25]	115,838	IVP	N 0.0, D 0.2	
Harkonen and Kjellstrand, 1977[20]	29	IVP	76	All with diabetic renal insufficiency (Scr $\geq$ 2.0)
Swartz et al., 1978[3]	109	Angiography	12.0	Most developing CN were severely ill
Harkonen and Kjellstrand, 1979[18]	24	IVP	0.0, DRI (Scr 1.5–1.8) 37.5	All with diabetes and Scr < 1.8
Martin-Paredero, et al., 1983[26]	400	Angiography	11.3 (N 8.2, RI 41.7)	
Prospective Studies				
Weinrauch et al., 1977[8]	13	Cardiac angiography	92.0	All with severe diabetic renal insufficiency (mean Scr = 6.8)
Shafi et al., 1978[16]	40	Drip IVP	70 (DRI 92.0, non-DRI 61.0)	All with renal insufficiency; prestudy i.v. hydration with 1.5L
Anto et al., 1981[23]	37	Drip IVP	21.6	All with renal insufficiency; prophylactic mannitol vs. historical controls[16]

Table 1
Reported Incidence of Contrast Nephropathy (CN) (Cont'd)

Author	Number of Patients	Procedure	Incidence (%)	Comments
Eisenberg et al., 1981[5]	537	Angiography	0.0	Vigorous i.v. hydration (800 cc/hr), 27% with renal insufficiency, 33% with diabetes
Kumar et al., 1981[6]	100	Angiography	1.0 (patient with Scr = 6.5)	24% with diabetes, 19% with nondiabetic renal insufficiency
Rahimi et al., 1981[27]	15	IVP	0.0	All with renal insufficiency, excluded diabetes
Teruel et al., 1981[17]	124	IVP	21.8 (RI 55, non-RI 15)	Prestudy dehydration 34% with diabetes, no
D'Elia et al., 1982[7]	378	Nonrenal angiography	1.6 (RI 23)	difference between diabetics vs. nondiabetics matched for renal insufficiency
Mason et al., 1985[28]	120	Angiography	31	Used creatinine clearance as marker
Der Shieh et al., 1982[19]	49	IVP	6.1	All with diabetes and Scr < 2.0
Taliercio et al., 1986[9]	139	Cardiac	23	All with Scr > 2.0

N = normal renal function; RI = renal insufficiency; D = diabetes, without renal insufficiency; DRI = diabetes with renal insufficiency; Scr = serum creatinine (mg/dL); IVP = intravenous pyelography study of noncardiac angiography, D'Elia et al.,[7] using the criteria of a 1 mg/dL increment in serum creatinine, observed acute renal failure in 6 of 378 patients monitored for 72 hours. Whereas the incidence in nonazotemic individuals was 2%, in patients with pre-existing azotemia (BUN $\geq$ 30 mg/dL, serum creatinine $\geq$ 1.5 mg/dL), the incidence was 33%.

Only a few studies address the incidence of contrast nephropathy following cardiac angiography. In a study of 13 patients with juvenile-onset diabetes and advanced diabetic nephropathy (mean serum creatinine = 6.8 mg/dL), who were undergoing coronary angiography for pretransplant evaluation, Weinrauch and co-workers[8] reported that 12 of 13 (92%) developed acute renal failure, with a mean increase in serum creatinine of 3.0 mg/dL (range: 1.2–6.5). Recognizing pre-existing renal insufficiency as a major risk factor for contrast media-induced renal dysfunction, Taliercio et al.[9] reported the incidence of renal dysfunction following cardiac angiography in this subgroup of patients. Of 139 patients with renal insufficiency (serum creatinine > 2.0 mg/dL) studied prospectively following cardiac angiography, 32 (23%) developed contrast nephropathy (1 mg/dL increment in serum creatinine) 1 to 5 days later. Thirteen (9%) developed anuria or oliguria and 2 required dialysis. Renal function subsequently returned to baseline in 25 of the patients.

In summary, the incidence of contrast nephropathy following angiography in the general patient population with normal pre-study renal function is probably less than 2%. However, the incidence in selected "high-risk" groups may be considerably increased, exceeding 90% in the presence of certain risk factors.

Characteristics of Contrast Agents

Conventional angiographic contrast agents are tri-iodinated derivatives of benzoic acid. All are extremely hyperosmolar compared with blood (1,350–1,700 mOsm/L). Currently, the most commonly used preparations consist of the diatrizoate or iothalamate anion as the iodine carrier in combination with sodium or meglumine as the cation. Both of these salts are highly water soluble and, because of the low pKa of the carboxyl group, are present in biologic fluids as the anion. Plasma protein binding is negligible; thus they are freely filtered at the glomerulus, neither secreted nor reabsorbed by the tubules, and rapidly excreted in the urine as the parent compound.

A major advance in recent years has been the development of contrast agents that do not dissociate into ionic particles in solution (nonionic media) and are, therefore, of lower osmolarity without a decrease in iodine content.[10] Owing to their lower osmolarity, these agents have less influence on renal blood flow and produce less osmotic diuresis than do conventional media. Animal experiments with these newer agents suggest that a lower incidence of contrast nephropathy might be expected. While not free from nephrotoxicity, the renal effects of these agents in humans is not yet understood due to limited experience. Examples of these nonionic agents include metrizamide, iopamidol, iohexol, and iopromide. All are considerably more expensive than conventional agents.

Pathogenesis

While the mechanisms of contrast-induced renal dysfunction remain unclear, experimental and clinical observations have produced several hypotheses. These include direct nephrotoxic tubular cell damage, intraluminal tubular obstruction, and renal ischemia related to hemodynamic alterations induced by contrast agents.

The direct tubular cell toxicity of contrast media is suggested by the work of Talner et al.[11] who reported increases in urinary enzyme excretion following renal artery injection in dogs. Enzymuria is generally thought to be a sensitive indicator of tubular cell damage. Enzymuria was also observed following renal artery injection with other hypertonic solutions, suggesting that cellular injury may be related to hyperosmolarity, rather than be a feature unique to contrast agents. The new low-osmolarity, nonionic contrast media produce less tubular enzymuria. Other evidence for nephrotoxicity include depressed renal extraction of para-aminohippurate, an index of tubular cell function. This effect is only partially related to contrast media osmolarity. In addition, vacuolization of proximal tubular cells and findings consistent with acute tubular necrosis have been described in renal biopsy specimens following contrast exposure.

Tubular obstruction due to the precipitation of proteinaceous or nonproteinaceous material has also been proposed as a mechanism for acute renal failure following contrast media administration. Intraluminal obstruction by paraprotein precipitation following intravenous pyelography in myeloma patients serves as the prototype. In addition, obstruction by the increased tubular secretion and subsequent precipitation of normal urinary mucroprotein (Tamm-Horsfall protein) following contrast agent administration has been suggested. Because of the known uricosuric and oxaluric effects of radiographic contrast agents, intraluminal obstruction due to enhanced crystalluria has also been postulated as a possible mechanism.[12]

Contrast media-induced alterations in renal hemodynamics are of particular interest and suggest that renal ischemia may play a prominent pathogenic role. Following intra-arterial injection of contrast media, a biphasic alteration in renal blood flow has consistently been observed.[13] A transient increase in renal blood flow due to the hyperosmolarity of the contrast is followed by a prolonged decrease in renal blood flow, as much as 30% below baseline. The reduction of renal blood flow is enhanced by sodium depletion and may be mediated by angiotensin II, saralasin blockade of which attenuates the vasoconstriction. Contrast-induced erythrocyte damage may lead to aggregation and sludging in the renal microvasculature, which could contribute to the depressed renal blood flow. With left ventricular injection of contrast material, Porter et al.[14] also found that initial renal vasodilation is followed by renal vasoconstriction. They noted, however, that when urine volume was simultaneously replaced, the initial vasodilatory response persisted but the vasoconstriction was abolished, suggesting that the physiologic stimulus for vasoconstriction may be extracellular volume depletion. Recognizing that the major group at increased risk for contrast nephropathy are those with pre-existing renal insufficiency—especially diabetics with nephropathy—one can postulate that these hemodynamic insults superimposed on an already compromised renal microvasculature may be sufficient to induce acute renal failure.

Finally, immunologically mediated renal injury has been proposed as a mechanism of contrast nephropathy; the evidence, however, is limited. While hypersensitivity reactions to contrast media occasionally occur, they are rarely associated with renal failure. Antibodies to iothalamate were reported in a single patient with acute renal failure following intravenous pyelography.[15]

Risk Factors

A number of prospective and retrospective studies have indicated that contrast media-induced acute renal failure is a significant risk for only a selected group of patients with readily identifiable predisposing factors. Early retrospective studies identified a wide range of clinical variables associated with contrast nephropathy (Table 2). However, subsequent prospective studies have failed to confirm many of these associations, resulting in considerable debate as to their importance as independent risk factors.

Renal Insufficiency: Both retrospective and prospective studies have convincingly shown that pre-existing renal insufficiency places an individual at increased risk for developing acute renal failure following contrast media exposure. Over 90% of patients with acute renal dysfunction following contrast media administration have pre-existing renal insufficiency. Van Zee et al.[2] reported that as pre-existing renal insufficiency became more severe the

---

Table 2
Possible Risk Factors for Contrast Nephropathy

Pre-existing renal insufficiency
Diabetes mellitus
Multiple myeloma
Volume depletion
Advanced age
Large or repeated doses of contrast media
Low renal perfusion states

  hypotension
  heart failure
  hypoalbuminemia
  renal vascular disease
  vasoactive drugs

Proteinuria
Hypertension
Hyperuricemia
Liver disease
Hypersensitivity reactions

incidence of contrast nephropathy increased in patients undergoing routine intravenous pyelography. In two prospective studies of renal function following pyelography, Shafi et al.[16] reported an incidence of acute renal dysfunction in nondiabetic patients with prior renal insufficiency (mean serum creatinine = 3.7 mg/dL) of 61% (17 of 28 patients), while Teruel et al.[17] reported an overall incidence of 55% in patients with prior renal insufficiency (serum creatinine ≥ 2 mg/dL). In addition, the latter report noted a direct correlation between the increase in serum creatinine and the initial serum creatinine level. In a prospective analysis of multiple risk factors in 378 patients undergoing angiography, D'Elia et al.[7] found the presence of underlying renal insufficiency (serum creatinine > 1.5 mg/dL) to be the sole independent risk factor for contrast nephropathy, observing a 17% incidence in this group compared with 0.6% in previously nonazotemic patients. Taliercio et al.[9] reported a 23% incidence of contrast nephropathy following cardiac angiography in patients with a baseline serum creatinine exceeding 2.0 mg/dL. Factors that appeared to increase the incidence in this group with pre-existing renal insufficiency included the presence of Class IV heart failure, insulin dependent diabetes mellitus, repeat contrast exposure within 72 hours, and increased contrast dose.

Diabetes Mellitus: While diabetes is frequently cited as a risk factor for the development of contrast nephropathy, in the absence of associated renal insufficiency the risk in diabetic patients is quite low and may not exceed that for the general population. Van Zee et al.[2] and Harkonen and Kjellstrand[18] reported no cases of contrast nephropathy following pyelography among diabetic patients with a baseline serum creatinine below 1.5 mg/dL, whereas Der Shieh et al.[19] found a 6% incidence (3 of 49 patients) in well hydrated type II diabetic patients with a pre-IVP serum creatinine below 2 mg/dL. Similarly, in diabetics with a serum creatinine less than 2.0 mg/dL, D'Elia and co-workers[7] observed only a 1% incidence of contrast nephropathy following angiography, a rate comparable to that in the nondiabetic, nonazotemic population.

On the other hand, diabetic patients with associated renal insufficiency are at significantly increased risk. This risk appears to exceed that present in patients with similar degrees of renal insufficiency from other causes. Harkonen and Kjellstrand[18] reported 3 of 8 diabetic patients with mild renal insufficiency (serum creatinine 1.5–1.8 mg/dL) sustained contrast-induced renal injury.

These same investigators had earlier reported a 76% incidence of acute renal dysfunction, half of which were oliguric, in 29 diabetic patients with initial serum creatinines of 2.0 mg/dL or greater.[20] Shafi et al.[16] observed contrast-induced renal dysfunction in 11 of 12 (92%) diabetics with a mean pre-IVP serum creatinine of 3.5 ± 0.5 mg/dL compared to 17 of 28 (61%) nondiabetic azotemic patients (mean serum creatinine of 4.0 ± 0.5 mg/dL). In the study of Van Zee et al.,[2] contrast nephropathy occurred in 5.6% of patients with nondiabetic renal disease and 23% of patients with diabetic nephropathy. Taliercio et al.[9] found type I insulin-dependent diabetes mellitus to be among the factors that increased the likelihood of renal dysfunction in patients with underlying renal impairment following coronary angiography. In diabetic patients with advanced renal insufficiency, the incidence of contrast nephropathy exceeds 90%, and the disorder may be irreversible. Weinrauch and co-workers[8] reported that 12 of 13 patients (92%) with juvenile-onset diabetes mellitus and a mean serum creatinine of 6.8 mg/dL developed acute renal failure following coronary angiography. Nine patients were oliguric and 6 of the 12 required temporary dialysis.

In contrast, some investigators have not found the presence of diabetes to be a significant risk factor. In a prospective study following angiography, D'Elia et al.[7] found no statistically significant difference in the incidence of contrast nephropathy between the diabetic versus the nondiabetic groups matched for the presence or absence of azotemia. Likewise, Teruel et al. [17] did not find diabetes mellitus to be a significant risk factor following pyelography.

Renal Hypoperfusion: Decreased renal perfusion may result from a variety of factors, including volume depletion, hypotension, low cardiac output states, and severe vascular disease. While not universally accepted as an important risk factor for the development of contrast nephropathy, renal hypoperfusion is believed by many to play a significant contributing role in patients with other risk factors. Although the role of volume depletion in the development of contrast nephropathy is not well defined, adequate hydration should probably accompany any contrast procedure in susceptible patients (discussed below). This may reduce both the incidence and severity of acute renal dysfunction. Renal hypoperfusion due to low cardiac output states or hypotension may also contribute to renal injury following contrast administration. In patients with pre-existing renal insufficiency who underwent cardiac angiography, Taliercio and coworkers found Class IV heart failure with low cardiac output to have the strongest association with contrast nephropathy.[9]

Multiple Myeloma: Patients with multiple myeloma have long been considered to be at increased risk of contrast-induced acute renal dysfunction caused by tubular obstruction resulting from the precipitation of abnormal urinary proteins by the contrast agent. While no prospective studies exist addressing the incidence of contrast nephropathy in myeloma patients, in the absence of pre-existing renal insufficiency the risk appears to be quite low.[21] This low incidence may be due, in part, to the low protein binding characteristics of current contrast media compared with earlier agents. Although contrast nephropathy is infrequent in myeloma patients without renal insufficiency, these patients are subject to renal failure for many other reasons, including light-chain nephropathy, hypercalcemia, hyperuricemia, and amyloidosis. Exposure to contrast media appears to be an added risk. When it occurs, contrast nephropathy in myeloma patients is often severe and irreversible.

Other Factors: In early retrospective studies, multiple other clinical variables have been associated with contrast nephropathy. In prospective studies, however, they have not been consistently reported as being significant risk factors. The presence of hypertension, proteinuria, and peripheral vascular disease are probably significant mainly as markers of underlying renal disease rather than as independent risk factors for contrast nephropathy.

In summary, there is general agreement among investigators that the major predisposing factor for the development of contrast nephropathy is the presence of pre-existing renal insufficiency. From the available data it appears that the greater the severity of underlying renal impairment the greater the risk of nephrotoxicity. Similarly, several authors emphasize the risk of contrast nephropathy in patients with diabetes mellitus, especially those with associated renal disease. Other risk factors have been suggested, but not reported consistently.

Clinical Features

Historically, the development of contrast nephropathy was heralded by the onset of oliguria within 24–48 hours following exposure to contrast media. However, numerous prospective studies have indicated that nonoliguric acute renal dysfunction, manifested as an asymptomatic transient rise in serum creatinine, is probably the most common presentation. Typically, the serum creatinine rises within 24 hours of the radiographic procedure, peaking by the third to fifth day, and returning to baseline in 7–14 days. Oliguria, if present, usually occurs abruptly following the procedure and is of short duration; urine output returns in 3–4 days. During the oliguric period, there is no response to volume replacement or diuretics, and the urine sodium concentration is often less than 30 mEq/L. The low urinary sodium concentration can mislead the physician into administering large amounts of intravenous saline solution for presumed volume depletion, leading to volume overload and pulmonary edema.

The most sensitive and practical method of diagnosing contrast nephropathy is by serial serum creatinine concentrations. An increase in serum creatinine of 1 mg/dL is generally accepted as sufficient criteria for the diagnosis. Urine output and urinary sediment changes are variable and insensitive as indices for contrast-induced renal dysfunction. An abdominal film at 24 hours showing a persistent nephrogram has been reported to be a sensitive, albeit nonspecific, screening test for contrast nephropathy.

In addition to contrast nephropathy, renal failure following angiography may result from atheromatous emboli that are dislodged during the procedure. While this may clinically resemble contrast nephropathy initially, the prognosis for recovery of renal function is not as favorable.[22]

Management

Since there is no specific therapy for contrast-induced nephropathy, prevention is desirable and depends on identifying individuals at excess risk. A prestudy serum creatinine determination is the simplest means of identifying underlying renal insufficiency. In such patients, there must be sound indications for performing the contrast procedure and a responsible likelihood of obtaining useful information that will impact on clinical management. This is particularly important in patients with advanced diabetic renal disease. If angiography is clearly indicated, prestudy volume depletion should be avoided and hydration should be maintained during the period of contrast-induced osmotic diuresis. In addition, the concomitant use of other potential nephrotoxins such as aminoglycoside antibiotics should be avoided, if possible. Consideration should be given to noninvasive isotopic or ultrasonic evaluation of left ventricular function in place of ventriculography. Following the procedure, the patient should be monitored for renal dysfunction by means of urine output and serial creatinine determinations at 24 and 48 hours. Such monitoring is probably not cost-effective for routine use in nonazotemic patients, in view of the low incidence of contrast-induced renal dysfunction in the general population. If acute renal failure does occur, management is the same as for acute renal failure from other causes, including maintenance of proper volume status, monitoring for hyperkalemia, serial BUN and serum creatinine determinations, nutritional support, and careful attention to the prevention and treatment of infection. Oliguria, if present, is invariably unresponsive to loop diuretics, mannitol infusion, or fluid challenges. Renal function in the vast majority of cases, including diabetic patients with advanced renal insufficiency, can be expected to recover. Temporary dialysis support may occasionally be required.

While fluid challenges and osmotic or loop diuretics do not appear to influence the course of established acute renal failure following contrast administration, several investigators have proposed these measures as a prophylaxis at the time the patient is exposed to the contrast agent. Human and animal studies in other nephrotoxic models of acute renal failure have suggested that such measures may be beneficial in reducing the incidence and severity of acute renal failure following contrast exposure. Eisenberg et al.[4] reported no instance of contrast nephropathy in 100 consecutive patients undergoing angiography, who were treated with a vigorous hydration regimen. It is noteworthy that of those 100 patients, 25 had renal insufficiency and 31 had diabetes. Their hydration protocol consisted of an average of 550 mL of intravenous 0.9% saline solution and 250 mL of heparinized saline solution given as flush solution for each hour of procedure time. These investigators subsequently expanded their experience to 537 consecutive angiographic procedures without a single incidence of renal dysfunction using this protocol, although one patient was inadvertently volume overloaded with resultant pulmonary edema. Unfortunately, seemingly adequate hydration does not invariably avoid renal toxicity.

Shafi et al.[16] hydrated patients with chronic renal insufficiency, using 1,500 mL of 5% dextrose in 0.45% normal saline, beginning the night prior to pyelography. Nonetheless, 92% of the diabetics and 61% of the nondiabetics sustained renal damage. However, all patients recovered renal function and did not require dialysis. Using these patients as historic controls, Anto et al.[23] studied 37 patients with chronic renal insufficiency, who were treated in a similar manner except for the addition of 250 mL of 20% mannitol given 60 minutes after the IVP, followed by a 24-hour infusion of 0.45% saline to match urine output. The overall incidence of acute renal dysfunction declined to 22% from the 70% incidence of the previous study, suggesting a protective effect with this protocol. Admittedly, the use of historic controls makes it difficult to assess the influence of other factors that may not have been controlled.

It is prudent to consider patients with a prestudy serum creatinine concentration exceeding 2.0 mg/dL to be at particular risk. The available data, while inconclusive, would favor the use of potentially prophylactic measures in these patients despite the lack of clinically proven efficacy. One such protocol, advocated by Berkseth and Kjellstrand[24] for patients with serum creatinine values greater than 2.0 mg/dL, involves a combined mannitol and furosemide infusion (Table 3). They recommend 500 mL of 20% mannitol solution to which furosemide is added in a dose of 100 mg for each

---

Table 3

Protocol for Contrast Nephropathy Prophylaxis in Patients with Serum Creatinine > 2.0 mg/dL

Solution:	500 mL 20% mannitol + 100 mg of furosemide for each mg/dL of serum creatinine (e.g., for a serum creatinine of 3.5 mg/dL, add 350 mg furosemide)
Rate:	20 mL/hr
Duration:	1 hour before and continuous for 6 hours following exposure
Urine output:	Replaced with D5 1/2 NS + 30 mEq KCl/L.

Modified from Berkseth and Kjellstrand[24].

mg/dL of serum creatinine. Infusion is begun at a rate of 20 mL/hr, one hour prior to contrast media exposure and continued during the procedure and 6 hours thereafter. Urine output is replaced with 5% dextrose in 0.45% saline with 30 mEq KCl/L. While this approach seems reasonable and we have employed this protocol at our institution, we have noted several instances of contrast-induced acute renal failure in high-risk patients despite its use.

In most patients a protocol for intravascular volume expansion and the induction of a diuresis, such as the one outlined above, is an appropriate prophylactic maneuver. However, the patient with severe congestive heart failure and oliguria may not tolerate volume expansion or respond with a diuresis. In such instances, prophylactic effects will be limited to measures that optimize cardiac output and renal perfusion. Following the angiographic procedure, dialysis may be needed to treat pulmonary edema resulting from the osmotic load represented by the contrast agent. While contrast media are readily dialyzable, there are no data available to suggest the use of prophylactic dialysis after contrast media exposure to prevent the development of renal failure.

Although the overall incidence of contrast nephropathy appears to be quite low, factors have been identified that increase the hazard of contrast administration, the most notable factor being the presence of pre-existing renal dysfunction. Appreciation of these factors, along with the prophylactic use of hydration and loop or osmotic diuretics, should minimize the occurrence and severity of acute renal dysfunction following cardiac angiography. While the clinical role of the newer "low osmolar" contrast agents is yet to be defined, their use in patients at increased risk for the development of contrast nephropathy can be considered prudent practice.

References

1. Hou SH, Bushinsky DA, Wish JB, et al: Hospital-acquired renal insufficiency: a prospective study. Am J Med 74:243, 1983.
2. Van Zee BE, Hoy WE, Talley TE, et al: Renal injury associated with intravenous pyelography in nondiabetic and diabetic patients. Ann Intern Med 89:51, 1978.
3. Swartz RD, Rubin JE, Leeming BW, et al: Renal failure following major angiography. Am J Med 65:31, 1978.
4. Eisenberg RL, Bank WO, Hedgcock MW: Renal failure after major angiography. Am J Med 68:43, 1980.

5. Eisenberg RL, Bank WO, Hedgcock MW: Renal failure after major angiography can be avoided with hydration. Am J Radiol 136:859, 1981.
6. Kumar S, Hull JD, Lathi S, et al: Low incidence of renal failure after angiography. Arch Intern Med 141:1268, 1981.
7. D'Elia JA, Gleason RE, Alday M, et al: Nephrotoxicity from angiographic contrast material: a prospective study. Am J Med 72:719, 1982.
8. Weinrauch LA, Healy RW, Leland OS, et al: Coronary angiography and acute renal failure in diabetic azotemic nephropathy. Ann Intern Med 86:56, 1977.
9. Taliercio CP, Vlietstra RE, Fisher LD, et al: Risk of renal dysfunction with cardiac angiography. Ann Intern Med 104:501, 1986.
10. Hanley PC, Holmes DR, Julsrud PR, et al: Use of conventional and newer radiographic contrast agents in cardiac angiography. Prog Cardiovasc Dis 28:435, 1986.
11. Talner LB, Roshmer HN, Coal MN: The effect of renal artery injection of contrast material on urinary enzyme excretion. Invest Radiol 7:311, 1972.
12. Mudge GH: Uricosuric action of cholecystographic agents: a possible factor in nephrotoxicity. N Engl J Med 284:929, 1971.
13. Russell SB, Sherwood T: Monomer/dimer contrast media in the renal circulation. Br J Radiol 47:26B, 1974.
14. Porter GA, Kloster FE, Bristow JD: Sequential effects of angiographic contrast agent in canine renal and systemic hemodynamics. Am Heart J 81:80, 1971.
15. Kleinknecht D, Deloux J, Hornberg JC: Acute renal failure after intravenous urography: detection of antibodies against contrast media. Clin Nephrol 2:116, 1974.
16. Shafi T, Chou S, Porush JG, et al: Infusion intravenous pyelography and renal function: effects in patients with chronic renal insufficiency. Arch Intern Med 138:1218, 1978.
17. Teruel JL, Marcen R, Onaindia JM, et al: Renal function impairment caused by intravenous urography: a prospective study. Arch Intern Med 141:1271, 1981.
18. Harkonen S, Kjellstrand CM: Intravenous pyelography in nonuremic diabetic patients. Nephron 24:268, 1979.
19. Der Shieh S, Hirsch SR, Boshell BR, et al: Low risk of contrast media-induced acute renal failure in nonazotemic type 2 diabetes mellitus. Kidney Int 21:739, 1982.
20. Harkonen S, Kjellstrand CM: Exacerbation of diabetic renal failure following intravenous pyelography. Am J Med 63:939, 1977.
21. Grainger RG: Renal toxicity of radiological contrast media. Br Med Bull 28:191, 1972.
22. Smith MC, Ghose MK, Henry AR: The clinical spectrum of renal cholesterol embolization. Am J Med 71:174, 1981.
23. Anto HR, Chou SY, Porush JG, et al: Infusion intravenous pyelography and renal function: effects of hypertonic mannitol in patients with chronic renal insufficiency. Arch Intern Med 141:1652, 1981.

24. Berkseth RO, Kjellstrand CM: Radiologic contrast-induced nephropathy. Med Clin N Am 68:351, 1984.
25. Diaz-Buxo JA, Wagoner RD, Hattery RR, et al: Acute renal failure after excretory urography in diabetic patients. Ann Intern Med 83:155, 1975.
26. Martin-Paredero V, Sherwood MD, Baker JD, et al: Risk of renal failure after major angiography. Arch Surg 118:1417, 1983.
27. Rahimi A, Edmondson RPS, Jones NF: Effect of radiocontrast media on kidneys of patients with renal disease. Br Med J 282:1194, 1981.
28. Mason RA, Arbeit LA, Giron F: Renal dysfunction after arteriography. J Am Med Assoc 253:1001, 1985.

Chapter 11

Surgical Management of Vascular and Cardiac Injuries Due to Catheterization Procedures

James L. McCullough, Jr. and Irving L. Kron

Introduction

With the present increase in coronary bypass surgery, increasing numbers of patients are undergoing cardiac catheterization. Despite continued technical improvements in retrograde arterial catheterization, significant numbers of patients have vascular complications related to these procedures that require consultation with a vascular surgeon. Most vascular injuries are related to the site of catheter introduction, usually the brachial or femoral artery. The most common types of complications are thromboembolic in nature and lead either to occlusion of the artery at the catheter introduction site or to embolism of thrombus distally in the extremity. Other complications include local hematoma, false aneurysm formation, and arteriovenous fistula. Vascular injury can also occur far from the catheter-introduction site, with injury to the arterial wall by guidewires or the catheter tip. There are also special considerations in treating vascular injuries in children. This chapter discusses the etiology of these different complications, emphasizing prevention.

From *Complications of Cardiac Catheterization and Angiography: Prevention and Management* edited by Jack Kron, M.D. and Mark J. Morton, M.D. © 1989, Futura Publishing Inc., Mount Kisco, NY.

The diagnosis and surgical treatment of vascular and cardiac complications of cardiac catheterization are also discussed.

Arterial Thrombosis and Embolism

Percutaneous Transfemoral Catheterization (Judkins Technique)

The most common vascular complications of percutaneous retrograde transfemoral catheterization are thrombosis of the common femoral artery and embolization of the thrombus distally in the lower extremity.

A review of several series shows an incidence of local vascular complications ranging from 0.5% to 1.5%.[1-6] These complications include femoral artery thrombosis, distal embolization, hematoma, false aneurysm formation, and intimal dissection. In a large study (11,402 patients) of the Seldinger percutaneous technique used for many types of angiographic procedures, the incidence of serious vascular complications was 0.7%.[6] The majority consisted of arterial thrombosis at the puncture site with a lesser number consisting of embolization from a dislodged atherosclerotic plaque or later embolization caused by intimal damage with thrombus formation. The most common cause of fatal complications in this study was also arterial thrombosis, in two cases involving the aorta and renal arteries and in one, the carotid artery. Green and associates reviewed a series of 445 cardiac catheterizations with five femoral artery thromboses.[2] In four of these five patients, predisposing risk factors were identified and included small femoral artery, preexisting aortoiliac occlusive disease, abdominal aortic aneurysm, and decreased cardiac output. Two patients had peripheral embolization with the loss of a distal pulse, but they did not require treatment.

There are several reasons for the variations in the incidence of vascular complications noted in different studies. Patient populations vary; some studies include a larger proportion of patients with such risk factors as preexisting peripheral vascular disease and cardiac valvular disease. The most important factors may be technical, such as the angiographer's experience, the length of of time required for the examination, and the number of catheters required during the study. The recognition of a vascular complication also varies, if physical diagnosis alone is used as compared to the more sensitive noninvasive vascular studies available. Barnes and colleagues used noninvasive vascular studies to detect the complications of catheterization; these included Doppler ultrasonic velocity detector and segmental Doppler pressures. Their complication rate was 14%, almost all of which was arterial thrombosis or embolism.[7]

Etiology

Several factors increase the risk of thrombotic vascular complications with the percutaneous transfemoral approach. In patients with preexisting peripheral vascular disease, there is a high incidence of atherosclerotic plaque in the region of the common femoral artery. During percutaneous arterial puncture, this abnormal endothelium tends to separate from the underlying media, thus creating an intimal flap. The resultant narrowing of the arterial lumen exposes underlying smooth muscle leading to platelet deposition and activation of the clotting mechanism. This clotting cascade results in local thrombus formation. Proximal arterial disease involving the aortic bifurcation and iliac vessels can lead to difficulty in passing the guidewire and catheter and can predispose to intimal damage and intimal dissection, both resulting in thrombosis and embolism. When arterial narrowing is located distal to the common femoral artery in the popliteal artery and runoff vessels, any emboli that reach the distal circulation of the extremity become more significant due to the already limited blood flow. In the previously cited study where complications were detected noninvasively, detectable complications occurred in 73% of the patients who had preexisting peripheral vascular disease.[7] Patients with cardiac valvular disease also have been shown to have a higher incidence of vascular complications following cardiac catheterization. In the same study, patients with mitral valve disease had a 32% incidence of vascular complications.[7]

Technical factors also play a significant role in the incidence of vascular complications. Judkins and Gander found that the complication rate in institutions that performed fewer than 100 cardiac catheterizations per year was 10 times that of institutions that performed more than 400 procedures per year.[8] This would appear to relate to the angiographer's experience. Other predisposing technical factors include: passage of multiple large catheters, multiple arterial punctures at a single site, relatively small femoral arteries (especially in women), intimal damage caused by the guidewire or the catheter tip, and the subintimal injection of contrast material. The length of the catheterization study also correlates with thrombus formation. When routine postcatheterization arteriograms were performed, thrombus was identified on the catheter in 54% of the patients.[9] When the length of the examination was less than 30 minutes, the incidence of thrombus formation on the catheter was 39% compared with 65% when the examination lasted longer than 30 minutes. Teflon-coated catheters were also found to be more thrombogenic than polyurethane catheters. Thrombus also accumulates at the puncture site as the catheter is withdrawn and can remain there, predisposing to local complete arterial thrombosis, or be carried proximally in the arterial tree on the tip of a second catheter, leading to embolization.

Inadvertent puncture of the superficial femoral or profunda femoris artery also increases the likelihood of a local arterial complication. A significant variation may exist in the distance below the inguinal ligament at which the common femoral artery divides into the smaller superficial femoral and profunda femoris arteries. In a review of complications following cardiac catheterization, McMilland and Murie found a 0.3% incidence (10 in 3,500) of femoral artery injury requiring surgical intervention.[4] Five of these 10 injuries occurred in either the superficial or the profunda femoris artery. These vessels are of relatively small caliber compared to the common femoral artery, and inadvertent puncture will carry a significantly higher risk of arterial thrombosis requiring surgical intervention (Fig.1).

Prevention

Several steps can be taken to decrease the incidence of vascular complications during cardiac catheterization. Patients with clinical evidence of peripheral vascular disease, such as intermittent claudication or decreased femoral pulses, can be studied through an alternate approach, such as the percutaneous transaxillary or the open transbrachial. Meticulous technique is also extremely important. The examination should be performed as rapidly as possible and with a minimum number of catheter changes. Catheter-tip

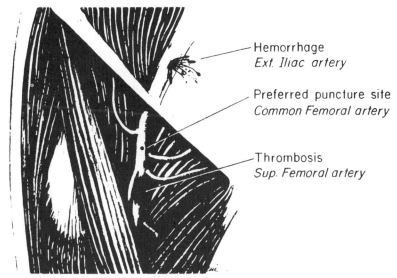

Hemorrhage
Ext. Iliac artery

Preferred puncture site
Common Femoral artery

Thrombosis
Sup. Femoral artery

Figure 1. *Percutaneous catheterization should be performed through the common femoral artery. Inadvertent puncture of the superficial femoral or profunda femoris artery can lead to thrombosis. Puncture of the external iliac artery above the inguinal ligament can lead to excessive hemorrhage.*

pressures should be monitored, and blood should be aspirated through the catheter intermittently to confirm that the catheter is in the arterial lumen prior to injection. The puncture site on the common femoral artery should be high on the vessel near the inguinal ligament to avoid injury to the superficial femoral or profunda femoris artery.

Some earlier reports suggested that morbidity and mortality were increased with the percutaneous retrograde transfemoral technique described by Judkins as compared with the Sones transbrachial technique. These techniques use different types of catheters; guidewires are used only with the Judkins technique. Both techniques employ continuous heparin-saline flushes through the catheters. One significant difference between the original descriptions of the two techniques is the intra-arterial injection of 5,000 units of heparin prior to study using the Sones technique. No systemic heparinization was originally used with the Judkins technique.

Walker and colleagues examined the use of systemic heparinization during cardiac catheterization by the Judkins technique.[10] In 135 patients who did not receive systemic heparinization, there were 24 thromboembolic complications and 5 deaths. In contrast, among 155 patients who received systemic heparinization, there were only two thromboembolic complications and 1 death. In this study, the heparin group received 3,000 to 7,000 units of intra-arterial heparin; however, the optimal dose has not been determined. The only other difference noted between the two groups was the longer period of compression required over the puncture site to control bleeding in the heparin group. There have been warnings in the literature concerning the increased risk of bleeding complications with systemic heparinization during cardiac catheterization,[11,12] but this does not appear to be well supported.[10] Other studies have confirmed the usefulness of heparin in preventing thrombus formation both in humans and in animals.[13,14]

Diagnosis

When a vascular complication does occur during cardiac catheterization, early diagnosis is the key to successful treatment. A careful postcatheterization examination of the patient and a high index of suspicion are most important. The patient may have symptoms of acute arterial insufficiency, such as numbness, pain, or decreased motor function, but these symptoms may be unreliable, owing to the sedation given during the examination. The patient should be examined frequently during the first 4 to 6 hours post catheterization because most vascular complications become apparent during this time. The most important findings are decreased skin temperature of the extremity and absent or decreased pulses. Examination should be performed repeatedly by the same examiner, if possible, because there could be variation in pulse detection between observers.

Special attention should be given to patients in the high-risk group for complications, such as previous peripheral vascular disease or valvular heart disease, and to those for whom the catheterization study was prolonged or difficult. In questionable cases, noninvasive vascular studies may be helpful.[2] The Doppler ultrasonic velocity detector is especially useful, and the study can be performed easily at bedside. The absence of a pulse by Doppler examination is indicative of a significant proximal arterial occlusion. Partial obstruction can also be detected by loss of the normal arterial multiphasic Doppler signal distal to an obstruction. Segmental Doppler pressures can also be determined to help localize the site of occlusion. It should be stressed that evidence of arterial insufficiency should not be attributed to arterial spasm. Arterial spasm following catheterization should be a very transient phenomenon that improves rapidly. In addition, studies of patients undergoing surgical exploration following cardiac catheterization have found arterial thrombosis to be the cause of ischemia in all cases.[15,16] Arteriography is rarely necessary to establish the diagnosis of a postcatheterization vascular injury and, indeed, may lead to an unnecessary delay in appropriate treatment. Once the diagnosis is made, prompt surgical exploration is indicated.

Surgical Treatment

Early diagnosis of an acute arterial thrombosis or embolus is one of the most important factors in achieving a good surgical result. Prompt restoration of arterial blood flow to the extremity will prevent permanent ischemic damage to nerves and muscle and also avoids the need for fasciotomies if compartment syndromes have not already developed. Early revascularization may also prevent significant systemic complications of reperfusion of ischemic or necrotic muscle. Systemic acidosis and hyperkalemia frequently occur following reperfusion after prolonged ischemia; the most serious side effects, hypotension and cardiac arrhythmias, can be especially devastating in patients who already have serious underlying cardiac disease. The release of myoglobin from infarcted muscle can precipitate acute tubular necrosis. Finally, early correction of an arterial thrombosis or embolus may avoid more complex vascular reconstructions that require longer operating times and possibly general anesthesia, both of which greatly increase the risk of cardiac complications.

The most common surgical complications after transfemoral catheterization are thrombosis of the common femoral artery and distal arterial embolism. Their correction is usually performed under local anesthesia. A longitudinal skin incision in the groin exposes the common femoral, superficial femoral, and profunda femoris arteries. All three vessels must be isolated so that thrombus can be adequately removed from all vessels. The smaller superficial femoral and profunda femoris arteries can usually be occluded by silastic vascular loops. These probably cause less intimal damage to the artery than vascular clamps. A vascular clamp is needed to occlude the proximal common femoral artery, and it is important to orient the clamp so that any plaque in the common femoral artery is not crushed.

In most cases the plaque will be located on the posterior wall of the common femoral artery, and therefore the clamp can be applied from the side of the vessel. Improper placement of the occluding clamp can lead to compression and fracture of the plaque and ultimately to intimal disruption and severe arterial damage, which could require a more complex vascular reconstruction such as replacement of the common femoral artery with a prosthetic graft. Systemic heparinization is often used prior to occlusion of the common femoral artery. The surgeon must work closely with the anesthesiologist to avoid severe systemic complications, which can be associated with revascularization of the ischemic extremity. The electrocardiogram, arterial pH, and potassium levels are monitored closely, and sodium bicarbonate can be given before blood flow is reestablished to counteract systemic acidosis. Adequate intravenous fluids, mannitol, and furosemide can also be given to promote diuresis, which protects against myoglobin-induced renal failure.

After the common femoral artery has been occluded, a transverse arteriotomy is made just proximal to the superficial femoral and profunda femoris arteries. The arteriotomy should incorporate the original puncture site, if possible. The thrombus at this site is removed, and the arterial lumen is inspected carefully for any evidence of intimal damage, especially on the posterior wall. The thrombus is removed from the distal arterial tree first via a Fogarty balloon catheter (Fig.2), which is passed distally through the arteriotomy, down both the superficial femoral and profunda femoris arteries. It is essential that catheter withdrawal and balloon inflation be performed by the same operator to avoid complications such as arterial wall perforation and intimal damage from an overinflated balloon. If the thrombus cannot be removed adequately, an operative arteriogram can be performed through the arteriotomy to locate the exact site of the occlusion. For emboli in the popliteal and distal runoff vessels, separate exposure of the popliteal artery may be necessary to adequately remove all thrombus. Good back-

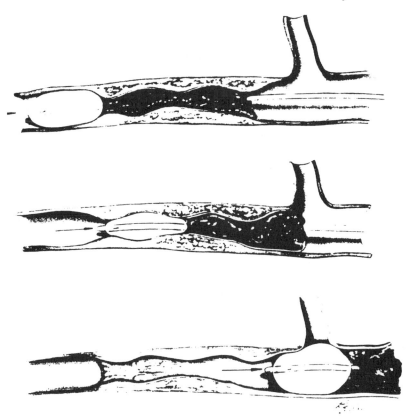

Figure 2. *Removal of thrombus using the balloon catheter. The balloon diameter can vary to match the changing size of the lumen of the artery.*

bleeding through the femoral arteriotomy is not a reliable indicator of adequate thrombus removal. An arteriogram should be performed if there is any doubt as to whether the distal arterial tree had been adequately cleared. The proximal iliac arteries are then cleared of thrombus, again via a Fogarty thrombectomy catheter. It is important that the catheter be passed carefully to avoid intimal dissection in areas of preexisting atherosclerotic plaque and to avoid dislodging thrombus in the proximal iliac artery, which would lead to embolism of the opposite leg. Following successful proximal and distal thrombectomy, the common femoral arteriotomy is closed transversely with either interrupted or running permanent monofilament suture. After the vascular clamps are removed, it is essential to confirm that adequate blood flow has been reestablished. The entire lower extremity should be included in the sterile operating field so that pedal pulses can be palpated or checked with the Doppler velocity detector. If there is any doubt concerning adequate blood flow, an arteriogram should be performed in the operating room. Absent pulses should not be attributed to arterial spasm.

If the common femoral artery is damaged severely, a local endarterectomy may be necessary or the common femoral artery replaced with a prosthetic graft such as knitted Dacron or polytetrafluoroethylene (PTFE). If adequate flow cannot be established through the superficial femoral or profunda femoris arteries, a femoropopliteal bypass graft may be required. In cases where adequate inflow cannot be established through the iliac arteries, blood flow can be reestablished by several routes, including femorofemoral bypass, axillofemoral bypass, and aortobifemoral bypass. If severe damage to the iliac vessels is suspected preoperatively, an arteriogram and noninvasive studies may be useful in planning the best operation for the patient.

Results

Many surgical series have demonstrated that, with early diagnosis and proper surgical management, excellent results can be obtained in treating postcatheterization vascular injuries. Bolasny and Killen reported 18 femoral artery thromboses managed by balloon-catheter thrombectomy under local anesthesia.[15] A femoropopliteal bypass was required in one patient, but distal pulses were restored in 17 of the 18 patients. After surgery, all patients were asymptomatic; there were no amputations. Two additional patients in this study had extensive intimal damage of the iliac vessels, which was caused as the angiography catheters were passed; endarterectomy was required as part of the definitive vascular reconstruction. The one patient who developed a distal embolus to the popliteal artery was treated by transfemoral balloon-catheter thrombectomy with good results.

In a similar study, Brener and Couch reported 5 patients with femoral artery thrombosis; 2 of the 5 patients also had distal thrombus in the extremity.[17] All 5 patients regained their pedal pulses following thrombectomy under local anesthesia. Eleven other patients had embolism to the popliteal artery. Three of the 11 patients were treated successfully by thrombectomy through a femoral artery approach under local anesthesia, and 3 required separate exposure of the popliteal artery for successful removal of the arterial emboli. The remaining 5 of the 11 patients with popliteal emboli did not undergo surgical treatment for various reasons. In 4 of those 5, pedal pulses returned within 24 hours, and the patients were asymptomatic.

This experience suggests that for small distal emboli that do not result in totally occluding the blood supply to the extremity, conservative treatment may be successful. One possible explanation for this is that small emboli undergo lysis in a short period of time with recanalization of the arterial lumen. In general, however, if acute arterial insufficiency is suspected following catheterization, prompt surgical exploration is required. The operative morbidity and mortality of these procedures performed under local anesthesia are small, and any unnecessary delay in treating a significant arterial occlusion can lead to irreversible damage to the extremity and serious systemic complications, as outlined above.

Brachial Artery Catheterization (Sones Technique)

Arterial thrombosis at the catheterization site is the most common complication of brachial artery catheterization. Hematomas, false aneurysms, and arteriovenous fistulas are less common, because this procedure is performed as an open technique with direct suture of the catheterization site in the brachial artery.

The incidence of arterial thrombosis of the brachial artery is higher than that with the percutaneous transfemoral approach. This complication ranges from 1.5% to 28%, but in most series the incidence of brachial artery thrombosis is approximately 5%.[4,16–20]

Etiology

The relative smallness of the brachial artery is probably the single factor most responsible for the higher incidence of arterial thrombosis, causing technical difficulties both in performing the arteriotomy and in subsequent closure. Several mechanisms lead to thrombosis and these include intimal disruption, thrombus formation at the arteriotomy site or on the catheter, and stenosis of the brachial artery caused by a technical problem with closure. Intimal damage is primarily caused as the angiography catheter is passed. The typical catheter injury involves the posterior wall of the brachial artery, usually within 1.5 cm of the arteriotomy. The intima is ragged and hemorrhagic, occasionally with an intimal flap or perforation. This area is the point of maximal pressure on the wall of the artery during catheter manipulation, which leads to endothelial cell loss, fracture of the internal elastic membrane, and pressure necrosis of the media.[16] Several studies showed a correlation between the arterial injury and the angiographer's experience, a prolonged procedure, and the number of catheter changes required.[17,18] The incidence of brachial artery thrombosis also appeared to be higher in female patients.[18]

Prevention

Most cases of brachial artery thrombosis are related to technical problems causing injury to the brachial artery. Meticulous technique is necessary when performing an arteriotomy with subsequent repair of this small artery. A small transverse arteriotomy should be performed with a scalpel or fine vascular scissors for minimal trauma to the intima and vessel wall at the site of the arteriotomy. The distal brachial artery should be flushed with heparinized saline solution after the arteriotomy. Catheters should be passed into the vessel under direct vision; care must be exercised to avoid undue pressure on the posterior wall. The length of the study and the number of catheter changes should be kept to a minimum. The arteriotomy should be closed with fine monofilament nonabsorbable suture, usually 6–0 polypropylene.

The transbrachial approach should be avoided, if possible, in patients who have small arteries, especially women. The transfemoral percutaneous approach may be better tolerated in these patients. Campion and colleagues recommended routine proximal and distal passage of a Fogarty thrombectomy catheter when the procedure is completed and before the arteriotomy is closed. These authors recovered unexpected thrombus in 48 of 328 patients.[18] A Fogarty catheter is not routinely recommended by most authors.

Diagnosis

It is most important to examine the patient frequently during the first 8 hours postcatheterization to detect thrombosis of the brachial artery. The patient may complain of decreased sensation, paresthesias, or pain in the hand. Symptoms may not be present at rest, however, due to the excellent collateral circulation around the elbow. Kitzmiller and colleagues found 68 of 100 patients with brachial artery thrombosis were asymptomatic at rest, 26 complained of some paresthesias, and only 6 complained of ischemic pain.[19] Physical findings appear to be more reliable. In the same series, almost all patients had pallor of the hand with elevation. Ninety of the 100 patients had an absent radial pulse, and in the remaining 10 patients the radial pulse was diminished. The Doppler ultrasonic probe is useful to detect flow in the radial artery, but this does not rule out a brachial artery thrombosis. Pulse volume recordings are very helpful in establishing the diagnosis of brachial artery thrombosis. Arteriography is usually not necessary in establishing the diagnosis. Surgical exploration of the brachial artery is indicated if a decreased pulse in the radial artery is noted during the first 24 hours following catheterization.[18] As stated earlier, a decreased pulse should never be attributed to arterial spasm.

Surgical Treatment

Once brachial artery thrombosis is suspected, immediate surgical exploration is indicated. In the original description of the transbrachial approach for catheterization by Sones, it was stated that brachial artery occlusion is well tolerated due to good collateral blood flow that will prevent ischemic tissue loss, and the majority of patients are asymptomatic after 3 months.[21] This has not been supported by subsequent experience, however. Several series have shown that 33% to 68% of patients discharged with decreased radial pulses following catheterization will have significant symptoms of ischemia.[16–18,20] Many of these patients will be asymptomatic at rest; however, they will have significant difficulty in the form of claudication during everyday tasks such as writing, combing hair, and other fine hand motions. These symptoms are exacerbated by cold temperatures.

The surgical procedure for repairing the brachial artery is relatively simple, carries minimal risk, and yields good results. The procedure can be performed under local anesthesia. A transverse incision is made in the brachial artery at the point of the original catheterization site. All collateral blood vessels should be preserved. To remove any thrombus, Fogarty balloon catheters are passed both distally and proximally and the vessels then flushed with heparinized saline. If there is minimal damage to the artery, the vessel can

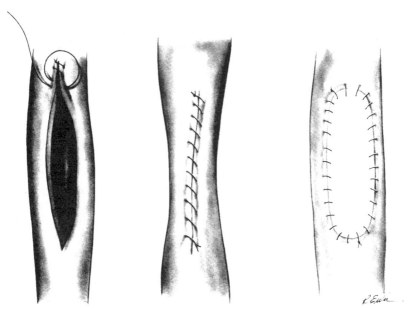

Figure 3. *Simple suturing of a longitudinal arterial defect can lead to significant narrowing of the lumen. This can be avoided by using a section of saphenous vein as a patch angioplasty.*

be debrided and closed primarily, or a vein patch may be required (Fig. 3). If there is more extensive damage, a segment of the artery must be resected. A primary reanastomosis of the vessel can usually be performed if less than 1.5 cm of vessel must be resected. An interposition reversed saphenous vein graft is necessary if larger segments of artery must be excised. Operative arteriography is indicated if radial and ulnar pulses are not reestablished. If there is distal thrombus in the radial and ulnar arteries that cannot be removed, then retrograde thrombectomy by separate arteriotomies in the radial and ulnar arteries may be necessary.

Results

Good long-term patency and functional results can be obtained with early surgical exploration following brachial artery thrombosis. Brener and Couch restored the radial pulse in 18 of 23 patients undergoing brachial artery repair.[17] Four of the five patients without palpable pulses were relieved of symptoms. Six additional patients who had previously been discharged with brachial artery thrombosis underwent delayed repair. Two of these were treated successfully with simple thrombectomy, but four required more complex reconstruction using interposition vein grafts. Kitzmiller and colleagues operated on 100 consecutive patients with brachial artery thrombosis at the Cleveland Clinic.[19] Eighty-seven patients had early successful results. Of the 13 patients who had early thrombosis of the repaired brachial artery, 11 achieved a good result with reexploration. Kitzmiller found an increased risk of early recurrent thrombosis of the brachial artery in female patients, as compared to males (25% vs 6%). Also, during late follow-up, 35% of the female patients had recurrent thrombosis, as compared to 12% of the male patients. Patients who underwent brachial artery repair more than 3 weeks after the original thrombosis required more extensive procedures, including resection of the artery and reconstruction with a saphenous vein graft.

Hematoma and False Aneurysm

A hematoma at the puncture site of the common femoral artery is one of the most common minor complications seen following percutaneous transfemoral cardiac catheterization. It can range from a small bruise at the puncture site to a large hematoma dissecting into the retroperitoneum that can cause life-threatening hemorrhage. Usually, however, hematomas are self-limiting and require no treatment. Serious bleeding complications are more likely to occur if the puncture site is proximal to the inguinal ligament and involves the external iliac artery, where there is less supporting tissue and it is more difficult to compress the puncture site after the catheter is removed (Fig. 1). The use of streptokinase also greatly increases the risk of serious postcatheterization hemorrhage.

Closely related to hematoma formation is the formation of a false aneurysm or pseudoaneurysm, which is an aneurysm at the puncture site on the femoral artery that does not contain the normal components of arterial wall. The initial event is a perivascular hematoma that occurs when all layers of the arterial wall are penetrated and that initially presents as an acute, pulsatile hematoma. Following this, there is gradual liquefaction and absorption of the

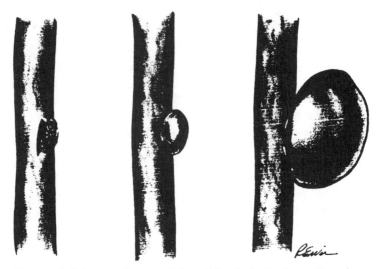

Figure 4. *Injury to the arterial wall leads to the formation of an acute pulsatile hematoma. With time, this develops into an enlarging pseudoaneurysm with risk of rupture or thrombosis.*

periarterial hematoma along with fibrosis of the surrounding tissue, leading to a chronic false aneurysm (Fig. 4). False aneurysms continue to enlarge with time. Several predisposing factors have been identified in their formation, the most important of which is inadequate compression at the puncture site after the angiography catheter is removed. Usually, it is necessary to compress the vessel for approximately 20 minutes to achieve good hemostasis. Other factors include the excessive use of heparin, the presence of intramural arterial calcifications, and hypertension. Rarely, infection at the puncture site can lead to the formation of a false aneurysm.[22]

The diagnosis of a false aneurysm is usually made after finding a pulsatile mass in a patient with a history of previous cardiac catheterization. A systolic bruit may be present, in contrast to the to-and-fro systolic-diastolic bruit heard with an arteriovenous fistula. There is usually a normal arterial pulse in the distal extremity. Ultrasonography or arteriography can be performed if the diagnosis is questionable.

Treatment

Perivascular hematomas or false aneurysms should be repaired as soon as possible, due to the possibility of early rupture or intravascular thrombosis. These can usually be repaired under local or regional anesthesia. The important principle is to obtain proximal control of the artery before dissecting the hematoma or false aneurysm. The aneurysm can be entered after the femoral artery is occluded and the defect in the artery, which usually is small, can be repaired with a few sutures. Rarely, is it necessary to resect a segment of the vessel to replace it with a prosthetic graft. If there is evidence of infection, it is usually necessary to ligate the artery and perform an extra-anatomic bypass to avoid placing a prosthetic graft in an area of infection.[22]

Arteriovenous Fistula

Arteriovenous fistula is a rare complication after percutaneous transfemoral cardiac catheterization. The mechanism of injury involves puncture through both the femoral artery and vein, commonly associated with a false aneurysm located between the artery and vein. With a chronic arteriovenous fistula, the proximal femoral artery becomes dilated and tortuous. Varicosities form in the proximal and distal veins (Fig. 5).

The diagnosis is usually suspected by the presence of a pulsatile mass in the groin. The temperature of the extremity may be decreased due to the high flow through the fistula; varicose veins may be present. The patient may also have symptoms of congestive failure, if the flow through the fistula is significant. On physical examination a to-and-fro murmur can be heard. A thrill is frequently present at the fistula site. The diagnosis can be confirmed by arteriography.

Flow through the arteriovenous fistula increases with time due to the dilatation of the veins. Symptoms of congestive heart failure and ischemia of the involved extremity will be noted as the flow increases. These patients are also at risk for infection at the fistula site and at subsequent risk for bacterial endocarditis. Spontaneous closure of the fistula is rare.

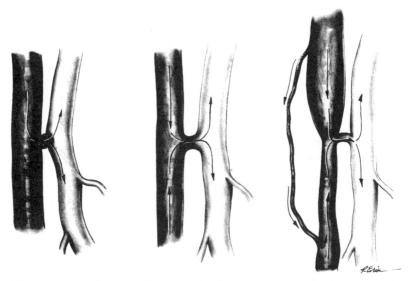

Figure 5. *Simultaneous injury to the femoral artery and vein can result in an arteriovenous fistula. With time, the proximal artery becomes tortous and dilated and flow is reversed in the distal artery, leading to ischemia. Varicose veins and chronic venous insufficiency can also develop.*

Repair of the arteriovenous fistula is indicated as soon as the diagnosis is made. Proximal and distal control of both the artery and the vein must be obtained before the fistula is divided. Suture repair of the defect in both the artery and the vein should be performed if possible. Occasionally, a segment of the involved artery must be resected and repaired with a vein patch or interposition graft.[22]

Vascular Injuries in Children

Iatrogenic vascular injuries caused by diagnostic or therapeutic procedures are the most common cause of arterial ischemia in children. Retrograde femoral catheterization is the most common method used to evaluate congenital heart disease. While thrombosis of the common femoral artery is an infrequent occurrence after percutaneous cannulation in older children and adults; it is relatively common in infants and small children. The most important predisposing factor is the small size of the femoral artery relative to the catheter used. In addition, children with cyanotic heart disease frequently have polycythemia, which increases the risk of vascular thrombosis. Arterial spasm is also much more severe in neonates. Loss of endothelial cells at the catheterization site has been showm to decrease the ability of the smooth muscle to relax after spasm of the artery.[23]

Villavicencio and colleagues[24] have given several recommendations for the treatment of neonates and small children with vascular occlusion secondary to catheterization procedures: (1) early intervention for severe ischemia in any age group; (2) in children with severe congenital heart disease with limited life expectancy operation can be deferred if the extremity appears viable; (3) if the initial revascularization attempt fails, a delay in subsequent repair may be appropriate due to the poor results obtained with reoperation; and (4) heparin is recommended as soon as the diagnosis is made and continued in the perioperative period. Flanigan and colleagues[25] stated that arterial spasm can be severe enough to cause actual vascular occlusion and severe, although transient, ischemia. They recommend systemic heparinization and observation for 6 hours. If the ischemia has not resolved by that time, operation is indicated. All children undergoing surgery after 6 hours were shown to have actual vascular thrombosis rather than spasm. In Flanigan's series, actual limb-threatening ischemia was rare. In most cases the extremity was obviously ischemic but viable. Another factor that must be considered in children is the significant risk of limb-growth retardation with chronic ischemia. In this series there was a 14% incidence of limb-growth retardation. They also advocate immediate operation in children with thrombosis of the abdominal aorta.

With nonoperative treatment, the mortality rate was 100% in this subgroup. Overall, 91% of the patients treated for iatrogenic vascular injuries eventually regained normal circulation; there were no amputations.

Direct Cardiac Injury

Left Heart

Occasionally, transseptal catheterization and left ventricular puncture can result in left atrial and left ventricular injury (Chapter 4). These injuries almost invariably present as hypotension due to cardiac tamponade. The diagnosis can be confirmed by echocardiography. Most patients can be managed with pericardiocentesis after which a catheter is left in the pericardial sac. Rarely this will not resolve the tamponade. Although a subxyphoid window can be used to evacuate tamponade, median sternotomy is the ideal operative approach for direct repair of such injuries, and better control of the circulation can be maintained than by thoracotomy. In the rare event that cardiopulmonary bypass is needed, either to resuscitate the patient or to repair the cardiac injury, then sternotomy is the ideal approach. If bypass is needed, then attention should also be paid to correcting the underlying cardiac lesion.

Right Heart

Rarely is the right atrium or pulmonary artery injured during right heart catheterization or pacemaker placement. A conservative approach that includes transfusion, relief of tamponade by pericardiocentesis, and observation almost invariably saves the patient.

Summary

Despite continued technical improvements in arterial catheterization, a significant number of patients will sustain vascular injuries. Arterial thrombosis or distal embolization are the most common injuries seen with both the percutaneous transfemoral (Judkins) and the open transbrachial (Sones) techniques. Less common complications include hematoma, false aneurysm, and arteriovenous fistula. Frequent examination of the patient and a high index of suspicion are the keys to early diagnosis of these injures. With early surgical treatment, excellent results can be obtained with minimal morbidity and mortality.

References

1. Judkins MP: Percutaneous transfemoral selective coronary arteriography. Radiol Clin N Am 6:467, 1968.
2. Green GS, McKinnon CM, Rösch J, et al: Complications of selective percutaneous transfemoral coronary arteriography and their prevention. Circulation 45:552, 1972.
3. Shah A, Gnoj J, Fisher VJ: Complications of selective coronary arteriography by the Judkins technique and their prevention. Am Heart J 90:353, 1975.

4. McMillan I, Murie JA: Vascular injury following cardiac catheterization. Br J Surg 71:832, 1984.
5. Spellburg RD, Ungar I: The percutaneous femoral artery approach to elective coronary arteriography. Circulation 36:730, 1967.
6. Lang EK: A survey of the complications of percutaneous retrograde arteriography. Radiology 81:257, 1963.
7. Barnes RW, Petersen JL, Krugmire RB, et al: Complications of percutaneous femoral arterial catheterization. Am J Cardiol 33:259, 1974.
8. Judkins MP, Gander MP: Editorial—Prevention of complications of coronary arteriography. Circulation 49:599, 1974.
9. Formanek G, Frech RS, Amplatz K: Arterial thrombus formation during clinical percutaneous catheterization. Circulation 41:833, 1970.
10. Walker WJ, Mundau SL, Broderick HG, et al: Systemic heparinization for femoral percutaneous coronary arteriography. N Engl J Med 288:826, 1973.
11. Swan HJC: Hemorrhage. Circulation 37 (Suppl III):52, 1968.
12. Braunwald E, Gorlin R, McIntosh HD: Summary. Circulation 37 (Suppl III):93, 1968.
13. Eyer KM: Complications of transfemoral coronary arteriography and their prevention using heparin. Am Heart J 86:428, 1973.
14. Nejad MS, Klaper MA, Steggerda FR, et al: Clotting on the outer surfaces of vascular catheters. Radiology 91:248, 1968.
15. Bolasny BL, Killen DA: Surgical management of arterial injuries secondary to angiography. Ann Surg 174:962, 1971.
16. Karmody AM, Zaman SN, Mirza RA, et al: The surgical management of catheter injuries of the brachial artery. J Thorac Cardiovasc Surg 73:149, 1977.
17. Brener BJ, Couch NP: Peripheral arterial complications of left heart catheterization and their management. Am J Surg 125:521, 1973.
18. Campion BC, Frye RL, Pluth JR, et al: Arterial complications of retrograde brachial arterial catheterization. Mayo Clin Proc 46:589, 1971.
19. Kitzmiller JW, Hertzer NR, Beren EG: Routine surgical management of brachial artery occlusion after cardiac catheterization. Arch Surg 117:1066, 1982.
20. Barabas AP, Bouhoutsos J, Martin P: Iatrogenic brachial artery injuries. Br Heart J 35:1080, 1973.
21. Sones FM, Jr, Shirey EK: Cine coronary arteriography. Mod Concepts Cardiovasc Dis 31:735, 1962.
22. Haimovici H: Vascular Surgery: Principles and Technique, 2nd Ed. Norwalk, Appleton-Century Crofts, 1984, p 389.
23. Franken EA, Girod D, Sequeira FW: Femoral artery spasm in children: catheter size is the principal cause. Am J Radiol 138:295, 1982.
24. Villavicencio JL, Gonzalez-Cerna JL, Velasco P: Acute vascular problems of children. Curr Prob Surg 22:14, 1985.
25. Flanigan DP, Keifer TJ, Schuler JJ, et al: Experience with iatrogenic pediatric vascular injuries. Ann Surg 198:430, 1983.

Chapter 12

Management of Knotted and Clotted Intravascular Catheters

Josef A. Rösch and Blaine E. Kozak

Knotting of intravascular catheters is a relatively rare complication but one that can occur with the use of both pressure monitoring and angiographic catheters. Flow-directed, balloon-tip catheters can become knotted during introduction, manipulation, or extraction.[1,2] Of the angiographic catheters, those with complicated curves and small diameters have the highest tendency to become knotted, particularly catheters with large reverse curves used for carotid artery catheterization.[3-6] However, knotting of left coronary and visceral catheters has also been reported.[7-9] The angiographic catheters mainly become knotted as they reform into their original shape in the thoracic or abdominal aorta. Knots most often involve the tip of the catheter.

Prevention, with adherence to basic catheterization techniques, is the best solution for this annoying complication. Careful introduction of flow-directed balloon-tip catheters, the use of early bedside chest radiographs to check their position, and catheter maneuvering under fluoroscopy if difficulties are encountered, help to avoid knotting of pressure monitoring catheters. Knotting of angiographic catheters with complicated curves can be prevented by their careful manipulation under fluoroscopic control and the use of sensible, unforceful rotation and careful advance during their reshaping. However, if knotting occurs, there is no need for panic or call to a friendly surgeon. Almost all knots on catheters can be

From *Complications of Cardiac Catheterization and Angiography: Prevention and Management* edited by Jack Kron, M.D. and Mark J. Morton, M.D. © 1989, Futura Publishing Inc., Mount Kisco, NY.

removed intravascularly with the help of guidewires and/or catheters. Common sense, an inventive mind and skillful catheter manipulation help to solve this complication without breaking the catheter or injuring the vessel.

With knots on *flow-directed catheters,* some angiographers suggest tightening the knot as much as possible, so it can be removed through the vein of insertion.[1] Introduction of a sheath over the catheter, large enough to take the knot, can simplify removal of the knotted catheter without risk of vein injury or catheter rupture, which can happen when the knot is pulled directly through the puncture tract. Most knots, however, can be loosened and untied and the catheter straightened by introducing a second (unwinding, untying) catheter containing a tip-deflecting guidewire (Cook, Inc., Bloomington, IN) (Fig. 1).[1,2,5,8,9] After the unwinding catheter is directed inside the knot, a deflecting guidewire is introduced through the catheter inside the knot, sharply curved to engage the knotted catheter loop, and used to unwind the knot. All manipulations are performed in one of the caval veins or the right atrium; if the knotted catheter is in the pulmonary artery or right ventricle, it is first pulled out into one of the preferred locations for untying. Prior to an attempt to untie the catheter knot, it is advisable to reproduce

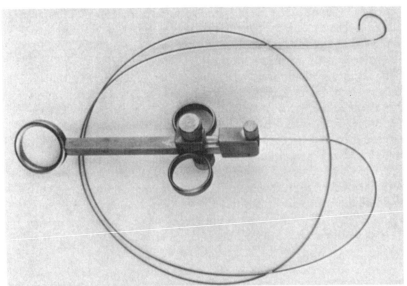

Figure 1. *Tip-deflecting guidewire system (Cook, Inc., Bloomington, IN).*

a similar situation in vitro and practice the technique selected. This makes unknotting a fast, successful, and safe procedure.[2]

A 6 French torque control catheter with a curved tip is usually used as the unwinding catheter. The site of its introduction depends on the size of the knotted loop. With a large loop knot, which is usually easy to unwind, the untying catheter can be introduced from the direction opposite to the knotted catheter (Fig. 2). After the unwinding catheter and deflecting guidewire engage the knotted loop, they are pulled, loosening and finally completely untying the knot.[1]

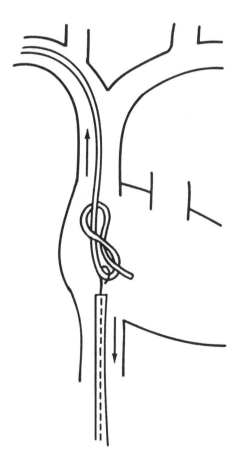

Figure 2. *Schematic drawing of the untying of a large loop knot of a flow-directed catheter introduced via the right subclavian vein. The untying catheter with a tip-deflecting guidewire, is introduced via a femoral vein. Untying is done by pulling on the knotted catheter and untying catheter in opposite directions.*

The situation is somewhat more difficult when a tight knot is present on the catheter. Such a knot tends to tighten rather than loosen if it is pulled from the opposite direction.[2] The unwinding catheter should, therefore, be introduced in the same direction as the knotted catheter (Fig. 3). The opposite femoral vein is used if the knotted catheter was introduced by the transfemoral approach. A jugular, subclavian, or arm vein is used to introduce the unwinding catheter when the knotted catheter comes from above. A strong guidewire with a rigid body (Lunderquist-type exchange wire) or transseptal needle-tip occluding wire is first introduced into the knotted catheter to the level of the knot. This stabilizes the position of the knot and prevents it from recoiling during the unknotting manipulations. The unwinding catheter is then directed inside the knot and the deflecting guidewire curved around the knotted loop and locked; unknotting is done mainly by pulling on the deflecting

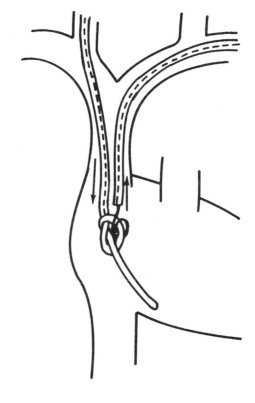

Figure 3. *Schematic drawing of the untying of a tight knot on a flow-directed catheter introduced via the right jugular vein. The knotted catheter is stiffened by introducing a rigid guidewire. The untying catheter with a tip-deflecting guidewire is introduced via a left antecubital vein. Untying is performed by holding and/or pushing the knotted catheter while pulling on the deflecting wire engaged in the knot. (From Dumesil JG, Proulx G: A new nonsurgical technique for untying knots in flow-directed balloon catheters. Am J Cardiol 53:395, 1984, with permission.)*

guidewire engaged in the knot. The knotted catheter, supported by the introduced guidewire, is held firmly or pushed against the deflecting wire to loosen the knot.[2] The entire procedure is done under fluoroscopic control, assuring that the knot is loosened and unwound rather than tightened further by the manipulations.

In case the unknotting manipulations are not successful and tightening the knot for its removal through the vein of insertion (via a sheath) is not possible, the knotted catheter can be managed like an unwanted intravascular foreign body.[1] A retrieval device (snare loop or basket) is introduced, usually through the femoral vein, and the knot firmly engaged into the retriever. The knotted catheter is then cut at its entrance into the vein, at its sterile portion, and is removed with the retrieval device via the femoral vein.

Knotted *angiographic arterial catheters* cannot be removed through a sheath after the knot has been tied more tightly, as in the venous system. The sheath would be too large for the artery at the puncture site. Several techniques can be used for unknotting arterial catheters. If the catheter tip is oriented against the aortic wall, it can be engaged in the left subclavian artery or lodged against the wall of the aortic arch (Fig. 4). Careful catheter advancment

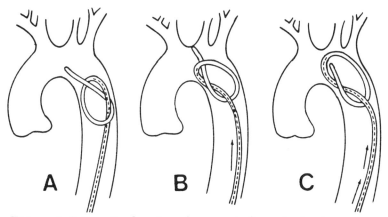

Figure 4. *Schematic drawing of an unwinding of a knot on an angiographic catheter in the aortic arch by catheter advancement. A. Knotted catheter in the thoracic aorta. B. Protruding tip of the knot is immobilized on the superior wall of the aortic arch. C. Catheter advancement enlarges the loop and loosens the knot. (From Thomas HA, Sievers RE: Nonsurgical reduction of arterial catheter knots. AJR 132:1018, 1979, with permission.)*

with a guidewire inserted to increase catheter stiffness can increase the size of the knotted loop until it opens completely or until the catheter tip turns inside the loop.[5] In the latter case, reinserting a standard guidewire is usually sufficient to straighten the catheter and eliminate the knot. This maneuver, however, should not be done in patients with atherosclerotic arch disease because of potential vessel injury and possible peripheral embolization due to dislodged plaques.

A deflecting guidewire inside the knotted catheter is another catheter unknotting technique effective mainly with larger loop knots (Figs. 5 and 6).[5,8] The deflecting guidewire is advanced until its tip begins to enter the first turn of the catheter knot. At this point the guidewire is slowly advanced with gradually increasing tip deflection. After it passes through the first turn of the knot, the deflecting guidewire is locked. Two possible manipulations can be done to unwind the knot and fluoroscopic control helps to select the more effective one. The knotted catheter can be gently retracted as the deflecting catheter is held in place (Fig. 5). The catheter is thus stripped from the guidewire, its terminal portion freed, and the knot released. Advancement of the catheter over the fixed de-

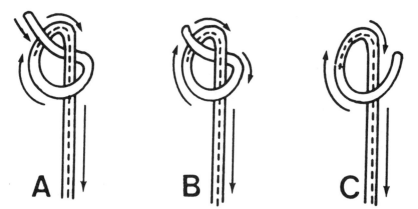

Figure 5. *Schematic drawing of unknotting a large loop knot on an angiographic catheter using a tip-deflecting guidewire. A. The tip deflecting guidewire is locked in the first turn of the knot. B. The catheter is gently retracted over the fixed guidewire. C. The knot is released. (From Hawkins IF, Tonkin A: Deflector method for nonsurgical removal of knotted catheters. Radiology 106:705, 1973, with permission.)*

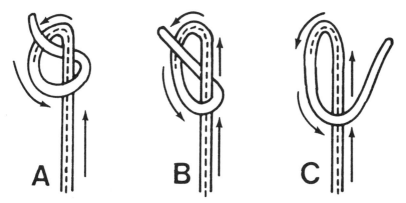

Figure 6. *Schematic drawing of the unknotting of a large loop knot on an angiographic catheter using a tip-deflecting guidewire. A. The tip-deflecting guidewire is locked in the first turn of the knot. B. The catheter advancement over the fixed deflecting wire results in widening the knot loop. C. The distal tip of the catheter is finally released. (From Hawkins IF, Tonkin A: Deflector method for nonsurgical removal of knotted catheters. Radiology 106:705, 1973, with permission.)*

flecting guidewire is another possibility; it results in widening the loop of the knot and eventually in its unknotting (Fig. 6).

If attempts with these techniques are not successful, a second, unwinding catheter, usually a 6 French torque control catheter, is used. It is introduced from the opposite femoral artery and used in combination with a deflecting guidewire to untie the knot in the same way as are intravenous flow-guided catheters (Figs. 7 and 8). The unknotting usually is done in the distal abdominal aorta. The knotted catheter is pulled down just above the bifurcation and the unwinding catheter, which is stiffened with a guidewire, is manipulated through the loop of the knot. Unknotting is usually achieved by withdrawing the knotted catheter, using gentle to-and-fro motion against the unwinding catheter (Fig. 7).[3–5] If this maneuver does not work, hooking the deflecting guidewire over a loop of the knotted catheter and holding or withdrawing it while the knotted catheter is advanced will open the knot (Fig. 8).[5] These manipulations, however, can be done only in patients with distal aortas free of atherosclerotic disease. Otherwise, the unknotting is done in the descending thoracic aorta and the untying catheter is introduced

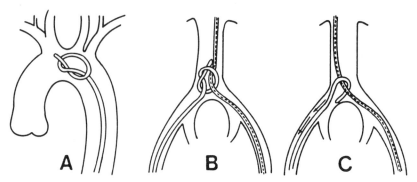

Figure 7. *Schematic drawing of the untying of a knotted angiographic arterial catheter with a second catheter introduced via the opposite femoral artery. A. Knotted catheter in the thoracic arch. B. Knotted catheter is withdrawn to the aortic bifurcation and the untying catheter, stiffened with a guidewire, is introduced through the knotted loop. C. Retraction and/or to and fro motions of the knotted catheter untie the knot. (From Thomas HA, Sievers RE: Nonsurgical reduction of arterial catheter knots. AJR 132:1018, 1979, with permission.)*

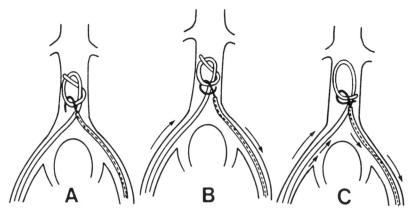

Figure 8. *Schematic drawing of the untying of a knotted angiographic arterial catheter with a second catheter and tip-deflecting guidewire. A. Tip of the deflecting guidewire is hooked and grasps a loop of the knot. B. The grasping hook is tightened to form a full curl. C. Simultaneous advancement of the knotted catheter and traction of the guidewire unwinds the knot. (From Thomas HA, Sievers RE: Nonsurgical reduction of arterial catheter knots. AJR 132:1018, 1979, with permission.)*

via a left axillary artery puncture. With all unknotting techniques, basic angiographic rules have to be followed; particularly, flushing both catheters with heparinized saline to prevent their occlusion by clots.

Clotted Catheters

Catheter clotting is an occasional, annoying complication of diagnostic and interventional angiography. It is often secondary to a guidewire that has remained inside the vessel and the catheter for a prolonged period of time. This usually happens during difficult catheter introduction or catheter exchange and the use of a guidewire for prolonged superselective catheterization or interventional procedures. Platelets and fibrin deposited on the guidewire are stripped during its removal, remain in the catheter, and result in its occlusion. Insufficient catheter flushing always has a contributory and sometimes a primary role in catheter clotting. When blood cannot be aspirated from the catheter after guidewire withdrawal or at any time during the procedure, the following steps are taken:

1. Using a catheter without sideholes, the catheter is moved, under fluoroscopy, up and down, rotated, or its tip curved to exclude the possibility that the inability to aspirate blood is due to a catheter-tip positioned against the aortic wall or wedged in a small branch. After this possibility has been excluded and after the operator is satisfied that the catheter is not kinked, twisted, or knotted, the catheter is pulled down in the distal abdominal aorta and attempts made to declot it. It is important to perform all declotting maneuvers below the level of the renal arteries so that an inadvertently dislodged, small broken clot does not cause renal infarction. If embolized in the leg circulation, a soft clot fragment rapidly lyses and does not cause significant damage. Attempts at declotting start with aspiration, using a small 2- or 3-mL syringe. Aspiration with a small syringe increases the effective force applied to the clot inside the catheter and is sometimes successful at breaking up a soft clot allowing it to be aspirated. If this happens, another forceful aspiration is performed to completely clean the catheter of residual deposits before flushing the catheter with heparinized saline.

2. An attempt to open the clotted catheter using a thin, 0.021-inch guidewire is the next step. The fibrin deposits and fragile clots are often located in the peripheral portion of the catheter close to the hub. Introducing a thin guidewire, 20 to 30 cm inside the catheter can break the clot and forecful aspiration with a small syringe may establish catheter patency. If this is not successful, the thin guidewire can be introduced farther, even closer to the tip to break up the more centrally located clots. The guidewire is small enough so as not to push the clots out of the catheter, particularly when used with 6 French catheters. However, to exclude this possibility completely, a Y adaptor is attached to the catheter hub and suction applied with a small syringe as the guidewire is advanced.[10]

3. If all declotting attempts are unsuccessful, the catheter must be removed. Prior to the widespread use of exchange sheaths, the catheter was withdrawn into the iliac artery and a hole punctured in the catheter wall close to the puncture site in the skin.[11] The tip of a standard guidewire was then introduced into the catheter, and both the catheter and guidewire advanced into the iliac artery. Once their intravascular position was established under fluoroscopy, the guidewire was withdrawn slightly from the catheter until its tip was free in the iliac artery; it was then advanced into the aorta. The clotted catheter was withdrawn and a new catheter introduced over the guidewire.

4. Presently, we prefer to retract the clotted catheter down into the pelvis and sever its distal half. If the deposits are close to the catheter hub, removal of the clotted catheter portion establishes spontaneous flow.[12] The guidewire is then introduced and the catheter exchanged for a new one. If, after this attempt, free blood flow is not obtained, we proceed to the final step, the introduction of a sheath with a self-sealing diaphragm over the clotted catheter and removal of the catheter.[13]

5. Catheter clotting can be minimized or completely avoided by following basic rules of angiography, particularly the use of systemic heparinization, frequent catheter flushing with heparinized saline, and avoiding prolonged insertion of a guidewire inside the catheter and vessel. Systemic heparinization is particularly important with prolonged diagnostic studies when multiple catheter exchanges are made, such as during left ventriculography with coronary angiography or subselective vis-

ceral angiography. It is essential for interventional procedures with prolonged use of coaxial catheters or leading guidewires, particularly with transluminal angioplasty. For diagnostic studies, we use a dose of 40 units of heparin for each kilogram of body weight and administer it intra-arterially after the catheter has been introduced into the abdominal aorta. A maximum of 3,000 units is used. With transluminal angioplasty, a full heparinization dose of 100 units/kg usually is given at the beginning of the procedure to a maximum total dose of 5,000 units.

6. The catheter is flushed every 1 to 2 minutes with heparinized saline. With systemic heparinization, the flushing solution contains 1,000 units of heparin in 500 mL of saline. In patients not treated with systemic heparinization (acute trauma, bleeding disorders), the flushing solution contains 3,000 units of heparin in 500 mL of saline. Double aspiration is done each time a guidewire is used or when a problem with aspiration is encountered. The initial aspirate is discarded. With the second aspirate, a small amount of blood is drawn into the syringe; with an endhole catheter, a small amount of flushing solution is injected to clean the blood out of the catheter. With a catheter that has both end- and sideholes, more forcible flushing is used to prevent clot formation between the end of the catheter and the most proximal sideholes.

7. Ionic contrast medium has been suggested as a flushing agent because of its clotting inhibition properties. It has proved to be more effective in preventing small clot formation than heparinized saline.[14] This, however, cannot be applied to the new nonionic, low osmolality contrast agents. They exhibit much less clotting inhibition than the ionic contrast media and with their use, catheters must be flushed more frequently; prolonged contact of blood with contrast medium in catheters and syringes should be avoided.[15]

References

1. Cho SR, Tisnado J, Beachley MC, et al: Percutaneous unknotting of intravascular catheters and retrieval of catheter fragments. AJR 141:397, 1983.
2. Dumesnil JG, Proulx G: A new nonsurgical technique for untying tight knots in flow-directed balloon catheters. Am J Cardiol 53:395, 1984.

3. Chinichian A, Liebeskind A, Zingesser LH, et al: Knotting of an 8 French "Headhunter" catheter and its successful removal. Radiology 104:282, 1972.
4. Cameron DC, Vaughan GT: A method of removal of knotted Headhunter catheter. Br J Radiol 50:211, 1977.
5. Thomas HA, Sievers RE: Nonsurgical reduction of arterial catheter knots. AJR 132:1018, 1979.
6. Lo WWM: Use of the Linderquist exchange guide wire for nonsurgical elimination of angiographic catheter knots. Radiology 145:835, 1982.
7. Stein HL: Successful nonsurgical removal of a knotted preshaped coronary artery catheter. Radiology 109:469, 1973.
8. Hawkins IF, Tonkin A: Deflector method for nonsurgical removal of knotted catheters. Radiology 106:705, 1973.
9. Holder JC, Cherry JF: The use of a tip deflecting guidewire in untying a knotted arterial catheter. Radiology 128:808, 1978.
10. Hawkins IF, Paige RM: Restoring patency of central venous catheters. AJR 140:391, 1983.
11. McKinnon CM, Kidd HJ, Robinson M: Simplified method of exchanging clotted intravascular catheters. Radiology 106:458, 1973.
12. Vinson AM, Wilcox CW, Knight MR, et al: The management of clotted angiographic catheters. Radiology 152:229, 1984.
13. Skolnick ML: A technique for exchanging a clotted intravascular catheter using the original arteriopuncture site. AJR 109:152, 1970.
14. Hawkins IF, Herbert L: Contrast material used as a catheter flushing agent: a method to reduce clot formation during angiography. Radiology 110:351, 1974.
15. Stormorken H, Skalpe IO, Testart MC: Effect of various contrast media on coagulation, fibrinolysis, and platelet function; an in vitro and in vivo study. Invest Radiol 21:348, 1986.

Chapter 13

Percutaneous Removal of Intravascular Iatrogenic Foreign Bodies

Josef A. Rösch, Blaine E. Kozak, and Fred S. Keller

Introduction

Cardiovascular catheterization has become an indispensable part of patient management. Various types of wires, catheters, and catheter devices are used in the heart and in both the venous and arterial systems for diagnostic studies, interventional therapeutic procedures, monitoring of central venous and pulmonary artery pressures, and cardiac pacing. Furthermore, intravenous catheters are employed for short- and long-term fluid management, feeding, and infusions of chemotherapeutic agents. Additional uses of catheters that lie partially intravenously include shunts for decompression of cerebral ventricles or peritoneal ascites. With such widespread use of intravascular wires and catheters, accidents and mishaps are bound to occur, even with careful attention to their insertion and removal. Accidents occur particularly with long-term venous catheterization. Wires occasionally break and catheters get cut, sheared, or fragmented. When catheters break or are sheared, the free fragments occasionally remain at the site of vascular entrance; however, the majority of them will usually embolize with blood flow. Fragments in the venous system lodge in the inferior or superior vena cava, the right heart, or pulmonary arteries. Catheter fragments in the arterial system, although relatively rare, can

From *Complications of Cardiac Catheterization and Angiography: Prevention and Management* edited by Jack Kron, M.D. and Mark J. Morton, M.D. © 1989, Futura Publishing Inc., Mount Kisco, NY.

embolize various distances, sometimes far peripherally from the site of their fragmentation.

Untreated intravascular foreign bodies carry significant risks, particularly those in larger vessels and the heart. They serve as a nidus for clot formation and infection and can lead to thromboembolism, endocarditis, septicemia, lung abscess, thrombotic occlusion of the involved vessel or vascular perforation resulting in a pseudoaneurysm or bleeding. When free fragments lodge in the heart, arrhythmias often occur, and even cardiac perforation with pericardial tamponade can develop. Removal of large fragments lodged in the heart or larger vessels of the venous, pulmonary artery, or systemic arterial circulations is, therefore, mandatory and should be done as soon as possible.

The majority of larger fragments of catheters and wires can be removed by relatively noninvasive percutaneous retrieval techniques. The risks and costs associated with surgical interventions can thus be avoided. This is of great importance because surgical removal almost always involves a major thoracic operation. The retrieval technique requires an inventive mind, knowledge of catheterization mechanics, and skillful catheter manipulation. Retrieval of intravascular foreign bodies should thus be reserved for experienced vascular radiologists or cardiologists.

History

Nonsurgical retrievals of iatrogenic intravascular foreign bodies were first performed by a cutdown approach. Thomas et al., in 1964, removed a broken guidewire extending from the inferior vena cava to the right atrium with a bronchoscopic forceps.[1] In 1966, Lasser et al.[2] retrieved a broken guidewire fragment from the descending aorta using a ureteral stone basket. Massumi et al., in 1967, used a snare loop technique to extract a sheared central venous catheter extending from the superior vena cava to the right ventricle.[3] In 1968, Henley et al. accomplished a similar removal percutaneously.[4] By 1971, Dotter et al.[5] reported a review of 29 transvascular foreign body retrievals, 6 done percutaneously. In the 1970s, multiple reports describing techniques used to retrieve unwanted foreign bodies from various parts of the vascular system were published, and in many of them the percutaneous approach was used.[6-17] In an international survey in 1977, Bloomfield found 180 cases of nonsurgical retrieval of intravascular foreign bodies with equal utilization of cutdown and percutaneous approaches; in the latter cases the femoral approach was most commonly used for introduction of the retrieval devices.[18] By now, it is not possible to determine the number of iatrogenic intravascular foreign bodies removed without surgery, but they probably number in the thousands. Retrieval has become a standard interventional procedure, and individual case reports are only rarely published. Occasionally larger series from one institution find the attention of editors of scientific journals such as that of Rubinstein et al. (1982: 13 cases), Cho et al. (1983: 12 cases), Endrys et al. (1985: 10 cases), or Uflacker et al. (1986: 20 cases).[19-22] Since 1970, we have been asked to retrieve intravascular iatrogenic foreign bodies in 25 patients and were successful in 24 patients. The youngest of our patients was 13 days old and 4 others were children 2 to 8 years old. The other 20 patients were adults 21 to 73 years of age.

Types of Foreign Bodies

Sheared fragments of central venous catheters for pressure monitoring and fluid management have formed the majority of intravascular foreign bodies that were retrieved during the 1970s; in the Bloomfield survey, 146 of the total 180 instances and 11 in our series. With extended use of long-term intravenous chemotherapy and total parenteral nutrition in the 1980s, we have more often recently faced the challenge of retrieving broken Silastic catheters (7 patients). Length of the retrieved broken fragments of central venous and Silastic catheters has varied over a wide range; in our series from 7 to 65 cm; Bloomfield found an average length of 12 cm. Broken ventriculoatrial shunts had to be recovered occasionally (12 in Bloomfield survey, 3 in our series). In addition, Bloomfield reported the recovery of 6 fragments of diagnostic catheters, 6 broken guidewires, 7 pacing catheters damaged during pacemaker replacement and 6 other items, ranging from bullets (presumably not iatrogenic) to a Swan-Ganz catheter sutured to the right atrial wall during prior surgery and broken during attempted withdrawal. If Bloomfield's collection were brought up to date, it would include

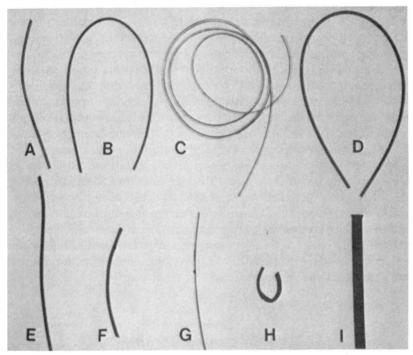

Figure 1. *Examples of the iatrogenic foreign bodies retrieved from our patients. A–C. Fragments of central venous pressure catheters and short-term infusion catheters. D and E. Fragments of long-term chemotherapy infusion catheters. F. Fragment of a ventriculo-atrial shunt. G. Fragment of a venous umbilical catheter. H. Fragment of a preshaped diagnostic catheter for selective pulmonary angiography. I. 18 French Teflon tubing used as a superior vena cava stent.*

several instances of Gianturco spring coil occluders being retrieved following their malplacement or subsequent displacement. Our series includes, in addition to the mentioned retrieved catheter fragments, a portion of an umbilical catheter, a fragment of a diagnostic catheter, and two tubular catheter stents placed in the superior vena cava for treatment of superior vena cava syndrome (Fig. 1).

Location of Foreign Bodies

The site to which the catheter fragment embolizes and the position of its ends are crucial for retrieval. Other important factors include the duration of intravascular catheter placement prior to and after its fragmentation. The final resting site of the fragment depends on the site of the original catheter entry, type of catheter material, particularly its stiffness and length of fragment. The majority of the venous catheter fragments lodge with their proximal end in the superior or inferior vena cava, its tributaries, or the right atrium (75% in Bloomfield's survey and 76% in our series). The fragments extend various distances centrally, depending on their length, with the distal ends frequently extending to the right atrium and lodging against its inferior wall or the tricuspid valve annulus. Sometimes the end of the fragment passes through the valve and lodges against the inferior wall of the right ventricle, or if it is long enough, it can extend into the pulmonary artery. One-fourth of the patients in Bloomfield's survey and 24% in our series, had the entire fragment embolized to the pulmonary arteries. The length of fragments in the pulmonary arteries in our 6 patients ranged from 3 to 25 cm. The 13-day-old child had an 8-cm long catheter fragment extending from the umbilical vein to the superior vena cava.

The distal end of the fragment usually rests against the wall of the vessel or the heart unless the proximal end is fixed at the site of the original catheter introduction, in which case the distal end is often free (Fig.2). The proximal end is sometimes free or can be manipulated from its position against the vessel wall into the vascular lumen (Fig. 3). A free position of one end of the fragment is important because it allows engagement of the fragment by the retrieval device and facilitates removal.

Stiff catheter fragments usually retain their position once they embolize, particularly when they are wedged with the distal end against the atrial wall. The position of soft, pliable, catheter fragments is often unstable early after separation has occurred. They often move during the cardiac cycle or with changes of intrathoracic pressure and patient motion. They can also be easily dislodged by retrieval maneuvers. This results in their embolization to a more central position in the heart or to the pulmonary arteries, making their retrieval more difficult (Fig. 4). Fragments located in the superior and inferior caval veins and the right atrium are relatively easy to remove with simple tools and little manipulation, especially when one of the ends is free. Retrieval of the fragments from the right ventricle and particularly from pulmonary arteries is more demanding. The selection of devices for retrieval of pulmonary artery fragments is limited, their manipulation through the heart

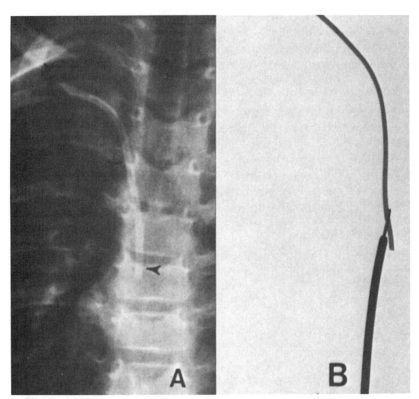

Figure 2. *A 5-year-old girl with malignant pelvic teratoma treated with long-term intravenous chemotherapy. The infusion catheter, which was in place for 5 months, broke during its removal. A. A 7-cm long fragment remained fixed with its proximal end in the right subclavian vein and extended almost to the right atrium (arrowheads). Preretrieval venogram showed intraluminal position of the catheter fragment and no clots around it. B. The fragment was retrieved with a snare loop after its caudal end was engaged in the loop.*

carries risk, and the final engagement of the embolized fragment often requires lengthy maneuvering.

Catheter fragments that have been allowed to remain against the walls of vessels or the right atrium usually cause reactive changes of the intima or endocardium with fibrotic tissue proliferation and neointimal formation. In a matter of months, the fragment end(s) and later the entire catheter fragment can become

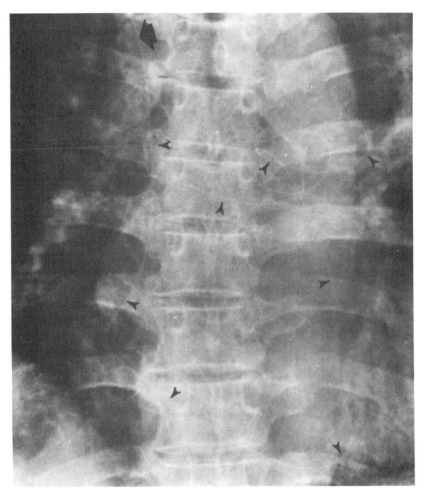

Figure 3. *A 60-year-old woman with massive upper gastrointestinal bleeding. A long intravenous catheter for transfusions was placed by cutdown into an antecubital vein. The catheter broke during its removal and a 65-cm long fragment remained in the venous system. It extended from the superior vena cava through the heart, looped in the left pulmonary artery, and ended in the right pulmonary artery. The ends of the fragment are indicated by arrows and the body by arrowheads. A snare loop retriever consisting of a 10 French Teflon catheter and a 3 French Teflon snare was used for retrieval. The end of the fragment has to be moved from the wall by a hook catheter prior to snaring.*

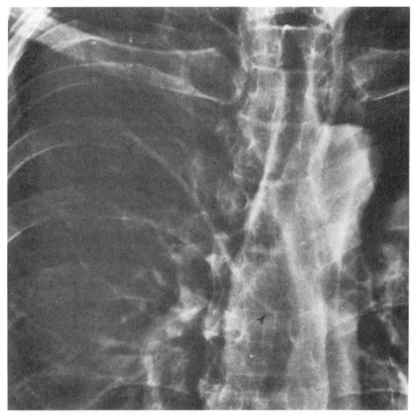

Figure 4. *A 62-year-old man with leukemia treated with long-term intravenous chemotherapy. The infusion catheter, which was in place for over 1 year, broke while the patient was doing yard work. An 11-cm long fragment embolized in the right pulmonary artery and its upper lobe branch (arrowheads). A snare loop was used to retrieve it.*

imbedded in the wall and completely covered by neoendothelium. Similarly, indwelling chemotherapy catheters left in a vein for long periods of time can become fully incorporated inside the vascular wall and lie outside the vascular lumen. These catheters are easy to break during their removal, but the retained catheter fragment cannot be retrieved by percutaneous techniques. We learned when treating one of our early patients who had a broken Silastic catheter that had been in place for 16 months. This patient has been the only failure in our series. A superior cava venogram performed after an unsuccessful attempt at retrieval showed that the broken catheter was extraluminal.

Retrieval Techniques

Retrieval of foreign bodies in the heart, particularly those causing cardiac arrhythmias, should be done on an emergent basis. Extracardiac fragments can be removed on an elective basis but without long delay. The incidence of complications increases in direct proportion to the length of time between embolization and retrieval.[23] Retrieval should be performed in angiographic or cardiologic laboratories equipped with a high quality fluoroscopic image intensifier, since some fragments are not very radiopaque. Radiographs of the area to which the broken catheter has embolized should be obtained in two projections prior to retrieval to confirm that the fragment has not migrated since its initial detection and to evaluate its position. With the patient under continuous cardiac monitoring, all manipulations are carried out under fluoroscopic control.[24] Retrieval of fragments of recently introduced catheters can be attempted without a preliminary angiogram. However, detailed angiograms of the structures containing the foreign body are necessary for broken catheters that have been in place for an extended period of time to detect possible thrombi around the fragment and to exclude an extraluminal position. An angiogram is also done to find nonopaque catheter fragments, which are extremely rare today.

Many tools and instruments have been developed and used to extract inravascular foreign bodies. The choice of instruments and techniques depends upon the size and location of the foreign body and its distance from the point of extraction. Of the basic retrievers, a loop snare catheter and a basket retriever have been used most often. Hook-tipped catheters or guidewires, grasping forceps and balloon catheters are also useful under special circumstances. Tip-deflecting guidewires and curved catheters can be useful aids, particularly for manipulating the fragment end away from the vessel wall. Vascular radiologists or cardiologists should become familiar with all retrieval systems and techniques and choose the one most suitable for a given case and with which they feel most comfortable.

The transfemoral approach is used for most retrievals, and both groins are usually prepared; the right for the introduction of the retrieval device because it gives straight access to the heart; while the left side is ready, if necessary, for introduction of a second catheter to aid in foreign body manipulation. If transfemoral venous access is not possible due to inferior vena cava obstruction, the internal jugular vein is a suitable alternative approach.

The percutaneous approach is suitable for introducing the majority of presently available retrieval devices, and with the use of sheaths it is possible to safely remove even relatively large foreign objects from the venous system. Cutdowns are usually indicated only for the final extraction of larger foreign bodies from the arterial system to prevent significant injury to the femoral artery. Vascular sheaths with self-sealing diaphragms at the hubs to prevent back bleeding are used to introduce large nontapered catheters. When using the transjugular approach, close attention should be directed toward the prevention of air embolism.

Loop Snare Catheters

The loop snare catheter is the simplest, safest and most effective retrieval device and has been used in a majority of catheter fragment retrievals.[3-6,8-10,12,15,16,19,20,22,25-33] It is the first choice for fragments lodged in the pulmonary arteries, and, in our opinion, it should be the first device attempted in any foreign body retrieval. We used it successfully in 16 patients. Loop snare catheters are commercially available (Cook, Inc., Bloomington, IN) but can easily be assembled from standard materials in the angiography laboratory (Fig. 5). The device consists of a nontapered Teflon-introducing catheter 45- to 100-cm long and 6 to 12 French in diameter, depending on the patient's age and the size and location of the object to be snared. It is usually introduced through a sheath. The snare is a 125- to 300-cm long, 0.015- to 0.025-inch stainless steel guidewire or a 3 French Teflon tubing (Fig. 6).

The technique of using a loop snare is as follows: the introducing catheter is first advanced to a point below the foreign body. When the intravascular foreign body is located in the pulmonary arteries, we always introduce a standard pulmonary artery catheter first to achieve safe passage through the heart. Once a selective position

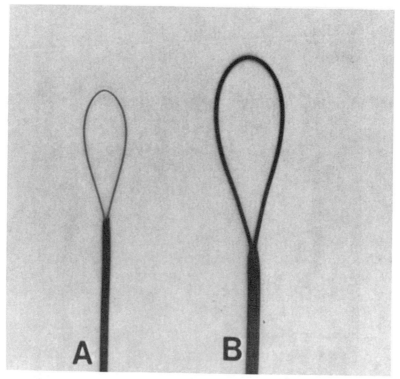

Figure 5. *Loop snare retrievers assembled in our laboratory. A. Snare loop for pediatric use consisting of a 6-French Teflon catheter and a 0.015-inch wire. B. Snare loop for adults consisting of a 9 French Teflon catheter and a 3 French Teflon tubing.*

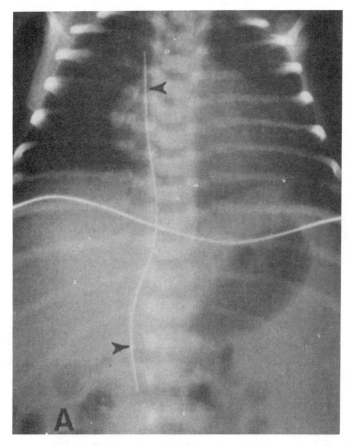

Figure 6A. *A 13-day-old girl weighing 2.2 kg. Her umbilical venous catheter became separated during removal. A. An 8-cm long segment remained in place, extending from the umbilical vein through the right atrium into the superior vena cava (arrowheads).*

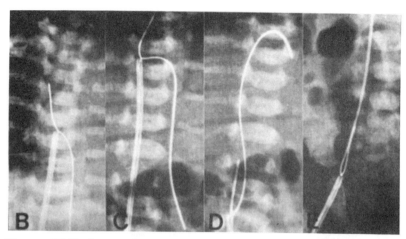

Figure 6B–E. *A snare loop consisting of 6 French Teflon catheter and a 0.015-inch wire was used for retrieval. The upper end of the fragment was engaged in the loop and the fragment was easily removed through the right femoral vein.*

in the pulmonary artery containing the fragment is established, we use a 260-cm long, 0.038-inch guidewire to exchange the pulmonary catheter for the Teflon-introducing catheter of the loop snare. Next, the snare guidewire or tubing is folded double and inserted through the Teflon catheter to a point just above the end of the introducer. With one limb of the snare being held, the other is advanced into the vessel to form a loop extending from the catheter tip towards the foreign body (Fig. 7). The size, configuration, and orientation of the snare loop is changed by advancing and withdrawing one limb of the snare. The introducing catheter can also be advanced or pulled down to engage the foreign body. Common sense, manipulative skill, and a bit of luck usually result in successful lassoing.

The lassoing is relatively easily achieved when the end of the fragment is free in the lumen of a large vessel. When the fragment end is firmly resting or wedged against the vessel wall, the snare loop may dislodge it from the wall, particularly if gently rotated; forming two snare loops may also help. However, a second catheter with a hook at the end, introduced from the left femoral approach, will almost always succed in freeing the wedged fragment end. Once

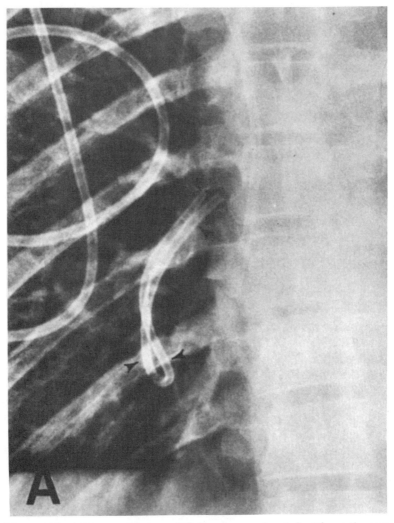

Figure 7A. *A 31-year-old man with lung cancer treated with continuous intravenous chemotherapy. A. His infusion catheter, which was in place for 3 months, broke during removal, and an 11-cm long segment (arrowheads) embolized to the right pulmonary artery and its lower lobe branch. A snare loop consisting of a 9 French Teflon catheter and 0.025-inch wire was used for retrieval.*

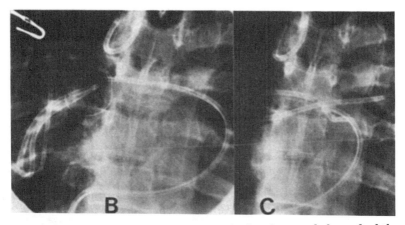

Figure 7B, C. *B. The wire loop is manipulated around the end of the fragment. C. The fragment is caught and pulled out.*

the lost fragment is lassoed, the snare is slowly withdrawn as the introducing catheter is carefully advanced so as not to lose the fragment. The snare is then drawn into the end of the catheter. Holding the snare tightly, but not so tight as to cut through a fragment of soft catheter, the fragment is locked to the catheter tip. Both the loop snare catheter and the foreign body fragment are then removed together through the introducing sheath.

When a fragment end is free inside the atrium, it is sometimes difficult to engage it with one snare loop, particularly when poor visibility impedes good three-dimensional control of snaring maneuvers. We found, in two such cases, that a compound loop consisting of several loops of 3-French Teflon tubing helped to successfully lasso the foreign body (Fig. 8).[5,24] The snare loop made of Teflon tubing is more pliable and easier to form than the stainless steel guidewire; however, one disadvantage is that a 9 to 10 French catheter is required for its introduction.

A number of snare loop catheter variations have been described as: (1) a combination of a 0.035-inch wire with nylon thread for the snare line, (2) a snare line with only one limb inside the catheter and the other limb attached to the catheter end, (3) a snare line with one limb exiting through a sidehole and the other through the endhole of the introducing catheter, or (4) both limbs exiting

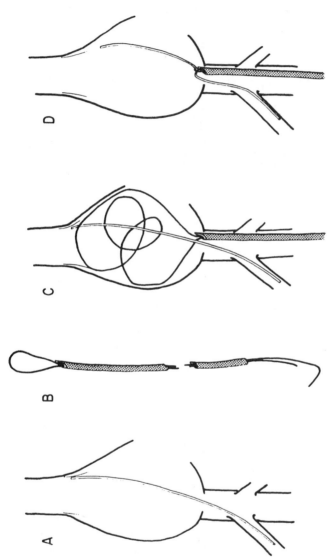

Figure 8. Retrieval of an 8-cm long fragment of a central venous catheter using a redundant loop snare in a 21-year-old female with septic abortion. A. The catheter fragment extends from the right hepatic vein into the right atrium. B. Homemade loop snare retriever consisting of a 12 12 French Teflon catheter and a 4 French snare. C. One convolution of a redundant loop has caught the foreign body. D. The fragment is securely held and about to be removed via the inferior vena cava and right femoral vein. (Reproduced with permission from Dotter CT, Rösch J, Bilboa MK: Transluminal extraction of catheter and guide fragments from the heart and great vessels: 29 collected cases. AJR 111:467, 1971.)

through the sidehole close to the catheter tip.[18,20,32] We have not tried these variations because we have found the original simple design quite satisfactory.

Basket Retrievers

Wire cage baskets used for ureteral and renal stone extraction (Dormia) or their modifications designed for intravascular use work well for entrapment of lost tubings lying within vessels (Fig. 9).[2,5,16,18,21,23,27,34-40] The urologic Dormia baskets, because of their small size, are particularly suitable for use in children and for retrieving foreign bodies from small vessels. The large-sized commercially available modifications (Cook, Inc., Bloomington, IN) are

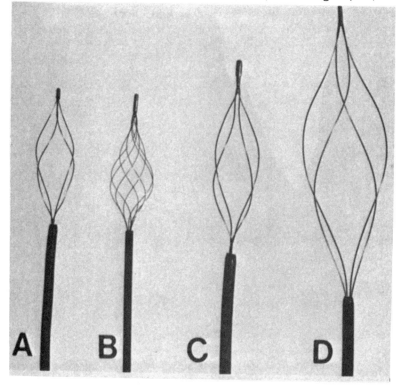

Figure 9. *Various types and sizes of basket devices for retrieval of intravascular foreign bodies (Cook, Inc., Blooimington, IN). A. A 3-cm long and 1.2-cm wide 4-wire basket. B. A 3-cm long and 1.3-cm wide 8-wire basket. C. A 4-cm long and 1.8-cm wide 4-wire basket. D. A 7.5-cm long and 3-cm wide 4-wire basket.*

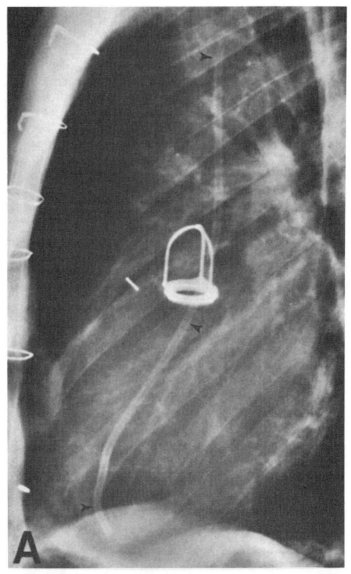

Figure 10A. *A 41-year-old man with subacute bacterial endocarditis and recent aortic valve replacement. An infusion catheter, which was in place for 2 weeks, broke during removal. A. A 21-cm long fragment lodged with caudal end in the right atrium and cranial end in the superior vena cava (arrowheads).*

used to retrieve catheter fragments from the caval veins. This large basket, however, should not be expanded and maneuvered within cardiac chambers because trabeculae or valves may be unintentionally caught and damaged.

A sheath is first percutaneously placed. The introducing catheter of the basket retriever is then advanced over a guidewire to just below the level of the foreign body. With a catheter fragment in the pulmonary arteries, a pulmonary catheter is first introduced through the heart in a similar fashion as with the snare loop technique. The guidewire is withdrawn and the basket is then advanced through the introducing catheter. Out of the catheter, it opens and is carefully manipulated to the level of or slightly above the lost catheter fragment (Fig. 10). With a free fragment end, the foreign

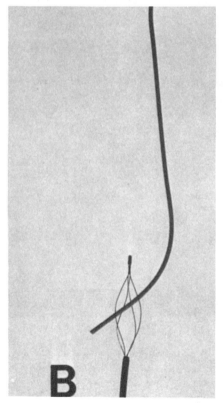

Figure 10B. *Basket retriever was used for removal, the end of the fragment had to be moved from the wall by a hook catheter prior to engagement into the basket.*

body usually is easy to engage between the basket wires. Sometimes several attempts with back-and-forth basket motion are necessary (Fig. 11). If the catheter fragment cannot be engaged with the introducing catheter tip pointing straight, the basket can be withdrawn and bent slightly at the base so as to form a 15 to 20° angle; this facilitates the fragment's capture.[23] A catheter fragment wedged against the vessel wall must be maneuvered into a free

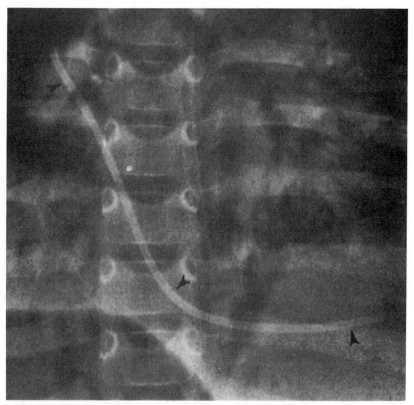

Figure 11. *An 8-year-old girl with intestinal pseudoobstruction and long-term intravenous hyperalimentation. The infusion catheter, which was in place for over 2 years, broke during attempted replacement. A 15-cm long fragment embolized into the heart and extended from the right atrium to the apex of the right ventricle (arrowheads), causing arrhythmias. A small basket was used for removal. The fragment broke into three pieces during removal; a 10-cm long piece was removed; 2-cm and 3-cm long pieces embolized to segmental pulmonary arteries and could not be retrieved.*

position; careful basket rotation may do the trick. Alternatively, a hook catheter can be introduced from the opposite femoral vein to push or pull the fragment away from the wall, thus allowing basket engagement. Once the foreign body is engaged, the introducing catheter is slowly advanced until the basket is closed with the foreign body entrapped inside (Fig. 12). The whole assembly is then withdrawn from the vascular system. External tension must be maintained on the basket against the introducing catheter during withdrawal so as not to lose the captured foreign body.

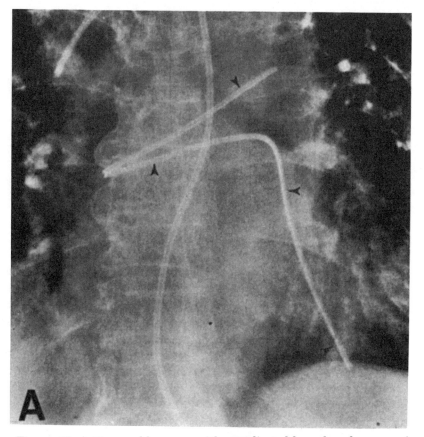

Figure 12. *A 70-year-old woman with complicated large bowel surgery. A central venous catheter broke during removal. A. A 24-cm long fragment embolized into the heart; it extended from the right ventricle and formed a loop in the right and left pulmonary arteries (arrowheads).*

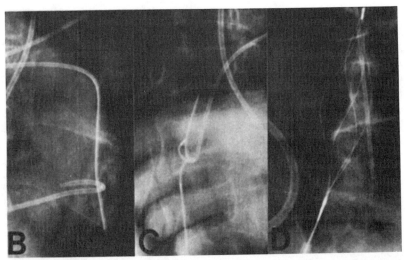

Figure 12B–D. *B. A hook catheter was used to move the ventricular end of the fragment into the right atrium. C. The atrial end was then caught with a tip- deflecting wire and pulled down into the inferior vena cava. D. The catheter fragment was then retrieved with a retrieval basket.*

Forceps

Endoscopic forceps used to remove foreign bodies from bronchi, the esophagus, or urinary tract have occasionally been used to retrieve intravascular catheter fragments (Fig. 13).[1,18,39–42] Introduced via a cutdown or through a sheath, the forceps is advanced with its jaws closed until it reaches the foreign body. The jaws are then opened and maneuvered around the broken catheter or guidewire. After being caught by the jaws, the foreign body is pulled out. Forceps have one major advantage; a free end of the fragment is not needed for retrieval, the fragment can be grasped at any contact point. Short length and relative rigidity, however, are major disadvantages of forceps, and limit substantially their use.

Relative rigidity of endoscopic forceps limits their introduction to those vessels with a straight route to the right atrium, usually the right internal jugular vein. Rigidity also decreases forceps maneuverability and poses an increased risk of vascular perforation.

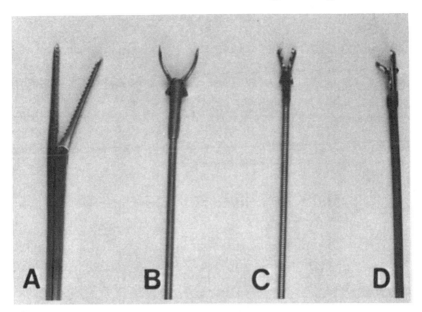

Figure 13. *Various types of grasping forceps. A and B. Rigid broncho-scopic forceps for removal of foreign bodies. C. Flexible bronchoscopic biopsy forceps. D. Myocardial biopsy catheter.*

Maneuverability is also compromised by the limited area that can be covered by opening the relatively short jaws and by difficulty in three-dimensional orientation during fluoroscopy, particularly if the foreign body is located in a large atrium.

Variants of the rigid forceps, such as the myocardial biopsy catheter and particularly the grasping forceps, have greater potential use for retrievals in selected cases. Myocardial biopsy catheters combine length, flexibility, and grasping force. However, their grasping cup-like ends are too small and only able to engage thin catheter fragments. The grasping forceps, a modification of flexible bronchoscopic forceps, consists of four stainless steel wires, 0.010 inch in diameter, arranged in the form of a claw and housed in a 5-French Teflon sheath (Medi-Tech, Inc., Watertown, MA).[23,41] The claw is opened and closed by advancing or withdrawing the wires through the sheath. When open, the claw measures 20 mm in diameter. The instrument is introduced through a steerable Medi-Tech catheter and handle (Medi-Tech, Inc., Watertown, MA), which gives excellent maneuverability to this retrieval system. For removal of an intravascular foreign body, the grasping forceps is advanced to meet the object with the claw closed. The claw is then opened by either sliding the wires forward or retracting the sheath. When the prongs engage the object, the sheath is advanced forward to tighten the grip. The assembly is then withdrawn.

The advantage of this soft, steerable catheter system in addition to its maneuverability, is its ability to grasp the lost fragment at any contact point. However, the risk of vascular laceration is present when the claw grasps the foreign body.

Hook-Tip Catheters or Guidewires

Hook-tip catheters or guidewires have been used in few cases to retrieve embolized fragments that did not present an accessible free end for snaring (Fig. 14).[7,8,11,14,20,22,26,35,38,46] A standard 7 or 8 French catheter, shaped with a sharp 180° curve at the tip, is in-

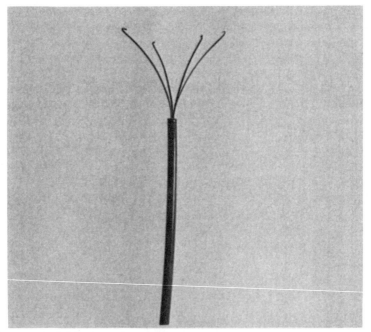

Figure 14. *Medi-tech grasping forceps (Medi-tech Inc., Watertown, MA).*

troduced through a sheath and over a guidewire above the level of the lost fragment. After guidewire withdrawal, the tip returns to the preformed curve, which is maneuvered over the fragment. The catheter is then rotated to securely grasp the fragment so it is not lost during withdrawal. This maneuver, however, works only with long pliable fragments; rigid fragments slip out of the hook. To prevent this, a hook-tip catheter can be combined with the Cook tip-deflecting wire system (Fig. 15) (Cook Inc., Bloomington, IN). The deflected wire tip, inside or outside the catheter, improves the grip of the hook-tip over the fragment and increases the chances it can be pulled down without being lost.

A cutdown and venotomy have usually been done for final removal of the fragment from the vessel of catheter entrance. The diameter of the hook is too large for percutaneous removal: at-

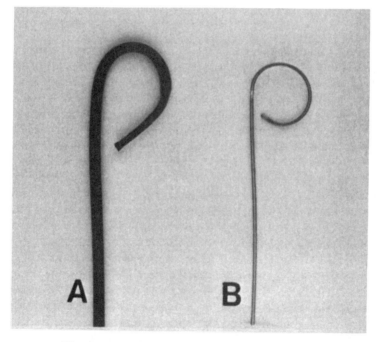

Figure 15. *A. Hook-tip 8 French polyethylene catheter. B. Curved tip of the Cook tip-deflecting wire system. (Cook Inc, Bloomington, IN).*

tempted percutaneous withdrawal of the hook would result in its straightening and loss of the fragment, and probable venous injury, particularly if the deflector system is used to enforce the catheter hook. To eliminate cutdown and venotomy in this case, it is preferable to introduce a snare loop or basket retriever through a puncture of the opposite femoral vein and grasp the foreign body in the inferior vena cava while it is held by the hook-tip catheter. The hook-tip catheter is also useful as an adjunct to primary retrievers to maneuver the fragment from the vessel wall and to facilitate its engagement into the snare loop or basket.

Balloon Catheters

A balloon catheter can be used as a primary retriever to remove larger tubular objects. We used it in two patients to remove Teflon stent tubes, 8 cm long and 16 and 18 French in diameter, which were placed in severely narrowed superior caval veins for relief of the superior vena cava syndrome. When, after 3 and 5 weeks respectively, the stents became occluded, they were removed using an 8 mm angioplasty balloon catheter. We dilated the right femoral vein puncture site to 16 and 18 French size, respectively and then used a large sheath to introduce the balloon catheter. After it was maneuvered through the occluded stent, the balloon was inflated above it, and the nonfunctional stent was removed by simply pulling it down and out the puncture hole together with the sheath (Fig. 16). Hemostasis was established without major problem.

Balloon catheters can also be useful as adjuncts to other primary retrieval devices. Introduced into a different vein than the primary retriever, the balloon catheter can be used to move an intravascular foreign body into a more favorable position for conventional catheter removal. Balloons could also be used to prevent undesired distal embolization of the foreign objects during their recovery.[24]

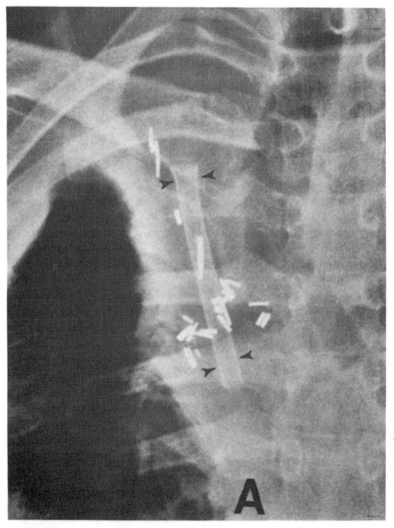

Figure 16A. *A 53-year-old man with recurrence of surgically treated lung carcinoma. A. He developed a superior vena cava syndrome and was treated by dilation of the severely stenosed superior vena cava and placement of an 18 French Teflon tubing as a shunt (arrowheads). When the shunt occluded, the stent was removed with an angioplasty dilation balloon catheter.*

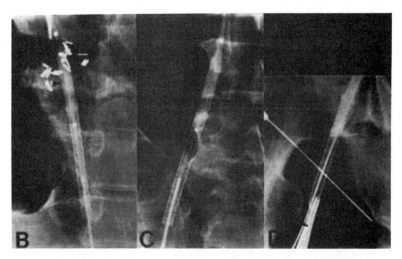

Figure 16B–D. *The balloon catheter was advanced through the stent and inflated above it (arrowheads). C. The stent was then pulled down through the right atrium and inferior vena cava. D. It was removed percutaneously via the right femoral vein with with the help of a hemostatic forceps (arrow).*

Retrieval Failures

The success rate of percutaneous removal of intravascular foreign bodies is quite high. Only 10% unsuccessful attempts (18 patients) were reported in Bloomfield's survey,[18] 5% in the Uflacker et al. report,[22] and 4% percent in our experience. Multiple factors can contribute to retrieval failure. Peripheral position of the foreign body is one, particularly if its location is in the pulmonary artery bed. Retrieval of a foreign body located in a lobar or central portion of a segmental pulmonary artery can be attempted with a reasonable chance of success. However, if a fragment is lodged in a more peripheral position, retrieval should not, in our opinion, be attempted.

Intravascular but extraluminal position of a lost catheter fragment can be another cause of removal failure (one patient in our series). Such a position, with complete incorporation of the fragment by neoendothelium, should be suspected with long-term indwelling Silastic catheters and if there has been a long-time interval between fragment loss and retrieval attempt. Angiography of the involved vessel or chamber helps to document the fragment position and avoid the frustration of prolonged unsuccessful attempts at removal. Angiography can also establish entirely extravascular positions of catheter fragments in patients who are occasionally referred for retrieval.[18]

Another cause of failure to remove an intravascular foreign body is unsuitable technique. One must realize that no retrieval system will be successful in every case. Common sense, experience, and a certain degree of ingenuity help in the selection of a suitable retrieval technique. However, if not successful, adjunctive techniques should be tried or another retrieval system used. Reasonable persistence, coupled with thoughts of the patient's surgical alternative in the event of failure of percutaneous retrieval usually pays off and results in successful removal of the foreign body.

Complications

The complication rate of percutaneous retrieval of intravascular foreign bodies is remarkably low. As far as is known, no one had died as a consequence of attempted catheter recovery, and no serious complications have been reported.[18]

There have been no perforations of vessels, even from the rigid endoscopic forceps, although this possibility has always been stressed. Lack of serious complications is quite striking, since a considerable number of foreign bodies were retrieved with minimal experience and often with homemade equipment.

Transient arrhythmias often occur with the introduction and manipulation of retrievers in the heart, during intracardiac transit of the foreign body being extracted from the pulmonary artery, and during removal of a fragment impinging on the right ventricular wall.[18] Careful catheter and retriever manipulation minimizes the arrhythmias, and fast but gentle removal of the retrieved catheter fragment from the heart restores cardiac rhythm to normal.

During retrieval, a catheter fragment that is not held tightly in a retrieval device can be lost. On the other hand, a catheter fragment held too tightly can be cut through and further fragmented. This can happen, particularly when the retriever device has thin wires. Fragments of soft, pliable indwelling catheters that have been left in place for long periods of time are particularly susceptible to further fragmentation. A lost fragment, and particularly a cut fragment, often embolizes to a more central position into the heart, to the pulmonary arteries, or to small peripheral vessels in the case of fragments in the arterial circulation. This makes their retrieval more difficult. In the case of fragmentation into small pieces that embolize quite far peripherally, retrieval is impossible.[22] In one of our patients, a catheter fragment originally lodged in the right pulmonary artery was lost during its retrieval by a snare loop, as it was being pulled through the heart; it embolized deep to a lobar branch of the left pulmonary artery. Luckily, we were able to retrieve it from this position with a snare loop. In another patient, an 8-year-old girl, a fragment of a long-term feeding catheter, which had been in place for over 2 years, broke into three pieces during retrieval with a small basket. We were able to retrieve the longest fragment but the other two small fragments embolized into subsegmental branches of the pulmonary arteries and could not be retrieved.

Clinically symptomatic pulmonary embolism from clots inside and around retrieved foreign bodies has not been reported, but asymptomatic embolism was documented by a lung perfusion scan following removal of a pacemaker that had been in place for 5 years.[18] In the venous system, there have been no problems of hemorrhage at the site of cutdown or percutaneous entry reported, despite the fact that relatively large catheters and sheaths have been used for the introduction of the retrieval instruments. In the arterial system, where the risk of local injury is much greater, intimal tear with thrombosis of the femoral artery close to the puncture site was reported in one case after successful removal of a lost guidewire from the abdominal aorta with a retrieval basket.[36]

Prevention

Prevention is the best solution for the problem of intravascular iatrogenic foreign bodies. Manufacturers have made great improvements in the safety of guidewires, angiographic catheters, and catheters used for pressure monitoring and fluid infusions. Intravascular iatrogenic foreign bodies can be prevented or their occurrence substantially decreased with attention to the following rules:

1. Adhere meticulously to instructions for catheter introduction and withdrawal.
2. Avoid inserting catheters near joints, particularly in areas of flexion and extension.
3. Avoid catheter insertion in uncooperative, combative patients.
4. Avoid catheter withdrawal through sharp needles to prevent their shearing.
5. Establish safe time limits for the use of intravascular catheters.

References

1. Thomas J, Sinclair-Smith B, Bloomfield D, et al: Non-surgical retrieval of a broken segment of steel spring guide from the right atrium and inferior vena cava. Circulation 30:106, 1964.
2. Lassers BW, Pickering D: Removal of an iatrogenic foreign body from the aorta by means of a ureteric stone catcher. Am Heart J 73:375, 1967.
3. Massumi RA, Ross AM: Atraumatic, nonsurgical technic for removal of broken catheters from cardiac cavities. N Engl J Med 277:195, 1967.
4. Henley FT, Ballard JW: Percutaneous removal of flexible foreign body from the heart. Radiology 92:176, 1969.
5. Dotter CT, Rumosch J, Bilbao MK: Transluminal extraction of catheter and guide fragments from the heart and great vessels; 29 collected cases. AJR 111:467, 1971.
6. Miller RE, Cockerill EM, Helbig H: Percutaneous removal of catheter emboli from the pulmonary arteries. Radiology 94:151, 1970.
7. Rossi P: "Hook catheter," technique for transfemoral removal of foreign body from right side of the heart. AJR 109:101, 1970.
8. Hipona FA, Sciammas FD, Hublitz UF: Nonthoracotomy retrieval of intraluminal cardiovascular foreign bodies. Radiol Clin N Am 9:583, 1971.
9. Bloomfield DA: Techniques of nonsurgical retrieval of iatrogenic foreign bodies from the heart. Am J Cardiol 27:538, 1971.
10. Randall PA: Percutaneous removal of iatrogenic intracardiac foreign body. Radiology 102:591, 1972.
11. Maxwell DD, Anderson RE: Transfemoral retrieval of an intracardiac catheter fragement, using a simple hook-shaped catheter. Radiology 103:213, 1972.
12. Enge I, Flatmark A: Percutaneous removal of intravascular foreign bodies by the snare technique. Acta Radiol (Diagn)(Stockh) 14:747, 1973.
13. Richardson JD, Grover FL, Trinkle JK: Intravenous catheter emboli. Experience with twenty cases and collective review. Am J Surg 128:722, 1974.
14. Fisher RG, Romero JR: Extraction of an embolized central venous catheter using percutaneous technique. Radiology 116:735, 1975.

15. Picard L, Roland J, Sigiel M, et al: Transluminal retrieval of ventriculoatrial shunt catheters from the heart and great vessels: a new method. Neuroradiology 10:159, 1975.
16. Aldridge HE, Lee J: Transvascular removal of catheter fragments from the great vessels and heart. Can Med Assoc J 117:1300, 1977.
17. Fisher RG, Ferreyro R: Evaluation of current techniques for nonsurgical removal of intravascular iatrogenic foreign bodies. AJR 130:541, 1978.
18. Bloomfield DA: The nonsurgical retrieval of intracardiac foreign bodies man international survey. Cathet Cardiovasc Diagn 4:1, 1978.
19. Rubinstein ZJ, Morag B, Itzchak Y: Percutaneous removal of intravascular foreign bodies. Cardiovasc Interven Radiol 5:64, 1982.
20. Cho SR, Tisnado J, Beachley MC, et al: Percutaneous unknotting of intravascular catheters and retrieval of catheter fragments. AJR 141:397, 1983.
21. Endrys J, Rubacek M, Podrabsky P: Percutaneous retrieval of foreign bodies from the cardiovascular system. Cor Vasa 27:36, 1985.
22. Uflacker R, Lima S, Melichar AC: Intravascular foreign bodies: percutaneous retrieval. Radiology 160:731, 1986.
23. Kadir S, Athanasoulis CA: Percutaneous retrieval of intravascular foreign bodies. In Athanasoulis CA, Pfister RC, Greene RE, et al (eds): Interventional Radiology. Philadelphia, WB Saunders Co, 1982, p 379.
24. Dotter CT, Keller FS, Rösch J: Transluminal catheter removal of foreign bodies from the cardiovascular system. In Abrams HL (ed): Abrams Angiography: Vascular and Interventional Radiology, 3rd Ed. Boston, Little, Brown and Co, 1983, p 2395.
25. Curry JL: Recovery of detached intravascular catheter or guide wire fragments. AJR 105:894, 1969.
26. Greenfield DH, McMullan GK, Parisi AF, et al: Snare retrieval of a catheter fragment with inaccessible ends from the pulmonary artery. Cathet Cardiovasc Diagn 4:87, 1978.
27. Grand M, Harry G, Rémy J, et al: Extraction non chirurgicale de corps étrangers iatrogenes intravasculaires. J Radiol 59:479, 1978.
28. Khaja F, Lakier J: Foreign body retrieval from the heart by two catheter technique. Cathet Cardiovasc Diagn 5:263, 1979.
29. Zollikofer C, Nath PH, Castaneda-Zuniga WR, et al: Nonsurgical removal of intravascular foreign bodies. ROFO 130:590, 1979.
30. Hubert JW, Krone RJ, Shatz BA, et al: An improved snare system for the nonsurgical retrieval of intravascular foreign bodies. Cathet Cardiovasc Diagn 6:405, 1980.
31. Schmidt G, Wirtzfeld A, Busch U, et al: Pervenose Entfernung von Schrittmacherelektrodenfragmenten. Herz Kreisl 12:503, 1980.
32. Vaeusorn N, Burodom N, Harnchonboth A, et al: Modified loopsnare for percutaneous removal of intravascular catheter fragments. Radiology 145:839, 1982.
33. Morse SS, Strauss EB, Hashim SW, et al: Percutaneous retrieval of an unusually large, nonopaque intravascular foreign body. AJR 146:863, 1986.

34. Harinck E, Rohmer J: Atraumatic retrieval of catheter fragments from the central circulation in children. Eur J Cardiol 1:421, 1974.
35. O'Neill G, Joseph SP: Pervenous retrieval of embolized catheters from the right heart and pulmonary arteries. Am Heart J 98:287, 1979.
36. Fälling M, List AR: Transvascular retrieval of an accidentally ejected tip occluder and wire. Cardiovasc Interven Radiol 5:34, 1982.
37. Huang TY, Abaskaron M: Nonsurgical removal of intravascular fragmented catheter. Am Fam Physician 30:177, 1984.
38. Clouse ME, Costello P, O'Leary DH: Removal of intravascular foreign bodies using modified Grollman catheter and Dormia basket. J Can Assoc Radiol 35:305, 1984.
39. Glatter TR, Scott CA, Early G: Percutaneous removal of intracardiac catheter fragment: unique internal jugular venous approach. Am Heart J 108:408, 1984.
40. Chuang VP: Nonoperative retrieval of Gianturco coils from abdominal aorta. AJR 132:996, 1979.
41. Smyth NPD, Boivin MR, Bacos JM: Transjugular removal of foreign body from the right atrium by endoscopic forceps. J Thorac Cardiovasc Surg 55:594, 1968.
42. King JF, Manley JC, Zeft HJ, et al: Nonsurgical removal of foreign body from right heart. A new percutaneous approach. J Thorac Cardiovasc Surg 71:785, 1976.
43. Millan VG: Retrieval of intravascular foreign bodies using a modified bronchoscopic forceps. Radiology 129:587, 1978.
44. Shaw TRD: Removal of embolised catheters using flexible endoscopy forceps. Br Heart J 48:497, 1982.
45. Kim MS, Horton JA: Intra-arterial foreign body retrieved using endoscopic biopsy forceps. Radiology 149:597, 1983.
46. McSweeney WJ, Schwartz DC: Retrieval of a catheter foreign body from the right heart using a guide wire deflector system. Radiology 100:61, 1971.

Chapter 14

Value of Two-Dimensional / Doppler Echocardiography and Cardiac Scintigraphy in Avoiding Complications of Cardiac Catheterization

Robert T. Palac and Richard A. Wilson

Patient characteristics associated with increased morbidity and mortality during cardiac catheterization include: age greater than 65 years; Class IV functional status; presence of severe coronary artery disease, especially left main coronary artery involvement; presence of valvular heart disease, especially aortic stenosis; severe left ventricular dysfunction, left ventricular ejection fraction less than or equal to 30%; and associated severe noncardiac disease.[1]

Two widely available noninvasive cardiac imaging techniques— two-dimensional / Doppler echocardiography and nuclear cardiac scintigraphy may be useful to identify patients at high risk of complications during cardiac catheterization and to tailor the catheterization protocol to reduce risk in patients who fall into a high-risk category. Each imaging method offers specific advantages depending on the clinical questions being addressed during the pre-catheterization patient evaluation. Table 1 lists the various measurements that are obtainable with each of these techniques.

This chapter discusses the value of two-dimensional / Doppler echocardiography and nuclear cardiac scintigraphy in the avoidance of cardiac catheterization complications in high-risk patients. Spe-

From *Complications of Cardiac Catheterization and Angiography: Prevention and Management* edited by Jack Kron, M.D. and Mark J. Morton, M.D. © 1989, Futura Publishing Inc., Mount Kisco, NY.

Table 1
Quantitative and Qualitative Noninvasive Measurements

2-D Echocardiography/Doppler	Nuclear Cardiology

A. M-mode echo
  1. Cardiac chamber dimensions
  2. Myocardial wall thickness/thickening
  3. E-point septal separation
  4. Valve motion
B. 2-dimensional echo
  1. Left ventricular function (segmental wall motion, thickening, and calculated ejection fraction)
  2. Left ventricular volumes
  3. Valvular pathology/motion
  4. Other cardiac chamber sizes
  5. Interventional studies (exercise and pharmacologic left ventricular wall motion analysis)
  6. Coronary artery imaging
  7. Complications of coronary disease (left ventricular aneurysm or pseudo aneurysm, thrombus, ventricular septal defect, torn chord)
  8. Congenital anomalies
  9. Pericardial disease
C. Doppler flow
  1. Valvular gradients (peak instantaneous and mean)
  2. Flow mapping (regurgitant lesions, turbulence)
  3. Stroke volume/cardiac output
  4. Shunts
  5. Assessment of intracardiac pressures
	A. Radionuclide angiography (gated blood pool imaging)
	  1. Left and right ventricular ejection fractions
	  2. Left ventricular regional wall motion
	  3. Left ventricular volumes
	  4. Left-sided valvular (LV/RV stroke count ratio)
	  5. Tricuspid insufficiency
	  6. Left ventricular functional response to exercise (ischemic or nonischemic dysfunction)
	B. Thallium-201 myocardial perfusion imaging (with exercise stress testing or pharmacological stress testing (dipyridamole or dobutamine infusions)
	  1. Transient ischemia (extent and severity)
	  2. Infarction
	  3. Transient left ventricular dysfunction with exercise (increased lung Tl-201 uptake)
	C. Positron emission tomography
	  1. Rubidium-82 transient deficits with exercise (= ischemia)
	  2. Increased 18-flurodeoxyglucose myocardial uptake (= ischemia)
	  3. Slow fatty acid palmitate clearance (= ischemia)

cific areas of importance in this regard are: quantitation of left ventricular function, identification of the high-risk coronary disease patient, and quantification of valvular stenosis and / or regurgitation. Important questions to be addressed in each of these specific areas include: how accurate and reproducible is the technique?; how often can the exam be performed?; what parameters can be evaluated by each technique?; and in what patients is the noninvasive evaluation most appropriate?

Left Ventricular Function Evaluation

Echocardiographic Technique

Measurements commonly obtained from left ventriculography include a measurement of left ventricular size at end-diastole and end-systole usually expressed as a volume calculation. These measurements are based on the application of volume formulae for particular geometric figures that approximate the configuration of the left ventricle. In most instances this is a prolate ellipsoid.[2] Additionally, left ventricular ejection fraction can be calculated from these volumes using the equation: End-diastolic volume—end-systolic volume / end-diastolic volume. Finally, from left ventriculography a qualitative or quantitative assessment of regional left ventricular wall motion may be performed. In addition, if mitral regurgitation or aortic regurgitation is present, a qualitative assessment of its severity is attempted from evaluation of the appropriate angiogram, left ventricular or supravalvular, respectively. The importance of each of these measurements is dependent on the clinical situation. Left ventricular ejection fraction and regional wall motion may be the most relevant to patients with coronary disease; whereas left ventricular volumes are more important in patients with valvular heart disease. How well, then, does two-dimensional echocardiography perform in evaluation of left ventricular function?

Unlike contrast ventriculography where left ventricular wall position is based on the observed edges of the contrast-containing left ventricle, two-dimensional echocardiography provides a series of tomographic images of the left ventricle from standardized imaging planes. The usefulness of two-dimensional echocardiography to assess left ventricular function is dependent on the ability in a given patient to accurately identify left ventricular endocardium. For quantitation of global left ventricular function, the most important views are the apical long-axis and apical four chamber views. In a prospective series from the Mayo Clinic, of 200 consecutive patients in whom multiview echocardiograms were performed, 99% were able to have an apical four-chamber view obtained and 93% either had an apical long-axis or two-chamber view.[3] Although visually interpretable echocardiograms may be obtained from the apical window in a high proportion of patients, in our experience adequate views to allow tracing of endocardial outlines for ejection fraction determination can be obtained in approximately 70% of patients. However, other centers with different patient populations may not have such a favorable experience. As with contrast ventriculography, the determination of echo-derived volumes from these orthogonal views is based on geometric models. The three most commonly used models are: (1) the prolate ellipsoid, (2) a combination of shapes such as a cylinder and truncated cone, or (3) the Simpson's rule. According to the Simpson's rule, the volume of a complex structure is estimated by summation of the volumes of multiple but geometrically simple figures that make up the complex structure. The ease and application of any of these approaches is enhanced by the availability of a computer-based digitizing device to assist in tracing and quantifying areas from the two-dimensional echo images. Studies comparing echo volumes using each modeling method have been performed.[4-6] These have highlighted problems that the clinician must be aware of when using this noninvasive technique to evaluate left ventricular function. At our hospital we use the Simpson's algorithm in combination with apical biplane views. Starling used a similar method to compare echo volumes and ejection fractions to these obtained during left ventricular angiography.[7] There was good agreement between echocardiographic and angiographic end-diastolic volumes (r = 0.80, SEE = 34 mL). Similar results were obtained for end-systolic volume (r = 0.88, SEE = 27 mL). Reproducibility for end-diastole and end-systolic volumes was excellent within observers (r = 0.97 and r = 0.98, respectively) and between observers (r = 0.85 and r = 0.98, respectively). In general, left ventricular volume was underestimated by 7%–27%. However, angiographic left ventricular volumes systematically overestimate true left ventricular volume. This underestimation has been a common finding in any echo method evaluated. Low echocardiographic volumes can be explained by four factors: "beam width," which leads to a widening of endocardial echoes with encroachment into the ventricular cavity, "foreshortening" of the ventricular long axis because of inability to place the transducer at the true left ventricular apex, inability to account for movement through the apex to base plane, and finally the inclusion of the spaces between the trabeculae during angiography and the exclusion of these during echocardiographic evaluation of LV volumes. In many laboratories these limitations are overcome by developing a regression relationship between calculated echo volumes and angiographic volumes. This results in excellent echo estimates of left ventricular volume that can effectively be substituted for angiographic volumes in the evaluation of patients. As previously mentioned, a significant limitation to the determination of echocardiographic volumes and left ventricular ejection fraction is the need for computer assistance. Quinones has developed a simple approach that does not use traced outlines for a computer.[8] Instead, using calipers, short axes from multiple views at end-diastole and end-systole are measured and combined with a long-axis determination at end-diastole and end-systole. Areas can be calculated that can then be converted to end-diastolic volumes by using a regression formula. Progressive evaluation of this method for volume determination even in patients with asynergy was excellent, (r = 0.95, SEE = 19 mL). Since a regression formula is used, there is no systematic underestimation of volumes.

One of the most useful measurements of global left ventricular performance made during angiography is left ventricular ejection fraction. Ejection fraction is determined by the calculation of relative changes in ventricular volumes at diastole and end-systole. These volumes are underestimated by echocardiography. However, if the quotient of measured and real volume is a constant throughout the range studied, the errors will cancel out and ejection fraction will be correct regardless of errors in the measurement of volume. This, in fact, has been the case with echo estimates of left ventricular ejection fraction. Calculation of left ventricular ejection fraction from biplane apical images in one study gave excellent agreement with angiographic ejection fraction (r = 0.91, SEE = 7%).[7] These results have been confirmed using other algorithms.[4,9-11] In these studies the presence of significant wall motion abnormality did not appear to dramatically alter the accuracy of left ventricular ejection fraction. In addition, Quinones compared echo estimates of left ventricular ejection fraction with angiography and radionuclide ventriculography.[11] He found excellent correlation ($r = 0.91$, SEE $= 7.4\%$ and $r = 0.93$, SEE 6.8%, respectively). Clearly, the assessment of global left ventricular function using M-mode echocardiography is fraught with difficulties, primarily because of the limited views of the left ventricle by this technique. Massie and co-workers, however, found an inverse relationship between the E-point septal separation and angiographic ejection fraction.[12] The value of this measurement is confirmatory; it gives one more independent estimate of left ventricular ejection fraction. Also it would be useful in situations where a two-dimensional echocardiogram or radionuclide ventriculogram is unobtainable.

The assessment of regional wall motion using echocardiography is especially critical in patients with coronary artery disease. The advantages of two-dimensional echocardiography in assessing regional function stem from its ability to image the ventricle in multiple tomographic planes. In addition, endocardial motion and wall thickening can be qualitatively and quantitatively assessed. Although quantitative methods for assessing regional wall motion are available, these techniques are considered experimental with regard to clinical application.[13] When qualitative assessment of regional wall motion was compared with qualitative assessment during angiography, excellent sensitivity in the detection of regional wall abnormality was obtained.[14] Also, inter- and intraobserver variability is low using the qualitative approaches, with major discrepancies occurring in approximately 3% of the segments analyzed. One final advantage of two-dimensional echocardiography is its precise definition of structural integrity and anatomic relationships, which makes it useful in the detection of complications of myocardial infarction such as: aneurysm, infarct expansion, ventricular pseudoaneurysm, acquired ventricular septal defect, papillary muscle dysfunction, and mural thrombus.[15] These complications may not be recognized during routine left ventricular and coronary angiography; however, the catheterization protocol might be modified if one of these complications were known to be present prior to the study. For example, the presence of left ventricular thrombus might alert the catheterizer to be more cautious in entering the left ventricular chamber. Hence, two-dimensional echocardiography and left ventricular angiography can be complimentary in evaluation of the patient with a high probability for one of these complications.

Radionuclide Ventriculography

Radionuclide ventriculography (gated blood pool imaging) is a noninvasive method of imaging the cyclic changes in left ventricular volume during the cardiac cycle.[16] A small proportion of the patients' circulating red blood cells are labeled with technetium-99m which emits a 140-keV gamma ray.[17] These gamma ray emissions are collimated and imaged on a scintillation gamma camera. Data acquisition usually involves 16-32 image frames during the cardiac cycle beginning at the onset of the electrocardiographic QRS. Multiple views are obtained including the anterior, "best septal" left anterior oblique and 60° left posterior oblique (a mirror image of the 30° right anterior oblique used in contrast left ventriculography). Since the radioisotope is thoroughly mixed with the circulating blood, the absolute and relative changes in radioactivity within the left ventricle should be directly proportional to changes in the blood volume within the ventricle. Therefore, left ventricular volume and ejection fraction and regional wall motion measurements can be obtained. The major advantages of this technique are that: (1) it is noninvasive, (2) it is not associated with a risk for contrast reactions, and (3) it is not limited by an adequate echocardiographic "window" to obtain satisfactory images. The measurements for the calculation of left ventricular volume by radionuclide ventriculography do not assume a particular geometric shape and therefore have been called "nongeometric." However, the measurement of left ventricular volume requires a correction for the attenuation of the 140-keV gamma rays as they pass through the ventricular chamber and chest wall. Measurements of ejection fraction and regional wall motion do not require attenuation correction.

The measurements of left ventricular volume have been shown to be accurate and reproducible.[18-20] Similarly, left ventricular ejection fraction and regional wall motion have been shown to be reproducible.[21] A major reason for the reproducibility of the left ventricular ejection fraction is the use of a computer-based semiautomated edge-detection algorithm for the measurement. As with contrast left ventriculography, regional wall motion is usually interpreted qualitatively. The region with the most variability in qualitative interpretations has been the interventricular septum.[21]

Radionuclide ventriculography offers the ability to noninvasively measure left ventricular ejection fraction and volumes before catheterization. As a result, a left ventriculogram could be avoided or, in other cases, the catheterizer alerted to the presence of an aneurysm or rarely a pseudoaneurysm.

Myocardial infarction is a common cause of congestive heart failure. Patients who undergo cardiac catheterization for medically refractory angina have frequently had one or more infarctions. The resultant impairment of the left ventricular function is also frequently not known prior to coronary angiography and therefore a contrast left ventriculogram may precipitate pulmonary edema. Alternatively, a patient may not be considered a candidate for operation (or catheterization) if extremely poor left ventricular function is identified noninvasively, but may be identified as a patient who could benefit symptomatically from medical therapy directed toward occult or incipient heart failure.

Left ventricular ejection fraction is one of the most powerful predictors of survival after myocardial infarction.[22,23] Therefore, the noninvasive measurement of this parameter alone provides important clinical information. In addition, the precatheterization assessment of regional hypokinesis as opposed to akinesis or dyskinesis is more likely to identify a region that contains viable myocardium even though some of the myocardium may be infarcted.[24]

Since noninvasive tests can accurately assess left ventricular function, when should they be used in place of left ventriculography to reduce catheterization complications? One must be guided by the clinical situation of the patient. It would be easy to make a case for a noninvasive assessment in patients with Class III or IV heart failure, the patient with multiple myocardial infarctions, the patient with significant cardiomegaly on chest x-ray, perhaps the patient older than 65 years of age, the patient at high risk for contrast nephropathy, i.e., the patient with chronic renal failure or diabetes mellitus with elevated serum creatinine, and the patient with a suspected complication of myocardial infarction.

Are there particular advantages offered by a specific method (echocardiography vs radionuclide ventriculography)? In certain patients, echocardiography has a high likelihood of being unobtainable, e.g., in the presence of obesity and chronic obstructive lung disease. In these patients, radionuclear assessment would be the method of choice. In patients with suspected coronary disease, either technique is probably adequate for assessment of left ventricular volume and function. In patients with valvular disease, echocardiography is preferred because it allows precise definition of the structural abnormality involved.

Identification of the High-Risk Coronary Disease Patient

Increasing severity of coronary artery disease is associated with increased morbidity and mortality during cardiac catheterization. This is especially true when left main coronary artery obstruction is present. How useful are the noninvasive methods in predicting the severity of coronary artery disease? In many instances a patient coming to the cardiac catheterization laboratory will have had a noninvasive test. Proper interpretation of the results with regard to severity of the disease would alert the catheterizer to exercise particular care in cannulating the left coronary artery or perhaps to use a "soft-tipped catheter." Additionally, the dichotomous decision to catheterize or not catheterize the elderly patient with typical or atypical chest pain and the diabetic patient with renal failure might be avoided after integration of the diagnostic and prognostic information obtained from noninvasive testing.

Role of Two-Dimensional Echocardiography

The clinical application of echocardiography in establishing the prognosis and estimating the severity of coronary artery disease in patients with chest pain syndromes is in an experimental phase. However, some of the rapid developments in the areas of stress echocardiography and left main coronary artery imaging must be highlighted as these techniques will be applied clinically with increasing frequency.

In patients with multiple infarctions and chest pain the presence of moderate to severe depression of the left ventricular function as assessed by echocardiography would alert the catheterizer to the fact that the patient potentially has a high risk coronary anatomy. However, in patients without clinical infarction, a normal resting echocardiogram does not exclude important coronary artery disease. In this setting, exercise or pharmacologic stress may produce ischemic dysfunction in the affected coronary distribution. This will result in a regional abnormality in wall motion amplitude and wall thickening that can be detected and evaluated by echocardiography. The greatest limitation to exercise echocardiography is the inability to obtain adequate studies for interpretation. This can be difficult because of the technical aspects of obtaining echocardiograms during the exaggerated chest wall motion and increased respiratory effort that accompanies exercise. In spite of this limitation, a number of studies[25-32] have been performed evaluating 2-D echocardiography during bicycle stress, prior to and immediately following treadmill exercise stress, and during pharmacologic stress.[26] The results are shown in Table 2. Adequate studies were obtainable in 71%–100% of the patients evaluated. Overall sensitivity and specificity ranged from 63%–100% and from 75%–100%, respectively. Most patients with multivessel coronary disease or left main coronary disease had a positive exercise echocardiogram. Sensitivity was considerably less for single-vessel disease. It appears that this is an exciting new technique that may be utilized to assess the severity of coronary disease (Table 2).

Another area that is being evaluated is the ultrasonic imaging of the coronary arteries. Although coronary arteriography remains the only reliable method of identifying obstructive coronary lesions, initial attempts at imaging the left main coronary artery using echocardiography have been made.[33,34] In a retrospective study of 72 patients undergoing coronary angiography, high intensity echos in the walls of the left main coronary artery were detected in all 7 patients with left main coronary obstruction of at least 50%.[33] In a prospective study of 31 patients, 2 independent observers identified all 3 patients with significant left main coronary artery narrowing.[34] One observer reported one false-positive. Recently, the development of annular phased ray imaging has improved resolution in the left main coronary artery. Perhaps in the future this technique will allow precatheterization identification of the highest risk coronary patient—the patient with left main coronary obstruction.

Table 2

Utility of Stress Echocardiography in Patients Being Evaluated for Coronary Artery Disease

Author	# of Patients	Type of Stress	Success Rate (%)	SVD Sensitivity (%)	MVD Sensitivity (%)	All Patients Sensitivity (%)	Specificity (%)
Wann[27]	28	Bicycle (s)	71	50	92	67	100
Morganroth[28]	55	Bicycle (s)	78	57	64	63	91
Maurer[29]	48	Posttreadmill	85	50	92	83	92
Crawford[30]	25	Bicycle (u)	72	–	–	72	100
Limacher[31]	73	Posttreadmill	100	45	96	86	88
Armstrong[32]	95	Posttreadmill	100	–	–	80	87
Palac[26]	44	Dobutamine	87	57	94	84	86

SVD = single vessel disease; MVD = multi-vessel disease; s = supine; u = upright.

Role of Thallium-201 Scintigraphy and Radionuclide Ventriculography

Thallium-201 (Tl-201) is a radioactive monovalent cation that initially distributes to the myocardium in proportion to coronary blood flow when injected intravenously[35] because it has a high first pass myocardial extraction fraction of approximately 85%.[36] This potassium analog has been used in recent years in conjunction with exercise stress testing or with pharmacologic vasodilatation with dipyridamole or dobutamine to diagnose ischemia and/or infarction in patients suspected of having coronary artery disease. The Tl-201 is injected intravenously near peak exercise or during dipyridamole or dobutamine infusion, followed by cardiac imaging of the initial myocardial uptake of the Tl-201. Two to four hours later another set of cardiac images is obtained after the Tl-201 has had time to equilibrate into the potassium space in viable myocardial cells. The initial and delayed cardiac images are then compared. Myocardial regions deficient of Tl-201 on the initial images that show enhanced Tl-201 activity on the 2–4 hour delayed images are interpreted as representing regions of transient ischemia in areas of viable myocardium (Fig. 1).[37,38] Myocardial regions with a deficient uptake of Tl-201 on both initial and delayed images commonly are thought to represent an area of infarction. Recently, however, some of these areas have been shown to contain significant amounts of viable myocardium.[39,40] Tl-201 imaging has been shown to be more sensitive than the electrocardiogram for diagnosing coronary artery disease[41,42] with an overall sensitivity of 84% and a specificity of 88% in a pooled group of studies by various investigators. In these studies, coronary angiographic assessment was assumed to accurately represent the presence or absence of "significant" stenoses. Recently this "gold standard" has been challenged,[43,44] hence, it is not a faithful indicator of the physiologic amount of flow supplied to a region of myocardium. Tl-201 myocardial perfusion scintigraphy may better predict the physiologic significance of a coronary artery stenosis.[45] According to Bayesian analysis, the diagnostic value of Tl-201 scintigraphy will depend on the patient population being evaluated.[46,47] Tl-201 scintigraphy may be most helpful clinically in the group of patients who have an intermediate pretest probability of having coronary artery disease based on age, sex, character of the chest pain, and the presence of other risk factors.

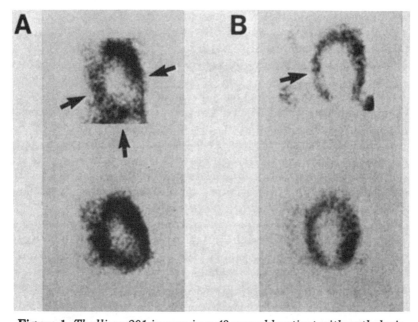

Figure 1. *Thallium-201 images in a 43-year-old patient with pathologic Q waves from multiple infarctions inferiorly and anteriorly with severe coronary disease and a left ventricular ejection fraction of 23%. Anterior (A, top) and 45° left anterior oblique (B, top), images immediately post-dipyridamole infusion and 4 hours later (bottom) show reversible Tl-201 defects in the anterior, septal apical and inferior walls (arrows) consistent with residual viable myocardium. After 3-vessel coronary artery bypass surgery, left ventricular ejection fraction rose to 54%.*

In this group of patients, Tl-201 scintigraphy may be the most cost-effective approach to the diagnosis of coronary artery disease.[48,49]

Precatheterization identification of the patient with significant left main or triple-vessel coronary artery disease may help to alert the catheterizer to the patient at a higher risk for a catheterization-related complication. Patients with left main or triple-vessel coronary disease may show multiple reversible Tl-201 myocardial defects involving anterior, septal, and posterolateral myocardial regions.[50] In addition, the presence of increased lung uptake of Tl-201 on the initial postexercise images usually indicates transient exercise-induced left ventricular dysfunction associated with a rise in pulmonary capillary wedge pressure.[51] This finding is a marker of multivessel coronary disease.[52] In addition, left ventricular cavity dilation seen on the initial postexercise images compared to the 4-hour delayed images also suggest severe left ventricular dysfunction with exercise.

Tl-201 scintigraphy has been shown to be of considerable clinical value in risk stratification of the uncomplicated postmyocardial infarction patient. Gibson et al. demonstrated a superiority of the Tl-201 exercise stress testing over electrocardiographic stress testing alone or cardiac catheterization for predicting future cardiac events postinfarction.[23] Similarly, dipyridamole Tl-201 scintigraphy predicted future cardiac events in postinfarction patients better than electrocardiographic stress testing or ejection fraction.[53]

Risk stratification for coronary events in patients undergoing noncardiac surgeries is also desirable. High-risk patients may have coronary revascularization first or elective noncardiac surgery may be deferred if the potential benefits do not outweigh the risks. Screening coronary angiography with its attendant risks could be avoided in these patients if a reliable noninvasive test were available to identify high- or low-risk patients. The dipyridamole Tl-201 test involves an intravenous injection or oral ingestion of dipyridamole followed by Tl-201 injection and subsequent serial myocardial imaging. Recently there have been several studies[54-56] that have demonstrated the ability of dipyridamole Tl-201 scintigraphy to identify a high-risk group of patients who were to undergo peripheral vascular disease surgery. In all three studies, the presence of Tl-201 myocardial redistribution identified a group of patients who were at high risk of a perioperative cardiac event (death, myocardial infarction, or unstable angina). These studies also demonstrated that the absence of Tl-201 myocardial redistribution stratified patients into a very low-risk group. For this low-risk group, noncardiac surgery can be performed without preoperative coronary angiography with the expectation that cardiac complications will be uncommon. This approach has been prospectively studied by Eagle et al.[55] They confirmed the earlier findings of low operative risk in patients without Tl-201 myocardial redistribution. They also extended these findings by showing that patients without clinical findings of angina, myocardial infarction, congestive heart failure, or diabetes mellitus were at low risk and did not need Tl-201 scintigraphy or cardiac catheterization. Conversely, Leppo et al. demonstrated that the presence of extensive areas of Tl-201 myocardial redistribution identified patients at high risk of cardiac complications from noncardiac surgery.[56]

Rest and exercise radionuclide ventriculography has been a sensitive and specific test to diagnose coronary artery disease when other cardiac conditions that can alter the normal rise in ejection fraction with exercise can be excluded.[57] The usual response is a greater than 5 ejection fraction unit increase from rest to exercise.[57] Conditions other than coronary artery disease that alter the normal rise in ejection fraction include: age greater than 60, elevated resting ejection fraction, atrial fibrillation, hypertension, and valvular or myocardial disease.[58,59] Patients with these conditions are probably best evaluated with thallium-201 scintigraphy for the diagnosis of concomitant coronary disease. Applications of exercise radionuclide ventriculography without recognition of these limitations results in a marked reduction in the specificity of the diagnosis of coronary artery disease.[60]

In summary, exercise thallium scintigraphy and exercise radionuclide ventriculography are extremely useful in the identification of patients with extensive myocardial ischemia or patients who are at low risk for subsequent coronary events. This information can reduce catheterization complications by alerting the angiographer to the possibility of high-risk anatomy or by eliminating the need for catheterization in low-risk patients. The role of exercise or pharmacologic stress echocardiography in risk stratification should still be regarded as experimental. As experience with these echocardiographic techniques increases, they may also become important in the noninvasive risk stratification of patients with coronary artery disease.

Two-Dimensional / Doppler Echocardiography in the Evaluation of Acquired Valvular and Congenital Heart Disease

The use of two-dimensional / Doppler echocardiography in the evaluation of acquired valvular and congenital heart disease perhaps provides the greatest opportunity to eliminate cardiac catheterization or selected aspects of catheterization and thereby reduce risk. The strengths of the ultrasound techniques are their ability to accurately define cardiac anatomy, ventricular function, valvular function, and shunts in patients with acquired valvular or congenital heart disease. In this section the utility of two-dimensional echocardiography and Doppler ultrasound in assessing the severity of stenosis or regurgitation involving the aortic and mitral valve is discussed. However, the principles outlined in this section can be easily applied to hemodynamic derangements across the pulmonic and tricuspid valves, and in shunt lesions, ventricular septal defect, and atrial septal defect.

Aortic stenosis is a common problem, especially in the elderly patient, and once symptoms are present in patients with severe aortic stenosis, prognosis without aortic valve replacement is poor. Additionally, patients with severe aortic stenosis represent one of the most challenging cardiac catheterizations because of the rapidity with which a transient episode of hypotension may evolve into a life-threatening or even fatal complication. Prior knowledge of the degree of aortic stenosis and the presence or absence of left ventricular dysfunction might help the catheterizer identify a high-risk patient. In a patient where all other data are consistent with the diagnosis of severe aortic stenosis, noninvasive information may obviate the need for left ventriculography or determination of aortic valve gradient at catheterization.

Two-dimensional and M-mode echocardiography are extremely useful in evaluating the aortic valve directly, and two-dimensional echocardiography can provide an accurate assessment of left ventricular performance. Both techniques are useful in detecting the presence or absence of associated left ventricular hypertrophy. The identification of nonthickened mobile aortic valve leaflets in older patients with systolic murmurs virtually excludes the presence of significant valvular aortic stenosis. However, examination of the leaflets and ventricular wall for hypertrophy is less specific for the presence of severe aortic stenosis, especially when heavy leaflet calcification prevents assessment of valve mobility or if ventricular hypertrophy is present due to systemic hypertension. Finally, once a gradient across the aortic valve is present, very small changes in cross-sectional orifice area, which is difficult to measure even if the aortic valve anatomy is well visualized, can result in large increments in transvalvular gradient. In spite of these limitations, severe aortic stenosis can be eliminated reliably by using a measurement known as maximal aortic cusp separation, which is determined from two-dimensional imaging.[61] In a study of Godley et al.,[62] maximal aortic cusp separation greater than or equal to 13 mm was associated with mild aortic valve disease with one exception. Thus, this particular measurement had a 96% predictive accuracy for mild stenosis. By contrast, when the maximal aortic cusp separation was less than 2 mm, all patients had severe aortic stenosis and the majority of those with a cusp separation of less than 8 mm had severe aortic stenosis. In this regard, a maximal aortic cusp separation of less than 8 mm was found to be predictive of critical aortic stenosis in 97% of the patients. One should be cautious in using this measurement since heavy calcification of the aortic valve may prevent accurate assessment of its true opening. Additionally, there is considerable overlap in hemodynamic severity with excursions between 9–12 mm. For these reasons, we have been reluctant to recommend aortic valve replacement based solely on two-dimensional echocardiographic appearance of the aortic valve.

In addressing the issue of substituting the noninvasive assessment of aortic stenosis for invasive assessment prior to valve replacement, heavy emphasis must be placed on determining transvalvular gradient. Transvalvular gradient or other measurements based on gradient have become the most important parameters for clinical decision making. With continuous wave Doppler, which may be guided by color flow imaging, transvalvular gradient can be measured and integrated with the structural and functional data gained from two-dimensional imaging resulting in an extremely powerful noninvasive technique to evaluate valvular disease. The potential to use this technique to modify the catheterization protocol then exists. For instance, in a patient with a Doppler gradient of 100 mmHg, severe cusp calcification and leaflet immobility, moderate hypertrophy, and normal symmetrical wall motion with normal ejection fraction based on two-dimensional echocardiography and Doppler studies, the catheterization protocol could be modified accordingly. Contrast left ventriculography and aortic valve gradient determination could be eliminated. If indicated, the sole catheterization procedure would be coronary angiography utilizing nonionic contrast.

$$V = \frac{C \times F}{2\,(TF)\,\cos\theta}$$

Figure 2. *The equation used to calculate blood flow velocity by the Doppler principle is shown. Most machines do this internally and display frequency shifts as velocities. The equation demonstrates the importance of the intercept angle for which the cosine is near 1 until the angle is greater than 20° when the value of the cosine drops rapidly. This emphasizes the importance of interrogating parallel to flow to reduce velocity calculation errors. V = velocity; C = speed of ultrasound in the medium; F = frequency shift in kHz; TF = transmitted frequency of ultrasound; Cos θ = cosine of the intercepting angle between the blood flow to be recorded and the transmitted ultrasound beam.*

There are three basic types of Doppler examinations: pulsed, continuous wave, and color flow. All Doppler techniques are based on measurements of the frequency shift of transmitted versus received ultrasound. From this shift, blood flow velocity can be calculated using the equation shown in Figure 2. With pulsed Doppler, the ultrasound is transmitted by a single crystal that is also used to receive the back scattered signal. This results in the ability to sample flow velocity at different depths by varying the time interval of the transmit and receive cycles, known as range gating the sample volume. Therefore, pulsed Doppler allows localization of the flow signal and is useful for detecting sites of abnormal flow, i.e., mapping of regurgitant and shunt lesions. The shortcoming of pulsed Doppler is that if the Doppler shift exceeds one half of a pulse repetition rate it cannot be accurately measured. Hence, there are limits on the maximum velocities that can be measured using pulsed Doppler. This limits its usefulness, particularly in assessing stenotic lesions with high velocities of flow. With continuous wave (CW) Doppler, ultrasound is continuously transmitted from one crystal and received by another, separate crystal. Because ultrasound is being continuously transmitted and received, virtually any clinically relevant maximal velocity can be measured. The trade-off in comparison to pulsed Doppler is that velocities are sampled irrespective of depth. Hence, range gating is lost. Recently, color flow Doppler mapping has been added to the echocardiographer's armamentarium. Color flow imaging is a technique in which regional blood flow pattern can be evaluated to allow assessment of flow patterns. Shades of gray are still used for imaging tissues; however, colors are assigned to display the flow data. Typically, blood flowing toward the transducer is displayed as blue; blood flowing away is red. Color brightness is increased in proportion to flow velocity. Green represents flow variance and is added proportionally to the directional colors red and blue in the presence of disturbed flow. Thus, color of disturbed flow toward the transducer appears yellow and that of disturbed flow away from the transducer appears purple. Using this approach, the extent and size of regurgitant jet, for instance, can be evaluated. In the stenotic lesions, color flow might allow an observer to precisely direct the continuous wave transducer to sample a particular area of high flow. More detailed discussions of the technical aspects of creating these images are available.[63]

The principal on which Doppler assessment of stenotic valvular lesions rests is based on the fact that these lesions produce discrete jets of high velocity laminar flow surrounded by areas of disordered or turbulent flow. When considering the flow through a stenotic valve, the magnitude of velocity change through a stenotic valve can be related to the pressure difference across the valve by the modified Bernoulli equation. Extensive discussion of this principle can be found in a standard Doppler textbook.[64] For clinical purposes, peak instantaneous gradient in millimeters of Hg can be related to peak blood flow velocity in meters per second by the modified Bernoulli equation, pressure gradient $= 4 \times (\text{velocity})^2$. Hence, a peak velocity of 5 meters per second is equal to a peak instantaneous gradient of 100 millimeters of Hg.

In addition to peak gradient calculation from Doppler, the Doppler flow velocity can be integrated over time to determine a mean gradient. Finally, by using Doppler flow and measuring the cross-sectional area at the site that the Doppler flow is sampled, a cardiac output can be determined. Cardiac output can be used in conjunction with the Doppler mean gradient calculation and the Gorlin formula to calculate a valve area. Alternatively, a thermodilution cardiac output can be substituted for Doppler output. This has been shown to result in a high correlation with catheterization-derived aortic valve areas.[65]

How well do Doppler-derived gradients compare with catheterization-derived gradients? Multiple studies have confirmed an excellent correlation between catheterization and Doppler-derived gradients with a range of correlation coefficients from .68 to .94, and a better correlation using mean gradients.[65–69] The standard errors in these studies were small. Thus there was an excellent correlation with catheterization; however, problems with these Doppler measurements must be understood. First, the peak instantaneous gradient derived from Doppler is not the same as the peak-to-peak gradient determined at catheterization. In fact, the Doppler-derived gradient reflects the peak instantaneous gradient that occurs before and is greater than the peak-to-peak cardiac catheterization gradient (Fig. 3). A second problem is the underestimation of the valve gradient by Doppler because of the presence of an unknown angle between the Doppler beam and the high velocity jet. The true velocity is equal to the measured velocity divided by the cosine of the angle of incidence between the transducer and the jet. Thus, for a 30° angle between the transducer and jet, the error is about a 13% underestimation of velocity. Because the gradient is related to the square of the velocity measurement, the underestimation of gradient by incident angulation is magnified. This problem should be reduced as the technologist's experience with the Doppler exam in a given laboratory increases. Multiple windows must be interrogated to measure the highest velocity jet. Additionally, color flow-directed continuous wave examination potentially can reduce this problem by visually demonstrating the jet orientation. Finally, the importance of the morphology of the aortic flow packet has been emphasized.[70] Severe aortic stenosis is associated with a mid to late peaking Doppler flow velocity packet. Therefore, in evaluating the severity of aortic stenosis by Doppler, the clinician must not only be concerned with the peak Doppler gradient but also the shape of the Doppler packet. This is especially true in patients with depressed left ventricular function. Doppler is very useful in the quantification of aortic valve gradient. In order to minimize underestimation of true gradient, it is required that multiple transducer windows be used to guarantee recording of the highest peak flow velocity. In the high-risk catheterization patient in whom aortic stenosis is suspected, rational substitution of Doppler-derived gradients is possible if the shortcomings of the technique are understood. An example is shown in Figure 4.

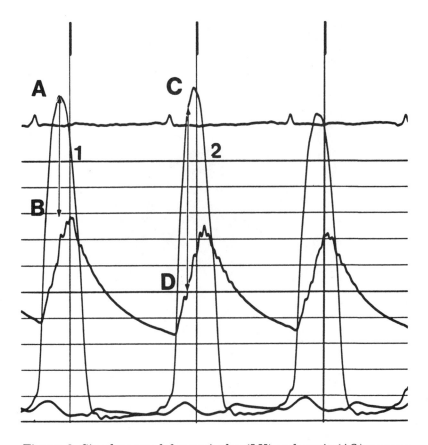

Figure 3. *Simultaneous left ventricular (LV) and aortic (AO) pressure tracings are shown from a patient with aortic stenosis. The difference between peak to peak (A–B beat 1) and maximum instantaneous pressure gradients (C–D beat 2) are demonstrated. Doppler peak gradients measure maximum instantaneous pressure gradients.*

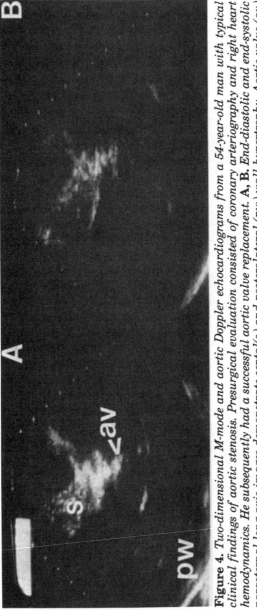

Figure 4. *Two-dimensional M-mode and aortic Doppler echocardiograms from a 54-year-old man with typical clinical findings of aortic stenosis. Presurgical evaluation consisted of coronary arteriography and right heart hemodynamics. He subsequently had a successful aortic valve replacement.* **A, B.** *End-diastolic and end-systolic parasternal long-axis images demonstrate septal(s) and posterolateral (pw) wall hypertrophy. Aortic valve (av) is densely calcified and demonstrates little opening in systole* (**Panel B**).

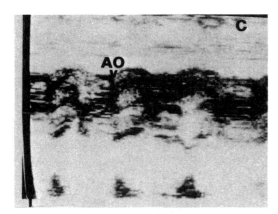

Figure 4C. *M-mode echocardiogram through the aortic root (AO) demonstrates markedly thickened and immobile aortic valve.*

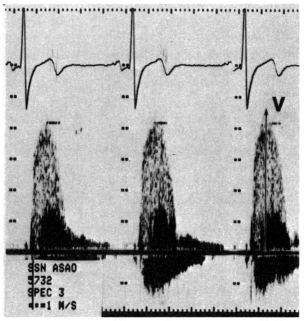

Figure 4D. *Continuous wave Doppler velocity recording of aortic flow is shown from the suprasternal (SSN) view. Peak instantaneous aortic flow velocity (V) was measured to be 4.6 meters per second, which is equivalent to a peak instantaneous gradient of 84 mmHg. The area of the flow velocity packet can be planimetered and divided by the ejection time to provide a mean velocity and therefore a mean gradient.*

In the evaluation of mitral stenosis, both two-dimensional echocardiography and Doppler have dramatically enhanced the ability of the clinician to diagnose mitral stenosis and to give accurate estimates of stenosis severity. These estimates compare extremely well with mitral orifice areas calculated at catheterization or surgery.[71,72] Echocardiography can be reasonably substituted for catheterization if necessary. Two techniques that are used are: planimetry of the valve area from the two-dimensional echo short-axis view, which contains the mitral valve and Doppler-derived indices of gradient or area. These techniques have been shown to be highly accurate in predicting the severity of mitral stenosis. To measure the mitral orifice, the orifice is placed in the center of the long-axis parasternal plane and the transducer is rotated 90° to allow visualization of the short-axis orifice area. The smallest mitral valve orifice during early diastole is identified, the images frozen, and the inner border at the black-white interface is traced. Planimetry of this circumference yields a cross-sectional area. Studies by Henry, Nichol, and Schweizer have shown excellent correlation (0.89 to 0.95) with catheterization-determined areas.[71-73] These estimates have a small standard error. Shortcomings include the inability to obtain a high quality short-axis view in as many as 25% of the patients, and overestimation or underestimation from plane misalignment or non-"optimal" settings of gain and reject. Importantly, correlation appears to be unaffected by the presence of mitral regurgitation. Doppler complements two-dimensional echocardiography and is an alternative when the parasternal window is not available. Continuous wave Doppler is necessary to make accurate peak velocity measurements. The principles outlined in the section on aortic stenosis also apply to the calculation of peak and mean gradients from continuous Doppler wave measurement of mitral inflow velocity. Gradients calculated by Doppler and catheterization have a high degree of correlation (r = .92).[64] Another technique used to estimate mitral valve area is based on the observation by Libanoff and Rodbard from cardiac catheterization data that the time required for mitral pressure gradient to decrease to one half its initial peak reflects the severity of mitral stenosis.[74] This measurement has been referred to as the pressure halftime. It was found by these investigators to be relatively independent of cardiac output, heart rate, and mitral regurgitation. The pressure halftime can be estimated from continuous wave Doppler recordings as the time required for calculated peak gradient to fall 50%. Because of the quadratic relationship between pressure gradient and velocity, the pressure halftime will occur at 71% of the initial peak velocity. Increasing halftime, therefore, is associated with increased severity of mitral stenosis. The proposed formula that relates pressure half-time to mitral valve area in square centimeters is 220 divided by the halftime in milliseconds. The correlation between pressure half-time and catheterization-determined mitral valve area has been excellent.[75]

In summary, a variety of methods utilizing two-dimensional and Doppler echocardiography have been outlined for quantification of the severity of mitral stenosis. Ideally these techniques are complementary and can result in highly accurate estimates of mitral valve stenosis. Effective use of these measurements in the precatheterization evaluation of the patient with suspected mitral stenosis can establish the role for further detailed hemodynamic evaluation by cardiac catheterization. In the young patient with severe mitral stenosis and a low likelihood of coronary disease, echocardiography has the potential to be substituted for catheterization evaluation prior to commissurotomy, valve replacement, or valvuloplasty.

In the regurgitant lesions, aortic or mitral, the role of two-dimensional echocardiography and Doppler echocardiography in the precatheterization evaluation of patients is still evolving. Certainly, the state of left ventricular systolic function can be ascertained using two-dimensional echocardiography, following the principles outlined in the section of this chapter on assessment of left ventricular function. Patients with poor left ventricular function who would not be candidates for surgical therapy can be identified by echocardiography and spared further invasive testing. Investigations concerning the role of Doppler echocardiography for estimation of the severity of aortic or mitral regurgitation are being performed but no clear concensus has been reached. The most frequently used techniques for gauging the severity of regurgitant lesions involve mapping the extent of disturbed flow in the appropriate receiving chamber, e.g., left ventricle for aortic incompetence or left atrium for mitral regurgitation.[76,77] This is fraught with multiple problems since the regurgitant jets can occur in three dimensions, yet pulsed Doppler echocardiography is mapping the regurgitant jet in two dimensions. In addition, minimal regurgitation may be associated with high velocity jets that are trackable deep into the atrial chamber.[78,79] Another method involves the calculation of a regurgitant fraction. This correlates well with angiographic estimates of regurgitation but is technically difficult, has multiple sources of error, and is cumbersome to apply clinically. Color flow Doppler may have an important impact on the noninvasive quantification of regurgitant lesions. Since color flow Doppler allows a spatial display of regurgitant velocities, a quick estimate of area of regurgitation on multiple imaging planes is obtained. When the area of regurgitation is normalized for the receiving chamber size, color flow Doppler estimates of regurgitation correlate well with angiographic findings.[78,79] The width of the regurgitant jet at the valve orifice also gives accurate estimates of the severity of regurgitation.

The exact role of two-dimensional/Doppler echocardiography in the reduction of catheterization risks in patients with regurgitant lesions remains to be determined. It certainly is useful in the evaluation of left ventricular function and in establishing the etiology of the regurgitation by its exquisite ability to elucidate the pathoanatomy. This information has more bearing on the patient's ultimate prognosis and need for catheterization than does the severity of the regurgitant jet itself. Finally, color flow Doppler-derived indices of regurgitation severity may become most useful when a noninvasive estimate of regurgitation severity is required.

Nuclear Cardiology in The Evaluation of Valvular Heart Disease

Radionuclide ventriculography can provide a measure of ejection fraction and wall motion similar to contrast ventriculography without exposing the patient to the risks of that procedure. Additional information obtainable from radionuclide angiography includes a quantitative measure of left-sided valvular insufficiency (aortic and/or mitral insufficiency) and left ventricular end-diastolic and end-systolic volumes. The quantitative assessment of left-sided regurgitation frequently may provide complementary information to a contrast left ventriculogram and aortogram in patients with mixed valvular stenosis and insufficiency.[80] This information may be valuable in judging the reliability of the aortic valve area calculation that would underestimate true valve area if significant valve insufficiency were present.

Nuclear cardiology techniques cannot directly measure mitral valve area. Radionuclide ventriculography can assess left ventricular function (ejection fraction) as well as the presence and amount of concomitant mitral insufficiency (LV/RV stroke count ratio). These measurements may be of precatheterization value in patients with allergies to radio-opaque contrast agents (obviating the need for a left ventriculogram) and in patients with poor left ventricular function who would be at high risk of a contrast-related complication or may be excluded from catheterization because they would be poor surgical candidates due to severely impaired LV function.

Summary

Noninvasive evaluations may assist in the precatheterization evaluation of selected patients with heart disease. The judicious use of these tests may decrease some of the risks involved in catheterization. Avoidance of left ventriculography in patients with severely depressed left ventricular function or renal insufficiency may be helpful. Precatheterization knowledge of a high-risk likelihood of severe coronary artery disease or aortic stenosis also should help heighten the awareness of risk for catheterization-related complications. Further studies may more clearly identify high-risk patients and other groups of patients in whom noninvasive echocardiographic or radionuclide studies will complement catheterization in the evaluation of patients with heart disease.

References

1. Kennedy JW, Baxley WA, Bunnel IA, et al: Mortality related to cardiac catheterization and angiography. Cathet Cardiovasc Diagn 207:207, 1977.
2. Dodge HT, Sandler H, Ballew DW, et al: The use of biplane angiocardiography for the measurement of left ventricular volume in man. Am Heart J 60:762, 1960.
3. Bansal RC, Tajik AJ, Seward JB, et al: Feasibility of detailed two-dimensional echocardiographic examination in adults: prospective study of 200 patients. Mayo Clinic Proc 55:291, 1980.
4. Folland ED, Parisi AF, Moynihan PF, et al: Assessment of left ventricular ejection fraction and volumes by real-time, two-dimensional echocardiography: a comparison of cineangiographic and radionuclide techniques. Circulation 60:760, 1974.

5. Wyatt HL, Heng MK, Meerbaum S, et al: Cross-sectional-analysis of mathematical models for quantifying mass of the left ventricle in dogs. Circulation 60:1104, 1979.
6. Schiller NB, Acquatella H, Ports T, et al: Left ventricular volume by paired biplane two-dimensional echocardiography. Circulation 60:547, 1979.
7. Starling MR, Crawford MJ, Sorensen SG, et al: Comparative accuracy of apical biplane cross-sectional echocardiography and gated equilibrium radionuclide angiography for estimating left ventricular size and performance. Circulation 63:1075, 1983.
8. Tortoledo FA, Quinones MA, Fernandez GC, et al: Quantification of left ventricular volumes by two-dimensional echocardiography: a simplified and accurate approach. Circulation 67:579, 1983.
9. Gveret P, Meerbaum S, Wyatt HL, Uchiyama T, et al: Two-dimensional echocardiographic quantitation of left ventricular volumes and ejection fraction. Importance of accounting for dyssynergy in short-axis reconstruction models. Circulation 62:1308, 1980.
10. Stamm RB, Carabello BA, Mayers DL, et al: Two-dimensional echocardiographic measurement of left ventricular ejection fraction: prospective analysis of what constitutes an adequate determination. Am Heart J 104:136, 1982.
11. Quinones MA, Waggoner AD, Reduto LA, et al: A new, simplified and accurate method for determining ejection fraction with two-dimensional echocardiography. Circulation 64:744, 1981.
12. Massie BM, Schiller NB, Ratshin RA, et al: Mitral-septal separation: new echocardiographic index of left ventricular function. Am J Cardiol 39:1008, 1977.
13. Moynihand PF, Parisi AF, Feldman CL: Quantitative detection of regional left ventricular contraction abnormalities by two-dimensional echocardiography. I. Analysis of methods. Circulation 63:752, 1981.
14. Kisslo JA, Robertson D, Gilbert BW, et al: A comparison of real-time, two-dimensional echocardiography and cineangiography in detecting left ventricular asynergy. Circulation 55:134, 1977.
15. Weiss JL, Bulkley BH, Hutchins GM, et al: Two-dimensional echocardiographic recognition of myocardial injury in man: comparison with postmorten studies. Circulation 63:401, 1981.
16. Strauss HW, McKusick KA, Boucher CA, et al: Of linens and laces—the eighth anniversary of the dated blood pool scan. Semin Nucl Med 9:296, 1979.
17. Callahan RJ, Froelich JW, McKusick KA, et al: Modified method for the in-vivo labelling of red blood cells with Tl-99m: concise communication. J Nucl Med 23:315, 1982.
18. Massie BM, Kramer BL, Gertz EW, et al: Radionuclide measurement of left ventricular volume: comparison of geometric and counts based methods. Circulation 65:725, 1982.
19. Links JM, Becker LC, Shindledecker JG, et al: Measurement of absolute left ventricular volume from gated blood pool studies. Circulation 65:82, 1982.

20. Starling MR, Dell'Italia LJ, Walsh RA, et al: Accurate estimates of absolute left ventricular volumes from equilibrium radionuclide angiographic count data using a simple geometric attenuation correction. J Am Coll Cardiol 3:789, 1984.
21. Okada RD, Kirshenbaum HD, Kushner FG, et al: Observer variance in the qualitative evaluation of left ventricular regional wall motion and the quantitation of left ventricular ejection fraction using rest and exercise multigated blood pool imaging. Circulation 61:128, 1980.
22. Brown KA, Boucher CA, Okada RD, et al: Prognostic value of exercise thallium-201 imaging in patients presenting for evaluation of chest pain. J Am Coll Cardiol 1:994, 1983.
23. Gibson RS, Watson DD, Craddock GB, et al: Prediction of cardiac events after uncomplicated myocardial infarction: a prospective study comparing predischarge exercise thallium-201 scintigraphy and coronary angiography. Circulation 68:321, 1983.
24. Bodenheimer MM, Banka VS, Hermann GA, et al: Reversible asynergy—histopathologic and electrocardiographic correlations in patients with coronary artery disease. Circulation 53:792, 1976.
25. Appelgate RJ, Crawford MH: Exercise echocardiography. Echocardiography 3:333, 1986.
26. Palac RT, Coombs BJ, Kudenchuk PJ, et al: Two-dimensional electrocardiography during dobutamine infusion—comparison with exercise testing in the evaluation of coronary disease. Circulation 70(II):184, 1984.
27. Wann LS, Faris JV, Childress RH, et al: Exercise cross-sectional echocardiography in ischemic heart disease. Circulation 60:1300, 1979.
28. Morganroth J, Chen CC, David D, et al: Exercise cross-sectional echocardiographic diagnosis of coronary artery disease. Am J Cardiol 47:20, 1981.
29. Maurer G, Nanda NC: Two-dimensional echocardiographic evaluation of exercise-induced left and right ventricular asynergy: correlation with thallium scanning. Am J Cardiol 48:720, 1981.
30. Crawford MH, Amon KW, Vance WS: Exercise 2-dimensional echocardiography. Am J Cardiol 51:1, 1983.
31. Limacher MC, Quinones MA, Poliner LR, et al: Detection of coronary disease with exercise two-dimensional echocardiography. Circulation 67:1211, 1983.
32. Armstrong WF, O'Donnell J, Dillon JC, et al: Complimentary value of two-dimensional exercise echocardiography to routine treadmill exercise testing. Ann Intern Med 105:829, 1986.
33. Weyman AE, Feigenbaum H, Dillon JC, et al: Noninvasive visualization of the left main coronary artery by cross-sectional echocardiography. Circulation 54:169, 1976.
34. Rink LD, Feigenbaum H, Godley RW, et al: Echocardiographic detection of left main coronary obstruction. Circulation 65:719, 1982.
35. Strauss HW, Harrison K, Langan JK, et al: Thallium-201 for myocardial imaging. Relation of thallium-201 to regional myocardial perfusion. Circulation 51:641, 1975.

36. Weich H, Strauss HW, Pitt B: The extraction of Tl-201 by the myocardium. Circulation 56:188, 1977.
37. Pohost GM, Zir LM, Moore RH, et al: Differentiation of transiently ischemic from infarcted myocardium by serial imaging after a single dose of thallium-201. Circulation 55:294, 1977.
38. Beller GA, Watson DD, Ackell P, et al: Time course of thallium-201 redistribution after transient ischemia. Circulation 61:791, 1980.
39. Lui P, Kress M, Okada RD, et al: The persistent defect on exercise thallium imaging and its fate after myocardial revascularization: does it represent scar or ischemia? Am Heart J 110:996, 1985.
40. Gutman J, Berman DS, Freeman M, et al: Time to completed redistribution of thallium-201 in exercise myocardial scintigraphy: relationship to the degree of coronary artery stenosis. Am Heart J 106:989, 1983.
41. Ritchie JL, Zaret BL, Strauss HW, et al: Myocardial imaging with thallium-201: a multicenter study in patients with angina pectoris or acute myocardial infarction. Am J Cardiol 42:345, 1978.
42. Gerson MC: Noninvasive detection of chronic coronary artery disease. In MC Gerson (ed): Cardiac Nuclear Medicine, New York, McGraw-Hill Book Co., 1987, p. 316.
43. White CW, White CB, Doty DB, et al: Does visual interpretation of the coronary angiogram predict the physiologic importance of a coronary stenosis. N Engl J Med 310:819, 1984.
44. Paulin S: Assessing the severity of coronary lesions with angiography. N Engl J Med 316:1405, 1987.
45. Bateman T, Raymond M, Czer L, et al: Stenosis severity: analysis using Tl-201 scintigraphy and intracoronary pressure gradients. (Abstract) J Am Coll Cardiol 3:606, 1984.
46. Rifkind RD, Hood WB, Jr.: Bayesian analysis of electrocardiographic exercise stress testing. N Engl J Med 297:681, 1977.
47. Epstein SE: Implications of probability analysis on the strategy used for noninvasive detection of coronary artery disease. Role of single or combined use of exercise electrocardiographic testing, radionuclide cineangiography and myocardial perfusion imaging. Am J Cardiol 46:491, 1980.
48. Patterson RE, Eng C, Horowitz SF, et al: Bayesian comparison of cost-effectiveness of different clinical approaches to diagnose coronary artery disease. J Am Coll Cardiol 4:278, 1984.
49. Hung J, Chaitman BR, Lam J, et al: Noninvasive diagnostic test choices for the evaluation of coronary artery disease in women: a multivariate comparison of cardiac fluoroscopy, exercise electrocardiography and exercise thallium myocardial perfusion scintigraphy. J Am Coll Cardiol 4:8, 1984.
50. Dash H, Massie BM, Botvinick EH, et al: The noninvasive identification of left main or triple vessel coronary artery disease by myocardial stress perfusion scintigraphy and treadmill exercise electrocardiography. Circulation 60:276, 1979.
51. Boucher CA, Zir LM, Beller GA, et al: Increased lung uptake of thal-

lium-201 during exercise myocardial imaging: clinical, hemodynamic and angiographic implications in patients with coronary artery disease. Am J Cardiol 46:189, 1980.

52. Kushner FG, Okada RD, Kirshenbaum HD, et al: Lung thallium-201 uptake after stress testing in patients with coronary artery disease. Circulation 63:341, 1981.

53. Leppo JA, O'Brien J, Rothendler JA, et al: Dipyridimole thallium-201 scintigraphy in the prediction of future cardiac events after myocardial infarction. N Engl J Med 310:1014, 1984.

54. Boucher CA, Brewster DC, Darling RC, et al: Determination of cardiac risk by dipyridamole—thallium imaging before peripheral vascular surgery. N Engl J Med 312:389, 1985.

55. Eagle KA, Singer DE, Brewster DC, et al: Dipyridamole-thallium scanning in patients undergoing vascular surgery. JAMA 257:2185, 1987.

56. Leppo JS, Plaja J, Gionet M, et al: The noninvasive evaluation of cardiac risk prior to vascular surgery. J Am Coll Cardiol 9:269, 1987.

57. Borer JS, Kent KM, Bacharach SL, et al: Sensitivity, specificity and predictive accuracy of radionuclide cineangiography during exercise in patients with coronary artery disease. Comparison with exercise electrocardiography. Circulation 60:572, 1979.

58. Port S, Cobb FR, Coleman RE, et al: Effect of age on the response of the left ventricular ejection fraction to exercise. N Engl J Med 303:1133, 1980.

59. Chen DCP, Rapp JS, Lindsay JL, Jr., et al: Cardiac response to exercise in the hyperkinetic heart. (Abstract) Radiology 149:181, 1983.

60. Rozanski A, Diamond GA, Berman D, et al: The declining specificity of exercise radionuclide ventriculography. N Engl J Med 309:518, 1983.

61. Demaria AN, Bommer W, Joye J, et al: Value and limitations of cross-sectional echocardiography of the aortic valve in the diagnosis and quantification of valvular aortic stenosis. Circulation 62:304, 1980.

62. Godley RW, Green D, Dillon JC, et al: Reliability of two-dimensional echocardiography in assessing the severity of valvular aortic stenosis. Chest 79:657, 1981.

63. Omoto R, Kasai C: Basic principles of Doppler color flow imaging, Echocardiography 3:463, 1986.

64. Hatle L, Angelson B: Doppler Ultrasound in Cardiology. Philadelphia, Lea and Febiger, 1985.

65. Warth DC, Stewart WJ, Block PC, et al: A new method to calculate aortic valve area without left heart catheterization. Circulation 70:978, 1984.

66. Agatson AS, Chengot M, Rao A, et al: Doppler diagnosis of aortic stenosis in patients over 60 years of age. Am J Cardiol 56:106, 1985.

67. Stamm RB, Martin RP: Quantification of pressure gradients across stenotic valves by Doppler ultrasound. J Am Coll Cardiol 2:707, 1983.

68. Currie PJ, Seward JB, Reeder GS, et al: Doppler echocardiographic assessment of severity of calcific aortic stenosis: a simultaneous Doppler-catheter correlative study in 100 patients. Circulation 71:1162, 1985.

69. Smith MD, Dawson P, Elion J, et al: Comparative correlation of continuous wave Doppler spectral measurements with hemodynamic parameters in patients with aortic stenosis. Circulation 70(II):116, 1984.
70. Hatle L, Angelsen BH, Tromsdale A: Non-invasive assessment of aortic stenosis by Doppler ultrasound. Br Heart J 43:284, 1980.
71. Nichol PM, Gilbert BW, Kisslo JA: Two-dimensional echocardiographic assessment of mitral stenosis. Circulation 55:120, 1977.
72. Schweizer P, Bardos P, Krebs W, et al: Morphometric investigations in mitral stenosis using two-dimensional echocardiography. Br Heart J 48:54, 1982.
73. Henry WL, Griffith JM, Michaelis LL, et al: Measurement of mitral orifice area in patients with mitral valve disease by real time, two-dimensional echocardiography. Circulation 51:827, 1975.
74. Libanoff AJ, Rodbard S: Atrio-ventricular pressure half-time: measure of mitral valve orifice area. Circulation 38:144, 1968.
75. Hatle L, Angelsen B, Tromsdale A: Noninvasive assessment of atrio-ventricular pressure half time by Doppler ultrasound. Circulation 60:1096, 1079.
76. Veyrat C, Ameur A, Gourtchiglouian C, et al: Calculation of pulsed Doppler left ventricular outflow tract regurgitant index for grading the severity of aortic regurgitation. Am Heart J 108:507, 1984.
77. Veyrat C, Ameur A, Bas S, et al: Pulsed Doppler echocardiographic indexes for assessing mitral regurgitation. Br Heart J 51:130, 1984.
78. Helmcke, F, Perry GH, Soto B, et al: Correlation of angiographic and color Doppler parameters of aortic insufficiency. (Abstract) Clin Res 34:307A, 1986.
79. Sevitzer DF, Nanda NC: Review: Doppler color flow mapping ultrasound. Med Biol 11:403, 1985.
80. Sorenson SG, O'Rourke RA, Chaudhari TK: Non-invasive quantitation of valvular regurgitation by gated equilibrium radionuclide angiography. Circulation 62:1089, 1980.

Index